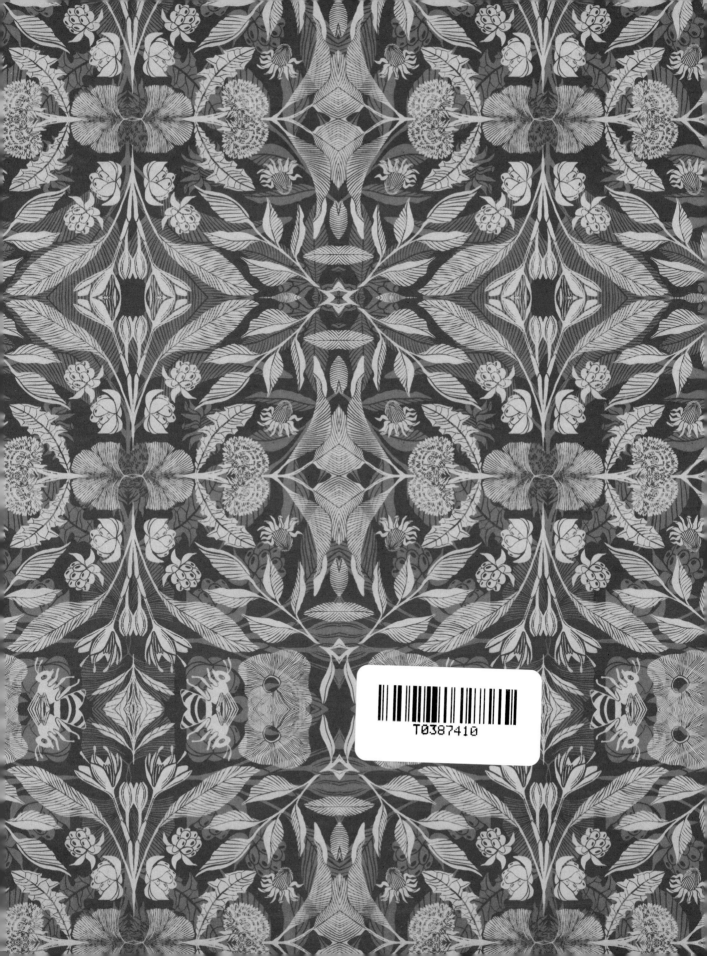

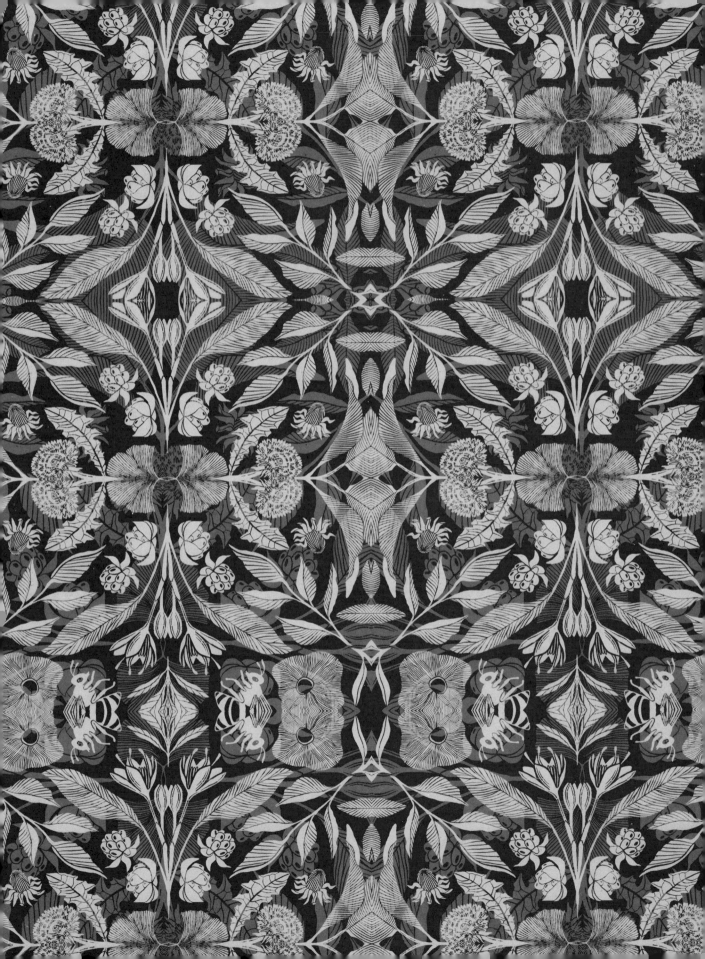

PLANT POWER

"Dutch anthropologist Wouter Bijdendijk marries healing knowledge with culinary art, magic with science, and active molecules with plant spirit and soul. *Unio mystica* of plant power. This book is filled with knowledge and broadens horizons."

— CLAUDIA MÜLLER-EBELING, Ph.D., anthropologist and coauthor of *Witchcraft Medicine, The Encyclopedia of Aphrodisiacs*, and *Pagan Christmas*

"I have been a fan of Joris's work, as he always is at the edge and pushing himself and his teams in that new direction, exploring the vast possibilities of food. This book is a testimony to his work in pushing vegetables to the forefront, not from a sustainability point of view but for their medical virtues. *Plant Power* is promising not only to deliver delicious recipes but like Hippocrates does, Joris and his brother, Wouter, explain how to let food be thy medicine."

— RICHARD EKKEBUS, three-Michelin-star chef and director of culinary operations and food and beverage at Amber at The Landmark Mandarin Oriental in Hong Kong

"A beautiful book packed with tasty knowledge and respect for plants. 'Knowledge Increases Pleasure' could be its motto."

— JEREMY NARBY, anthropologist and author of *The Cosmic Serpent* and *The Psychotropic Mind*

"Wouter and Joris Bijdendijk have put together an important and timely volume filled with easy-to-follow recipes for a variety of ailments and nutritious living. As faith in both the food and pharmaceutical industries deteriorates, books like this one will prove paramount in providing healthy alternatives to the chemical-ridden products that often pass for sustenance in the 21st century."

— THOMAS HATSIS, historian and author of *The Witches' Ointment* and *Psychedelic Mystery Traditions*

"An elegant intermingling of the culinary and the curative, *Plant Power* entices readers to nourish both body and spirit through the medicinal magic of the natural world."

— COBY MICHAEL, author of *The Poison Path Herbal* and *The Poison Path Grimoire*

"A visually stunning exploration that bridges rigorous science with cultural heritage and ancient wisdom. By thoughtfully integrating contemporary research with time-honored knowledge, this book invites critical engagement, compassionate stewardship, and a holistic relationship with our natural world. *Plant Power* offers a path back to the nourishing, transformative magic of our interconnected existence with the plant kingdom."

— J. DEREK LOMAS, Ph.D., assistant professor of Human-Centered Design at TU Delft University

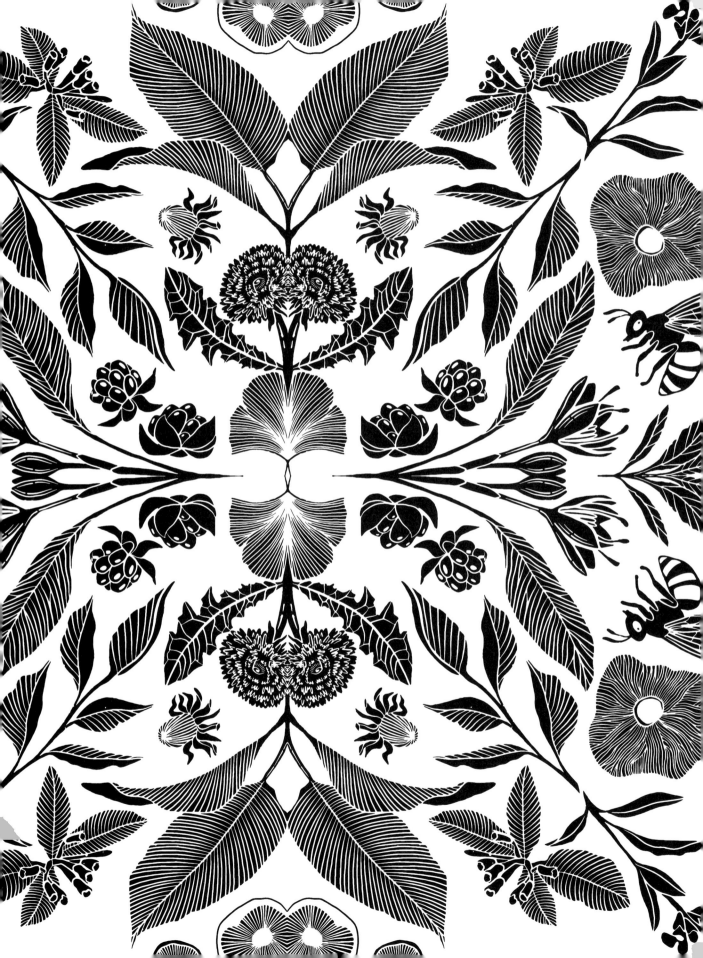

WOUTER
BIJDENDIJK

PLANT POWER

Heal Yourself with
Medicinal Mushrooms,
Roots, Flowers,
and Herbs

With
60 RECIPES
by Michelin Star Chef
JORIS BIJDENDIJK

Translated by
Suzanne Heukensfeldt Jansen

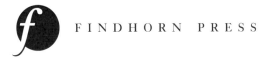

Contents

Preface 6
Our Immune System 10
How to Use This Book 18
Working with Medicinal
   and Ritual Plants 22
Methods 26

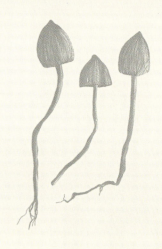

1

MUSHROOMS

Chaga 34
Button Mushroom 40
Ink Cap 46
Reishi 50
Shiitake 54
Lion's Mane 60
Further Plant Journeys
   Fly Agaric 64
   Psilocybin 67

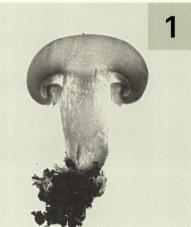

2

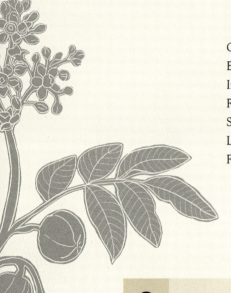

FRUIT & NUTS

Papaya 74
Grape 80
Bilberry 88
Olive 94
Walnut 100
Cloudberry 106
Further Plant Journeys
   Kola Nut 113
   Crabwood 114

5

3

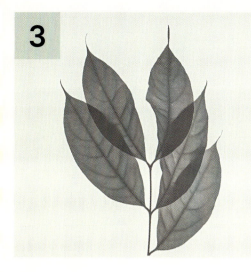

HERBS AND SPICES

Clove	120
Parsley	126
Sage	132
Verbena	140
Saffron	146
Valerian	150
Further Plant Journeys	
Cannabis	156
Sweetgale	158

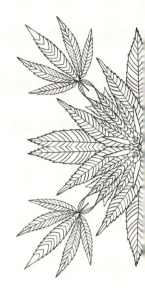

4

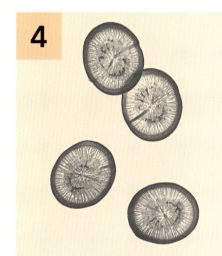

LEAVES AND FLOWERS

Nettle	166
Ginkgo	174
German Chamomile	180
Matcha	186
Meadowsweet	192
Dandelion	200
Further Plant Journeys	
Coca	206
Blue Lotus	208
Huachuma Cactus	210
Peyote Cactus	212

BULBS AND ROOTS

Ginger	218
Ginseng	224
Garlic	230
Turmeric	238
Horseradish	244
Black Radish	250
Further Plant Journeys	
Maca	254
Kava	255
Tepezcohuite	257
Tabernanthe Iboga	259

Afterword	261
Glossary	262
Notes	267
Resources	271
Recipe Overview	276
Food Glossary	277
Index	278
About the Authors	284

PREFACE

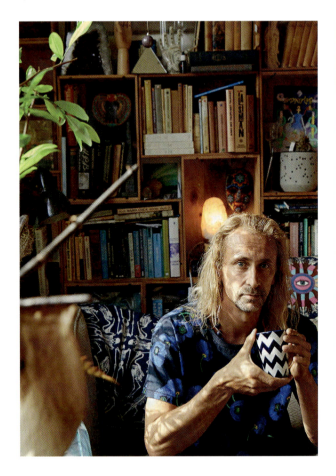
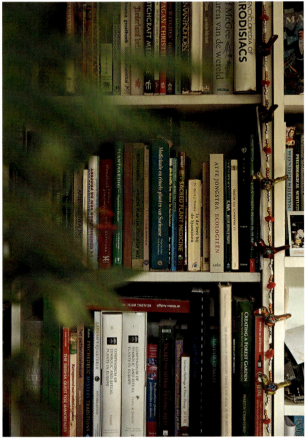

Evolutionarily, plants are much older than animals and, therefore, humans. Plants have had to deal with natural pathogens such as fungi and bacteria for millennia, and during that time have learned to successfully defend themselves by producing natural bactericides and fungicides among other important substances. These defensive substances not only benefit plants but humans as well, as we can use them for our own defense and other purposes.

During my fieldwork as a cultural anthropologist and museologist in South India, I discovered that all the medicines used in the Indian martial art of Kalaripayattu come from plants. In the martial temples, the teachers (*gurukkals*) work with various medicinal plants, which they process into oils and use in steam baths and compresses. The plants help heal muscles, bones, joints, and tendons and keep them flexible.

In Kerala, I was introduced to the medicinal art of Siddha, which is also based on medicinal plants. Siddha originated from the Dravidian culture and is older than the better-known Ayurvedic medicine. I decided to stay in India for six months to learn more about medicinal plants. The Siddhar sage and alchemist I was apprenticed to, Swami Siddha Anand Nataraj, told me that he produced the supreme, most powerful medicine in the universe entirely from plants and minerals. That naturally excited me. I was also apprenticed to a magician, who taught me to levitate, an ancient Indian magical act. This greatly excited me as well.

Once back in the Netherlands, I began performing as a magician. During a levitation act over the Amsterdam Spui, I had an accident at a height of 12 meters, resulting in serious back injuries. I tried all kinds of treatments;

PREFACE

physical therapy, mensendieck, orthobionomy, manual therapy—I did it all. Nothing helped; in fact, it only got worse. That is, until I met Paké, a Surinamese medicine man. He believed that he could help me heal by using medicinal plant knowledge he had learned from his African ancestors.

Before my treatment with Paké started, I had X-rays taken of my injury. After completing the treatment, I had a fresh set of X-rays taken. I had already felt it, but now I saw it in black and white: the bone and tissue of my vertebrae had healed. It felt like a miracle and made an incredible impression.

I immediately decided that I wanted to study medicine and enrolled in pharmacognosy, a branch of pharmacy focused on the study of the physical, chemical, biochemical, and biological properties of medicines of natural origin. It also focuses on the search for new medicines obtained from natural sources. I not only gained knowledge about active ingredients in plants but also learned how to extract and dose them. Thanks to this study I acquired over 2,000 years' worth of pharmaceutical knowledge.

After college, I focused on study tours, writing articles on medicinal plants, and started a business in ethnobotany. I also went back to working as a magician. I perform abroad several times a year, often in countries where medicinal plants are used. In 2011, I was invited to Suriname, my first visit to the country. In the jungle around Paramaribo, I met Carib Indians who showed me how they made medicinal oil with plants from the Amazon jungle. They called this medicine "body pain medicine."

This book also contains monographs on plants from other countries and cultures. While traveling for my fieldwork, I found myself in the Canary Islands, Hong Kong, Jamaica, and other countries around the Caribbean, North America, India, Egypt, Lapland, and the Middle East.

Even in the Netherlands I still deepen my knowledge. For many years, I have been working at the Free University of Amsterdam's Botanic Garden Zuidas. I learned a great deal about cultivating plants there, and via the botanical garden I came into contact with various living plant libraries, which has been incredibly useful. Eighty percent of the world's population depends on traditional medicine in which plants play an important role.

Plant Power is a precious testimony to ancient herbal medicine knowledge from various cultures. It features familiar and less familiar plants, fruits, nuts, bulbs, roots, flowers, and mushrooms that have an effect on the immune system, overall health, stamina, digestion, vitality, and improve your brain. In addition, you will find a number of plants that have played an important role in our rituals and ceremonies and have enabled humans to get in touch with their own deeper layers for more than 10,000 years.

The descriptions in this book are based on interdisciplinary studies; anthropological, botanical, pharmacognostic, and historical research; and the plants' effects have been demonstrated and substantiated by the latest scientific studies. All the chapters in the book, except for Further Plant Journeys, include two vegetarian recipes by my brother, celebrity chef Joris Bijdendijk.

Plant Power is part personal quest and part the story of our human urge to harmonize with, and get (and keep) a grip on, our environment, body, mind, and the "unknown," alongside the discovery of plants and mushrooms able to keep in check unknown forces, oxidative stress, and mental and physical discomforts.

At a time of great environmental pollution, a pandemic, climate change, lifestyle diseases, cancer, and modern, uprooted urban humans detached from nature, it is good to reflect on the age-old connection between man and nature, particularly the plant and fungal kingdom. Above all, in this book I hope to take you on a beautiful and sometimes provocative journey of discovery into powerful medicinal and ritual plants and mushrooms from all over the world.

Wouter Bijdendijk, M.Sc.

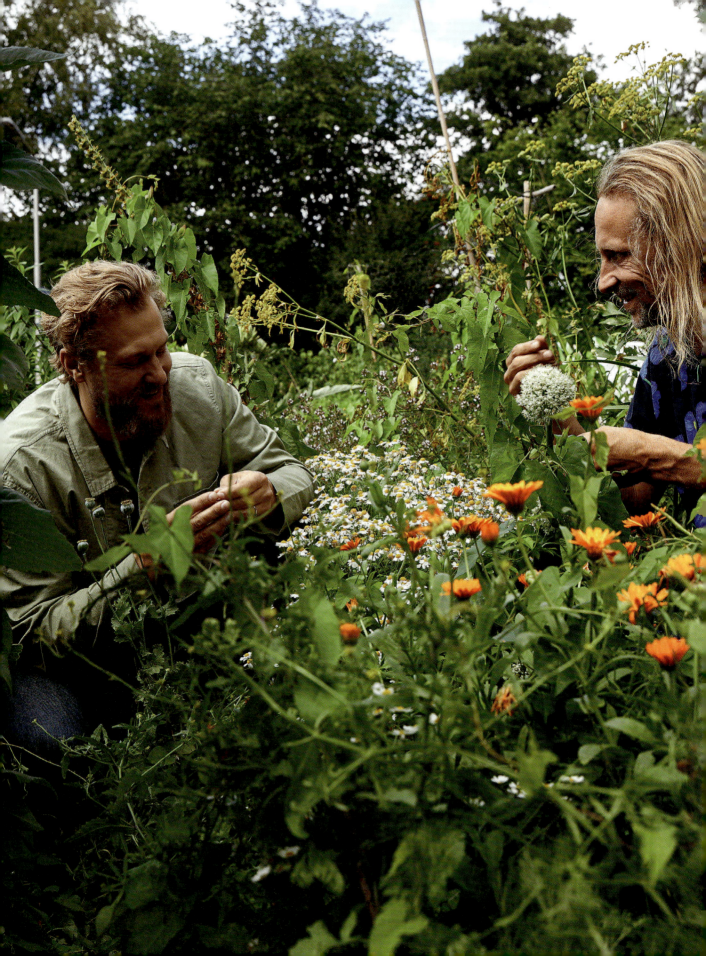

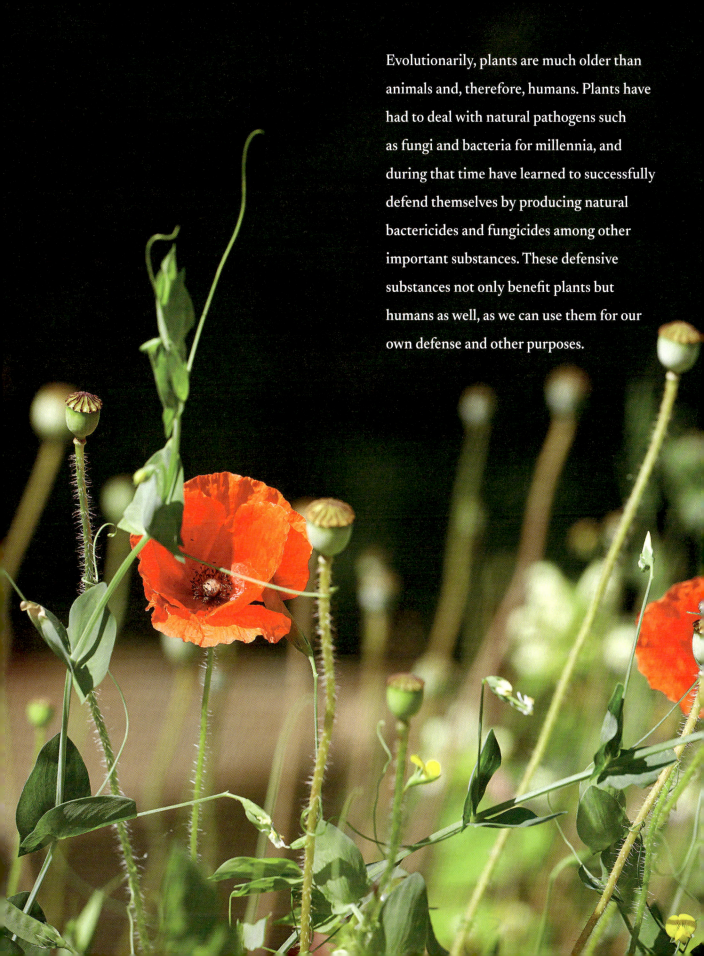

Evolutionarily, plants are much older than animals and, therefore, humans. Plants have had to deal with natural pathogens such as fungi and bacteria for millennia, and during that time have learned to successfully defend themselves by producing natural bactericides and fungicides among other important substances. These defensive substances not only benefit plants but humans as well, as we can use them for our own defense and other purposes.

OUR IMMUNE SYSTEM

People are living longer and longer, so we might expect them to be healthier. And yet the opposite is true.

A critical component of good health is our immune system, which is made up of an acquired and an innate part and is present throughout our body. Relatively simple measures can strengthen our immune system, such as getting enough exercise, quitting smoking, sleeping well, getting enough rest, and eating healthily.

It is preferable to consume at least 25 different types of plant-based foods a week, including organic fruits and vegetables, herbs, nuts, seeds, and mushrooms; there are even studies showing that you should aim for a minimum of 30 different plant foods per week.[1] A diet lacking in variety weakens the immune system.

The environment in which you live, your genetic predisposition, how you live, and what you eat play an important role in your health. It is important to know that these different factors interact, and that you can view your health holistically.

Our immune system is one of the fundamental pillars of our health. It is not only important for keeping harmful bacteria, viruses, fungi, and other microorganisms at bay but also for our overall health. I am very taken by immunologist Jenna Macciochi's idea that we should see the immune system as a kind of sense that you can train, fine-tune, and boost as you can with your other senses.[2] If you want to stay healthy, try to support it throughout your life.

As mentioned, exercise, good sleep, plenty of fresh air, varied organic food (including 300 grams/10.5 ounces of fresh plant-based foods each day, such as vegetables and fruits) and the use of beneficial plants and mushrooms are a good first step to boosting your immune system. Taking a cold shower has also been proven to improve our resistance.[3] In Europe's earliest hospitals, often in monasteries, the (monastery) garden was considered an essential part of the healing process.

Gut Flora

Consuming plenty of omega-3 fatty acids (such as from walnuts) and specific plant substances such as polyphenols has a positive effect on our immune system. Polyphenols have an anti-inflammatory and anticarcinogenic effect and protect the body's cells against free radicals. Well-known examples are anthocyanins from wild blueberries, blackcurrants, and raspberries; sulforaphane from broccoli; resveratrol from grapes; ECGC from green tea and matcha; vitamins A, C, and E; fiber; and probiotics.

Fiber, in particular, feeds the good bacteria in your intestines and is essential for healthy gut flora—there may be a relationship between imbalanced gut flora and obesity, depression, Alzheimer's disease, and allergies. Most of your immune system is, in fact, located in your gut. As Swiss physician Alfred Vogel put it, "Death sits in the intestines."[4]

Indeed, diseases often enter our bodies through the intestines, so it is extremely important to maintain good gut flora. Being conscious of what you put in your body, what you eat and drink, and the effects of diet on your health and resistance is essential. Billions of bacteria and viruses live in our intestines, most of which we need and are beneficial. A well-functioning immune system recognizes the good microbes and leaves them alone, while malicious intruders are blocked or dealt with. In fact, our immune system attacks anything that looks genetically different from us and, moreover, it has a "memory." If we experience a great deal of stress, take certain medications, and consume excess alcohol, a pathogen is more likely to be able to penetrate the intestinal mucosa. Our bodies also perceive extreme sport as stress, which means that insufficient energy goes to the core of resistance, our intestines.[5]

The good bacteria even pass on information to our immune system about new, still unknown microbes. Our brains and intestines are strongly connected. For example, 95 percent of the "happiness hormone" serotonin is produced in the intestines. It is also important to train your immune system and not spend all your time in a sterile environment. This works in the same way as vaccines, which are designed to trigger an immune response, thus protecting us against future exposure to certain diseases.

Inflammation

Many diseases are caused by inflammation. When your immune system is functioning well, it detects inflammation and clears it. Inflammation is an immune response that is crucial for our health but primarily intended as an acute short-term attack. If your immune system is not functioning properly, inflammation can become chronic, severe, and cause diseases.

One of the causes of inflammation is bacteria. Many people are frightened by the word bacteria, yet we live symbiotically with many bacteria that actually help us. In our intestines, especially, there are billions of bacteria that we should see as allies; our body is essentially an ecosystem with many different inhabitants. In fact, 99 percent of the bacteria that surround us at any given moment do not cause disease.[6]

Most people who are given antibiotics for a urinary tract infection, for example, do not realize that these will also kill the good bacteria in their gut. Although antibiotics are fantastic medicines that have saved millions of lives, you have to be careful with them. Using them too often weakens your overall immune system (especially in your intestines), making you much more susceptible to a flu virus, for example.

One of the disadvantages of a large number of chemical antibiotics is the long-term side effects. They also destroy the natural balance in our intestines by killing the good bacteria along with the bad, weakening our resistance in

> In our intestines, especially, there are billions of bacteria that we should think of as allies. Our body is essentially an ecosystem with many different inhabitants. In fact, 99 percent of the bacteria that surround us at any given moment do not cause disease.

the process. This is something we have only lately come to realize, as the long-term dangers were not previously known. If it is medically necessary to go on a course of antibiotics, I think it is important to simultaneously supplement with high-quality probiotics and prebiotics to replace any beneficial bacteria that are lost.

Your immune system uses short-lived but powerful inflammation to eliminate pathogens. It is used for defense; however, under certain circumstances, temporary inflammation can become chronic and weaken your immune system. On the other hand, you can also overstrain your immune system, allowing an allergy or autoimmune disease to develop, essentially an overreaction. Many people experience chronic inflammation that may not be evident but causes damage. You can do a great deal to prevent and counteract chronic inflammation, starting with adjusting your diet to include more antioxidants from fruits and vegetables.

Many people are deficient in nutrients because their diet is too limited and thus, lacks trace elements, minerals, vitamins, antioxidants, and other beneficial plant compounds, as well as good fats and enough healthy protein. As you probably already know, eating junk food, such as industrially processed and refined products, is the first thing that destroys our immune defenses. The "Standard American Diet" (SAD) is considered one of the unhealthiest in the world by physician and researcher Kris Verburgh, and many agree with this.

Verburgh believes that the body's own antioxidants, which are thousands of times better at neutralizing free radicals than antioxidant supplements, need the mineral selenium in order to function properly, as is the case with many of the immune system's proteins.[7] Most Europeans and Americans do not get enough selenium as soil in Europe and many parts of the United States of America is depleted of this mineral. Seafood, such as oysters, is high in selenium, as are some types of nuts and seeds.

One of the richest natural sources of selenium is Brazil nuts, with each nut containing 60–90 micrograms of selenium. Although it is essential, too much selenium is unhealthy, so don't eat Brazil nuts every day; instead, aim for no more than a few a week.[8] Nettles and spirulina also contain selenium.

When it comes down to it, you do not have to get too worked up about taking extra nutritional supplements if you eat a diet containing a variety of organic foods. However, since many people lack minerals, it may be a good idea to take an all-natural mineral supplement.

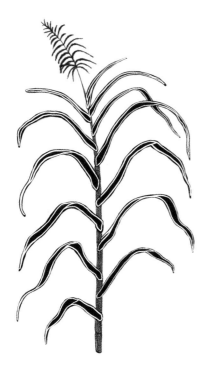

SUGAR CANE – Millions of people (mostly Africans) were exploited and died because of greedy Westerners who, using violence and slavery, put them to work on plantations. Many of these people did not even survive the journey from their own countries. In Europe, for years, sugar was reserved exclusively for the wealthy elite; now it is a billion-dollar industry, and everyone eats it. Not a good development, because excess white sugar has led to many diseases and obesity. But on a positive note, we have sugar to thank for the prolonged shelf life of food and medicinal herbs in syrups, for example.

One special mineral source is shilajit, also known as the "sweat or tears of Himalaya." It comes from prehistoric plant material released from the rocks of the Himalayan Mountains by pressure and the heat of the sun. It's also found in other places like the Altai mountains, and sometimes called *mumijo* in its purest form. Akin to ancient tar, it is a natural extract from the primeval forest that existed here millions of years ago. Shilajit is a complex natural mix of at least 85 minerals, five of which do not occur in natural form in any other substance on Earth. In Indian Ayurvedic medicine, shilajit is considered a *rasayana* ("path of essence" in Pali or Sanskrit), a substance that helps boost our strength, immunity, and vitality. Sanskrit scriptures that are 3,000 years old already mention shilajit as a "destroyer of weakness."

Shilajit's main bioactive component is fulvic acid. Fulvic acid helps our body to detoxify, regulates our body's pH value, and improves the absorption of nutrients, particularly minerals. Fulvates (the salts from fulvic acid) act as antioxidants that neutralize harmful free radicals, among other things, and help the body to get rid of free radicals. Animal studies have shown that shilajit improves cognitive function and blood supply to the brain.

Most people have elevated blood sugar levels from eating too much sugar. This causes the body to become "candied," as it were, and leads to the development of persistent inflammation. Eating too much sugar also accelerates ageing. In addition, pesticides found on non-organic foods weaken our immune system and can also cause inflammation, which you obviously do not want. It is common knowledge that obesity contributes to chronic inflammation. That's why eating well-balanced food and limiting "fast" processed carbs like white sugar, flour, and starch is important. It is better to consume minimally processed wholegrain products that release slower-acting sugars and to avoid soft drinks.

By now, most people know that white sugar is very harmful. My grandfather, August Bijdendijk, who also told me about the magical gardens of Findhorn and was a family doctor and dermatologist, told us that white sugar was the worst thing you could put in your body. This is not recent knowledge. One of the strongest men on Earth, Joseph L. Greenstein (1893–1977), better known as The Mighty Atom, noted in his biography of the same title that sugar was not nutrition but dead food, a vitamin-less, addictive drug that neither supports life nor your well-being.

As affirmed by many physicians, taking sufficient exercise (not extreme sports) is important for good health. Among other things, a healthy immune system activates your lymph nodes. Lymph nodes produce immune cells to fight infections and transport these via the lymphatic fluid to various locations in your body. But you have to move in order to activate the lymphatic system. Blood, of which an average adult human has five liters, is pumped around by the electrical impulses and muscle movements of the heart. Lymphatic fluid, of which you have on average 15 liters, can only move and flow through actual physical movement.

Aim to be on the move for at least 40 minutes a day. Being more physically active can reduce the risk of various diseases associated with ageing. A major reason for this is that physical exercise forces our cells to work harder and for longer. The damage they experience as a result makes them stronger for the future, a process known as *hormesis*.[9] You can achieve the same effect by taking a short cold shower alongside your regular warm shower in the morning, or by occasionally taking a sauna. Our bodies were never made to do so much sitting.

In addition, the abundance of light at night is not conducive to our functioning immune system and overall health, especially considering the short time in our evolutionary history in which we so fundamentally changed how we live. It simply does not match our constitution at all well.

Other Weakening Elements

Our immune system is weakened through drinking poor-quality water and ingesting airborne toxins. Particulate matter pollution emitted by industry, cars, airplanes, boats, and trucks weakens us, causing us to get sick faster and shorten our life.

Radioactive and other types of radiation can also weaken us, although some studies show that a very low dose of radioactivity can actually make us stronger, because radiation is believed to have a hormetic effect (see above paragraph).[10] Very little is known about some forms of radiation. Without realizing it, many people suffer from electromagnetic stress by spending all day in front of their laptop computers and on their phones.

Most people have elevated blood sugar levels from eating too much sugar. This causes the body to become "candied," as it were, and leads to the development of persistent inflammation. Eating too much sugar also accelerates ageing.

If, by now, you have decided to walk five kilometers every day, include a short distance barefoot on grass, a path, or stone floor to release some of this electromagnetic field (EMF) build-up. The stress hormone cortisol is also known to be pro-inflammatory. Remember that anxiety, like stress, is immunosuppressive, so meditation, moments of quietness, walking in nature, relaxing, and sleeping well are very important.

If you have never meditated, look at water in a natural environment and allow yourself to feel its flow. Taking time to become still so that you can experience first-hand the flow of nature, the flow of water, which is also the flow of your own organism, is just as good as meditating.[11] Following the fluid movement of your breathing can also help you to become still.

People who sleep six hours a night or less are four times more likely to catch a cold if they are exposed to a virus, compared to those who sleep more than seven hours a night.[12] Blue light from laptops and smartphones disrupts your sleep and disregulates your biological clock. It is best to avoid looking at your smartphone two hours before going to bed. You might also consider getting glasses with a blue light filter. Some foods contain tryptophan, the precursor to the relaxing hormone serotonin and sleep-inducing melatonin. Foods that contain this substance include bananas, broccoli, nuts, and spinach. Pistachios have the highest level of melatonin of all foods.
Also helpful are sufficient movement and natural light during the day, sleeping in a cool environment, and avoiding stimulating drinks such as coffee and black tea up to six hours before bedtime. There are obviously many more suggestions for improving your sleep that will boost your immune system in the process. You can find these yourself through various sources or you could ask your doctor for advice. But, in the words of Professor of Neuroscience and Psychology

Matthew Walker, the author of *Why We Sleep*, "The shorter you sleep, the shorter your life."[13]

Something else I want to make a case for is the use of old-school soap for washing skin. The hydroalcoholic sanitizer gels based on ethanol that we have started using so much during the past few years of the Covid pandemic should not, in fact, be used daily because they weaken the bacteria and lipid film on our skin that serves as a barrier against viruses and other microbes.[14] Many people suffer from a weakened immune system, and one reason for this is the excessive use of antibacterial products and a misunderstanding of the role of bacteria in protecting our immunity. With each passing year, our bodies become more sensitive. The more we use these alcohol-based gels, the more sensitive and thus accessible to viruses our epidermis becomes. Let's prioritize the use of simple soap again!

Boosting Your Immune System

As mentioned before, you help your immune system by training it and by not living too sterile a life. A scientific study conducted by the University of Pittsburgh in 1997 showed that people with a large and diverse social network (family, friends, work, neighborhood) are more resistant to an intentionally dispersed cold virus than people with a smaller social network. A large and diverse social network means a more powerful immune system! A small social network was found to have a greater negative impact on the immune system than smoking, poor sleep, alcohol consumption, and low intake of vitamin C.

Almost all ailments and diseases begin with inflammation at the cellular level. That's why I believe that, in addition to sufficient movement and rest, eating a varied anti-inflammatory diet that includes a wide range of (organic) foods is essential for remaining healthy. It ensures that we get sufficient different nutrients and antioxidants to help our body to detoxify and reduce inflammation, make enough white blood cells, and boost our immune system in other ways as well.

For instance, in addition to a range of medicinal plants and mushrooms that can help us stay healthy, it is good to know that asparagus contains the highest amount of glutathione of any food. Glutathione is a powerful antioxidant that is made in the liver (about 10 grams/0.35 ounces per day) from amino acids (proteins). Some orthomolecular physicians even call glutathione "the mother of all antioxidants." Orthomolecular physician Carel Hoffman once told me that glutathione is without question at the heart of protection against free radicals.

Glutathione binds to many different toxic substances, including heavy metals, solvents, and pesticides. It can convert these fat-soluble substances into water-soluble ones. Only water-soluble substances can be excreted via your liver, bile, intestines, or kidneys. Glutathione helps strengthen the immune system and keep it active. It protects your brain from deteriorating. A study from 2003 by Ralf Dringen and Johannes Hirrlinger showed that the antioxidant glutathione is essential for the cellular detoxification of reactive oxygen species in brain cells. Ageing and stress factors can cause glutathione production to drop. Supplementing it through nutrition seems like a good decision to me if you want to live healthily and longer. Avocados and walnuts are also naturally rich in glutathione.

Fasting is another thing that helps the immune system by allowing the body to clear out dead immune cells.[15] You should also know that there are some plants that can boost your resistance. When I have a cold or flu, I always use echinacea (*Echinacea purpurea*), and during the flu season, elderflower syrup (*Sambucus nigra*) is a great support for my resistance. Many essential oils have antiviral, antibacterial, and antifungal properties. We humans have a defensive and healing potential that is infinitely more powerful than any medication, which can be quickly activated by giving our body the right building blocks. Our body is a true healing machine.

You soon find that you have to do extensive research if you want to learn how to support your immune system in a natural way. When I was researching this topic, I could not find this knowledge gathered in one place, so that is what I have tried to do with this book. I dedicated myself to the pleasurable task of working through piles of scientific studies and some popular science books on the subject.

Dr. Jenna Macciochi's book on the immune system was the only place where I came across a good and accessible explanation of the immune system, but that was only after I had written this text.

In any case, the immune system is a complex entity that, rather than the occasional booster, needs regular maintenance and can be influenced and strengthened by various factors, such as sleep, exercise, and maintaining good gut flora and the right nutrition. I will not elaborate on autoimmune diseases here. The causes of these diseases remain vague and rarely have one single cause. Allergies tend to be linked to autoimmunity. They are often the result of an immune system that is over-reacting—not to ourselves but to benign nutrients and things in our environment.

Validation

These days, validation of a cancer drug up to the trial stage on humans on a sufficiently large scale costs between 500 million and a billion dollars. Such an investment seems justified if you know that a drug like Taxol earns its patent holder a billion dollars a year. But demonstrating the efficacy of broccoli, raspberries, or green tea is completely unthinkable, because these cannot be patented, and their commercialization will not recoup the initial investment. In order to prove the cancer-combatting properties of foodstuffs, we will never have human trials on the same scale as those for drugs. And that's why you often hear people say, "All these studies on mice do not prove anything for humans." And this is true, but they do make their efficacy more likely.[16] It is therefore essential to encourage public agencies to fund research into the cancer-combatting effects of foods on humans.

I believe this also applies to research into strengthening our immune system. There is ample evidence that exercise and healthy living reduce the risk of certain types of cancer, but reducing is not completely eliminating. We cannot dispel all risk, but we can influence it a great deal by boosting our immune system with resources and methods that maintain it, work preventively against diseases, and cost relatively little.

Fortunately, more and more scientific studies on this topic are being published, and we are becoming wiser about the effects of diet and lifestyle on our health. People are also gathering more information themselves and educating each other. Our countries would be greatly served by government bodies that encourage preventive medicine and support think tanks, thereby increasing knowledge and creating information services where people can voluntarily obtain and share information about how the immune system works. Likewise, in schools, children would benefit from being taught a subject covering healthy eating and natural ways to strengthen their bodies and immune systems.

Moreover, it is important to remain open-minded to other ways of eating and to nutrition and lifestyle knowledge from various cultures, and to be open to other viewpoints, because we can all learn a great deal from each other. Together we are stronger. Everything is *interconnected*. Much more is known that can unquestioningly help boost your immune system. To do this, embark on your own research. A starting point might be the books and other sources of information listed in the Resources section on page 271.

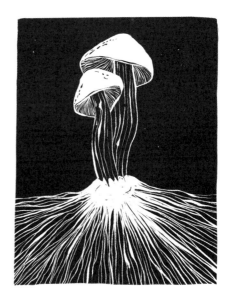

MYCELIUM – The mycelium network under the soil branches and forms in a manner that is similar to the natural phenomenon of electrically charged lightning. We have similar kinds of connections and branches in our own nervous system, brain, and brain cells.

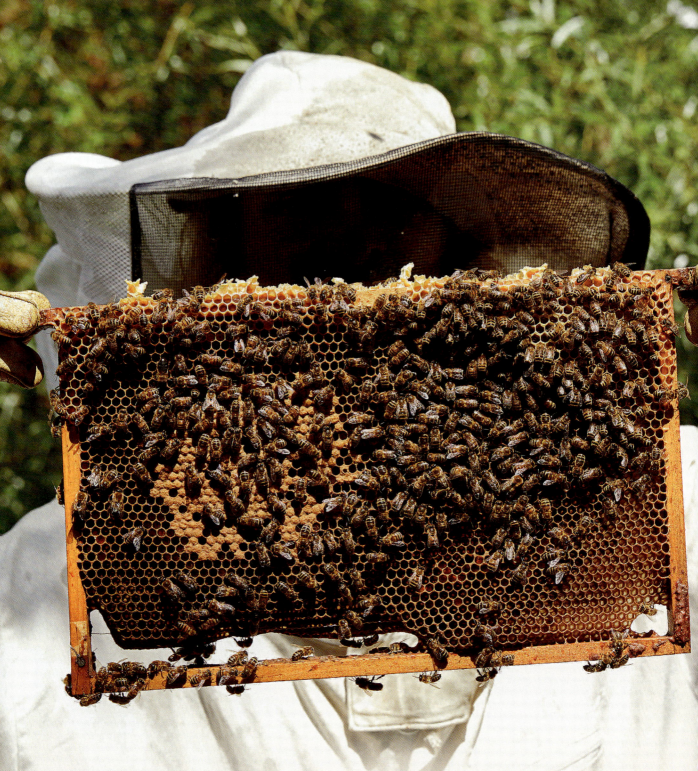

BEES – I keep a colony of black bees (Apis mellifera mellifera), the European original bee. Not only has this bee adapted well to the local flora and climate but also to living with other pollinators. Since the Pleistocene Era (1.25 million years ago), the European bee has coexisted with bumblebees and solitary bees, adapting to the flowers from which they gather nectar and pollen, and thus ensuring abundance for every species, even though they all live off the same pollen and nectar. Unfortunately, the introduction of artificially bred bee species, such as Buckfast and Carniolan bees, has led to an imbalance. The difference in spatial scale at which dark honeybees and solitary bees forage reduces competition for food. Groundwater pollution from years of artificial fertilizer and pesticide use, along with other soil contamination and agricultural monoculture, threaten the biodiversity of bees and, ultimately, the existence of humans.

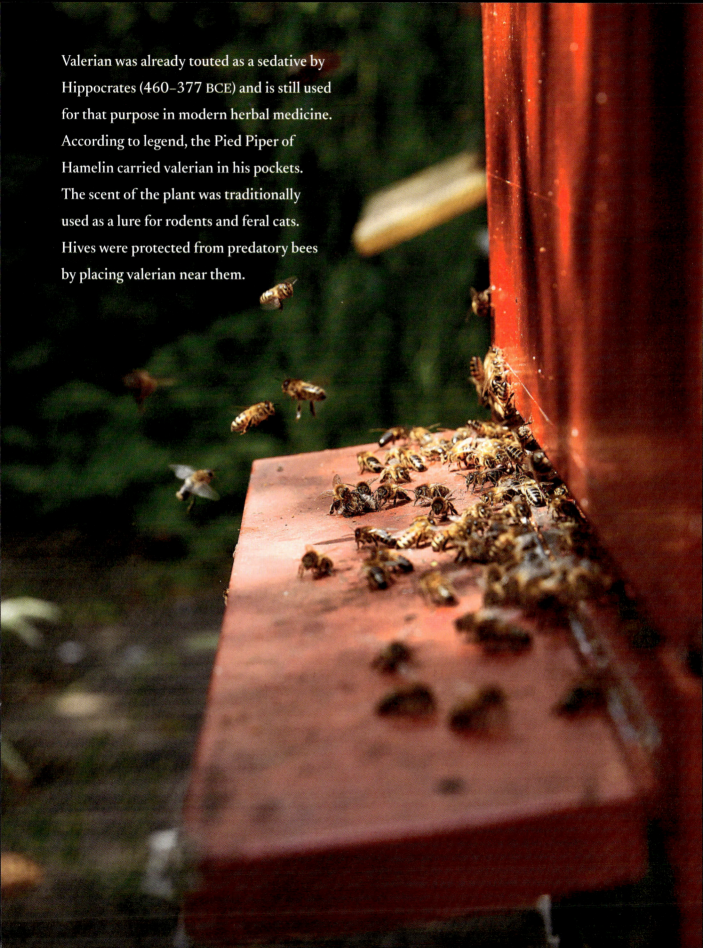

Valerian was already touted as a sedative by Hippocrates (460–377 BCE) and is still used for that purpose in modern herbal medicine. According to legend, the Pied Piper of Hamelin carried valerian in his pockets. The scent of the plant was traditionally used as a lure for rodents and feral cats. Hives were protected from predatory bees by placing valerian near them.

HOW TO USE THIS BOOK

Each chapter gives the Latin scientific name of the plant or mushroom, allowing you to explore beyond this book once you have finished reading it. There is a glossary in the back of the book with the most important active substances found in plants and mushrooms and their effects. The texts occasionally include complicated words, such as medical terms; these are also explained in the glossary. The book also has a bibliography listing sources.

You can read the chapters individually, but I recommend reading the book in its entirety first. The book is structured and organized around several categories. Each plant or mushroom covers a separate section within its category. Each section contains a comprehensive substantive description of a plant, mushroom, or plant-based product and their effects on the body and/or mind.

At the end of each chapter all kinds of practical details are given, such as a brief, clear summary of the properties and effects on the body, possible dosage, what you might need to be careful about, and how to get hold of the product. There are references to how you can make your own extracts or how to grow the plant yourself. The necessary tools are readily available in stores, or you will already have them. The pans and kitchen utensils needed for the dishes are listed alongside the recipe.

Further Plant Journeys

In this book, in addition to plants and mushrooms that support our physical health, I wanted to include particular plants I am interested in that I believe have helped humanity become what it is today. Over the centuries, through the intervention of priests and religious and state laws, attempts have been made to deprive us of the right to explore other worlds within our own consciousness. Western civilization is the only one on Earth where, for 500 years, the use of sacraments has been suppressed and demonized, driving all this knowledge and rituals underground; just like magic and other arts, it had to be hidden because practitioners were condemned. I believe that having psychedelic experiences should be a free choice, as a way to learn about other dimensions and your own mind as well as process trauma. Why, in the West, can we drink coffee *en masse* and as a result exist in a constant state of fight-or-flight consciousness, while there is often still a taboo on other states of consciousness? For instance, some plants and mushrooms can make you very empathetic.

Entheogenic (literally, "the divine within you") remedies help us understand our mind and consciousness and receive revelations. Personally, I have benefitted enormously from experimenting with these. I have taken them both in microdoses and slightly larger doses, trying these mostly in ritual settings, often in nature. But everyone is different, so the effects may also be different for you. Plant and fungi sacraments can open the door and be a bridge to an extraordinary, fascinating, and almost unearthly world. Because of this, they occupy a very important place in Indigenous magical-religious traditions worldwide. Today, they are known to us as psychotherapeutic vehicles.

Our deepest human ancestral tradition of the sacramental use, preparation, and intake of plants and mushrooms dates back to the Neolithic era, when people gathered in caves and left art that shows us that entheogens had been used, such as in the caves on the Tassili Plateau in Algeria. Exactly how these sacraments were prepared and what the precise dosages were is now being researched by psychonauts and historians. From archaeobotany and chemistry, more and more evidence is being found that psychoactive plants and mushrooms were commonly used and that they formed part of the sacraments drunk from (holy) grail cups.

Psychonauts are pioneers who have the courage to walk the path of poison and medicine. In ancient writings and works of art, we find numerous references to entheogenic substances, such as vision-inducing wines from ancient Egypt, Palestine, and Sumeria. When, in the Old Testament, strong wine is mentioned, I believe that this means wine made from visionary plants and mushrooms because, at that time, it was normal to include psychoactive plants in wine.

HOW TO USE THIS BOOK

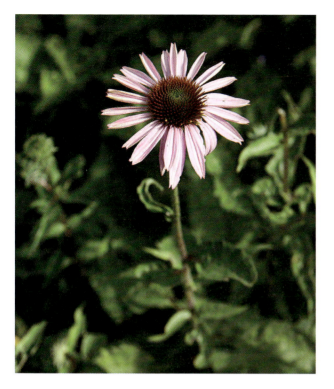
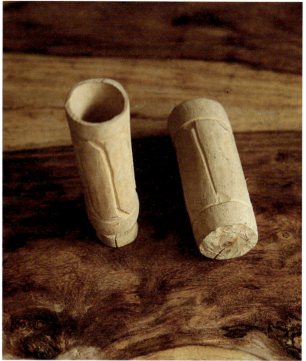
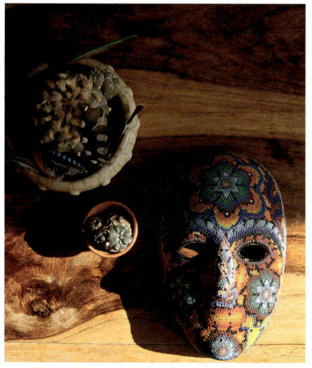
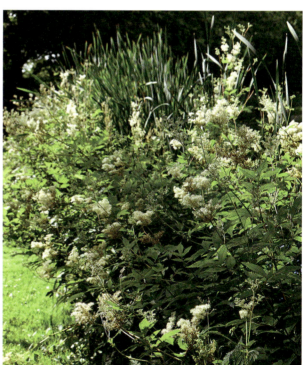

In the Bible, the use of visionary plants in the form of incense, potions, and food features frequently. With the advent of Christianity and the accompanying Inquisition in Europe, we largely lost the traditions in which entheogenic medicines played a role. We are fortunate that after the Inquisition and other (religious and colonial) expressions of power, some knowledge has been preserved in ancient writings and through oral tradition.

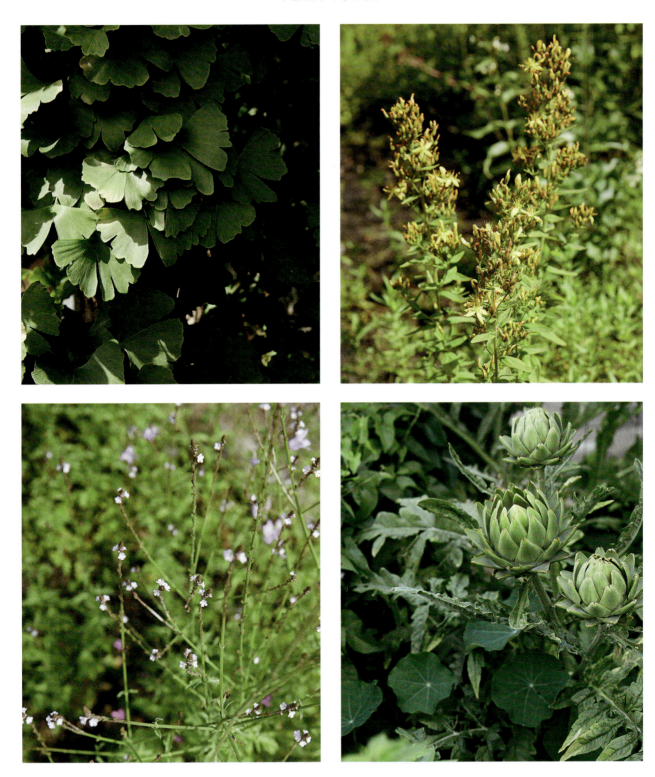

In Lapland, which I have visited several times, an even larger shamanic primal tradition existed that was more or less completely destroyed by the Church fathers. I consider it a great loss that the Sámi shamanic drums, which depicted the stories and ways of entering a state of trance, were almost all burned by Christian fanatics. Since the 1960s, more and more people have again become interested in entheogens.

It seems as if we have collectively gone in search of our spiritual roots. However, there is a difference between having a hallucinogenic trip now and having one in the past. Formerly, people sought confirmation and connection through the spiritual world and unity with their ancestors; these days, we undertake the spiritual journey primarily for ourselves, to connect with a group or with the cosmos, or as an end in itself, with society usually disapproving. Right now, in the West, we are in the midst of a psychedelic renaissance. Ever more people are taking part in ceremonies, such as the magical and sacred ayahuasca in the Amazon rainforest, or are experimenting with (microdosing) psychedelic substances.

The use of psychedelics is not recommended for people with a predisposition to psychosis, who present borderline personality disorder characteristics, and who are on antidepressants. Use psychedelics only under the guidance of experienced experts or professionals. When consuming these kinds of plants, you enter a realm that normally becomes known to us only after death. As the inscription above the gateway of the Pauline monastery on Mount Athos in Greece reads, "If You Die before You Truly Die, Then You Won't Die When You Die." Set (mindset), setting (environment), and proper preparation are important.

Plants and mushrooms have an extremely important role in all ancient shamanistic traditions and mystery schools. They teach you to live in wonder in the now. Through entheogens, many people experience blissful visions, feel reborn, and see the world and their lives through fresh eyes. In the words of one of my magic teachers, Eugene Burger: "Now I am on the way to the ultimate capital-M Mystery of life." Most people have only one psychedelic experience in their life, and that is death.

Warning

This is a literary non-fiction work and should be seen as an ethnobotanical journey aimed at preserving and passing on knowledge. The majority of information and knowledge set out in this book was found in scientific sources. We have done our utmost best to reference all these sources accordingly.

Plant Power is a journey of discovery on the path of medicinal plants. Remedies listed are purely informative and not intended to be used as self-medication. All plants and mushrooms in this book contain substances that can affect your body or mind. In some cases, incorrect dosage and/or unskilled use may result in undesired known and unknown health effects. It is the dosage that determines whether something is a medicine or a poison.

Many plants and mushrooms in this book have been used by humans for thousands of years; however, consuming plant material is entirely your own responsibility. Discuss everything you do with a physician from the conventional medical field. If you suspect that you have a medical condition, always go and see a regular doctor. Be cautious with the use of medicinal plants if you are pregnant or breastfeeding, and as above, always discuss this with a mainstream physician first.

This book is not intended to replace any medications you have been prescribed by a physician. It does not purport to be a self-help book and is intended only as a source of reference. Neither the publisher, nor the authors, nor anyone who has contributed to this guide accepts any liability for any actions by the reader. The author and publisher will be deemed innocent for any injury to the reader that may result from ingesting, using, sharing or reading information in this book. Avoid dangerous and illegal acts and always comply with the law.

All the knowledge set out in *Plant Power* is available throughout the world. In museums, living libraries such as forests and botanical gardens, archaeological sites, image and script libraries and bookstores, a treasure trove of knowledge can be found about the plants and mushrooms detailed in this book. This book is just the tip of the iceberg. I encourage you to explore further on your own.

WORKING WITH MEDICINAL AND RITUAL PLANTS

If you want to work with medicinal and ritual plants and mushrooms, it is important to know how to extract the plant ingredients and in what dosage. As mentioned earlier, it is the dosage that determines whether something is a poison or a medicine. It is also crucial to understand how to make an extracted substance from a plant or mushroom that can be absorbed by your body. Sometimes, you have to boil raw material for several hours to extract the substances so that they can be absorbed by your body. In other cases, it is more beneficial to consume the entire plant.

Essentially, many of the active substances are in fact defenses that plants use to keep natural enemies at bay. In the right dosage, these substances can work either as a drug or medicine due to their physiological effects.

A vast number of medicines available in your local pharmacy continue to be based on molecules and atoms found in plants. Sometimes molecules are recreated synthetically and at other times extracts are used. The plant and animal kingdom contain many more substances than we can recreate in a lab. That is one of the reasons why biodiversity is so important. The more diversity there is, the greater the chance of finding special and unusual substances with specific effects.

When phytotherapy, the science of herbal medicine, is mentioned, many people still confuse it with homeopathy. In homeopathy, substances are diluted to such an extent that sometimes they can no longer even be detected. In phytotherapy, you tend to work with extracts that contain actual molecules. When people tell me that they do not believe in it, I give them three cups of arabica coffee to drink. They soon notice the effect of the caffeine and then they usually understand.

During my studies, I discovered that in allopathic medicine—our most familiar, conventional form of medicine, which is based on symptom relief—double-blind studies must be able to prove the effectiveness of a medicine on the body or mind of 20 percent of patients before it can be approved. In phytomedicine in the Netherlands, a plant must show an effect in 80 percent of test subjects for it to be allowed to be sold as a medicine.

In the Netherlands, it is unfortunately illegal to provide knowledge about medicinal plants as well as to sell them. You may either sell or give information about them, but not both within the same company. Also, packaging cannot list what effect the plant may have. This also applies to risks. For example, a package of St. John's wort cannot state that it is an antidepressant, because that would be considered a "significant" medical claim, even though psychiatrists recognize the antidepressant properties of this herb. Just before all medical claims were banned, a number of phytotherapists and scientists managed to negotiate a list of the permissible claims to be drawn up. Therefore, the label on St. John's wort is permitted to say "uplifting for the mind." If you are interested in trading herbs and would like to put more than just the name of the plant on your packaging, I recommend you contact the following government agencies: In the Netherlands, the KOAG/KAG Inspection Council; in the United States, the Food and Drug Administration (FDA); in the United Kingdom, the Medicines & Healthcare Products Regulatory Agency; and in the European Union, the Committee on Herbal Medicinal Products, which makes recommendations on behalf of the European Medicines Agency.

It is also important to note that some plants can be extremely dangerous. Digitalis, which in the right dosage acts as a cardiac tonic, can be deadly if the dose is slightly too high. The plant can be picked in the wild.

Other plants or food crops, such as the goji berry, can cause a variety of unwanted symptoms if used incorrectly. When goji berries suddenly became popular in the superfood scene as an anti-ageing remedy, they were hard to come by. As it turned out, many people began to suffer from cramps due to the berries. In traditional Chinese medicine, the

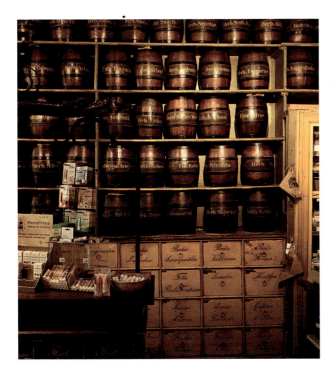 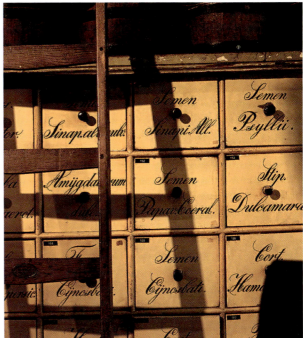

berry has been used for thousands of years, but only in very small doses; 5–10 berries a day (6 grams/0.2 ounces maximum). Now, people are throwing handfuls in their smoothies, because "they're so healthy." In other words, the correct dosage is always the key when working with plants. In traditional Chinese medicine, many medicinal plants are used for short periods of time, just long enough to activate the desired effect.

There are also plants that you need to use for a longer period before they achieve their proper effect. Ginseng, for instance, used by astronauts on the International Space Station to combat stress, only begins to work after three weeks of use.

If you want to experiment with the plants featured in this book, as noted, always do so in consultation with a mainstream physician, preferably a specialist. Also, use your own judgment (see also page 21). Furthermore, the information about the plants and mushrooms described here is not complete. Much more information about each plant is available elsewhere. If you want to conduct your own research, I recommend investigating traditional knowledge on the use of plants or mushrooms as well as scientific pharmacognostic publications on plants and monographs.

I myself try to consult at least three different sources. I find that alongside (my own) fieldwork and recent scientific research, ancient texts can offer extremely interesting and useful information. If a plant has long been used by various communities for specific purposes, this tends be an indication of clear medicinal properties. A good website for finding out what scientific and/or medical research has been conducted on certain plants is www.pubmed.gov. Search by the Latin name of the plant. For all the items in this book, I have used various research methods, including literature review, interviews, and fieldwork.

To conclude: Our bodies are part of nature and always seek a natural balance. We come from nature, and we are nature. We recharge by spending several hours in a natural environment. In addition to cleansing our body, as I mentioned earlier, sleep, rest, and regularity are also necessary to allow a healing process to run its course more effectively. Breathe sufficient fresh air, spend some time in the company of other people, and try to eat 300 grams/10.5 ounces of fresh fruits and organic vegetables per day. You may wish to supplement this lifestyle with medicinal plants and mushrooms. Each one of us is different, and each illness requires a different method to restore your unique body to top condition.

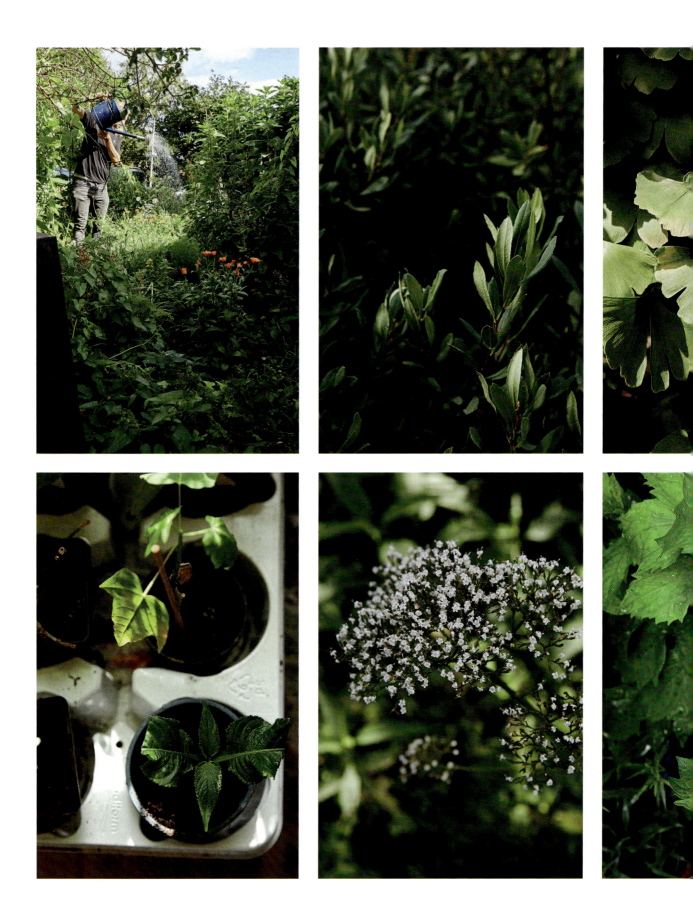

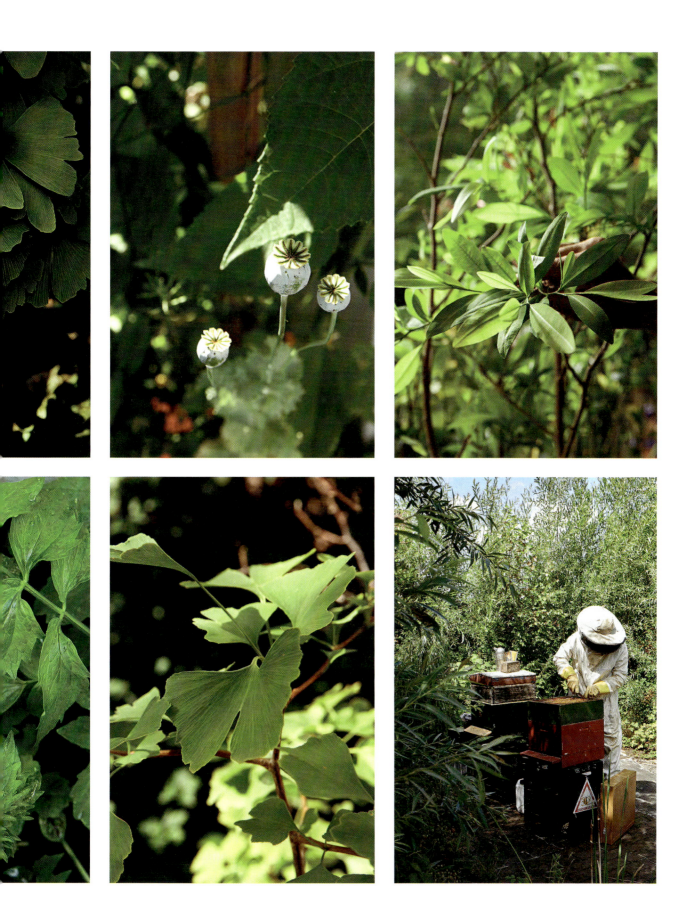

METHODS

Extraction

■ EQUIPMENT NEEDED
- coffee grinder
- pan (or 2)
- consumable alcohol, either 96% or 40% (gin, vodka)
- water
- coffee filter
- funnel
- dropper bottle
- large and small preserving jars with lids
- large and small preserving bottles with swing-top closure
- labels

In herbal medicine, various extraction methods are used to extract active substances from plants. Some substances are only soluble in alcohol, others only in oil. Some plants or mushrooms need to be boiled or cooked for a long time.

Ensure that all the equipment you use is perfectly clean: the pan, filter, and so on. If you need to filter something, use an unbleached paper coffee filter.

When making plant and mushroom extracts, or macerates, always label the container with the name of the plant or mushroom and the date. This is useful when you are making multiple extractions at the same time. This way, you can track precisely when your product will be ready. For preservation, plants are usually dried first.

A Few Rules of Herbal Medicine

Always remove plant materials from the ground with deep respect and gratitude. Ensure that you leave 75 percent of the plants in place so that the plant can continue to develop. Carefully observe the material and notice all the details.

Before You Begin, Sterilize All Bottles or Jars

Glass bottles or jars can be easily sterilized by boiling them for 15 minutes in a pan of water or by washing them in the dishwasher at the hottest setting.

Drying Plants

Many medicinal plants can be dried for later use as a tea or to make a macerate. To do this, stretch lines of hemp rope in a warm, dark, well-ventilated room. Hang the plants upside down from the lines and let them dry for 2 weeks. Put the dried plants in a plastic Ziplock bag and squeeze all the air out. You can put this bag into a larger bag. Write the harvest date and plant name on the bag. Store in a cool and dry dark space to best preserve the active ingredients.

If you have harvested roots, such as valerian or dandelion, first brush them clean under running water from the faucet. Dry them on a rack or in a dehydrator (no warmer than 40°C/100°F).

Mushrooms are best dried on an untreated wooden board in a dry space. Make sure that the fungi do not touch each other, so that enough air can circulate around them.

40, 70, or 96 Percent Alcohol Macerate

You can macerate fresh plant material in a sterilized jar with alcohol. Clean plant material thoroughly, and as noted, brush any roots clean under running water from the faucet. Finally, chop the material, and place it in the jar. Pour vodka or gin over it until all the material is submerged. Affix a label with the plant name, which part of the plant you used, and the date. Seal the jar tightly with the lid.

The more finely you chop the material, the better. This allows more of the material's surface area to come into contact with the alcohol. Let it sit for at least 14 days, shaking the jar occasionally, and then strain the contents through a cheesecloth or filter into a bowl or bottle. Make sure all your equipment is clean.

Because of the alcohol, this extraction will keep for quite a long time and can be used for 1–4 years. For easy dosing, transfer it from the jar or bottle into a dropper bottle with a pipette using a funnel.

METHODS

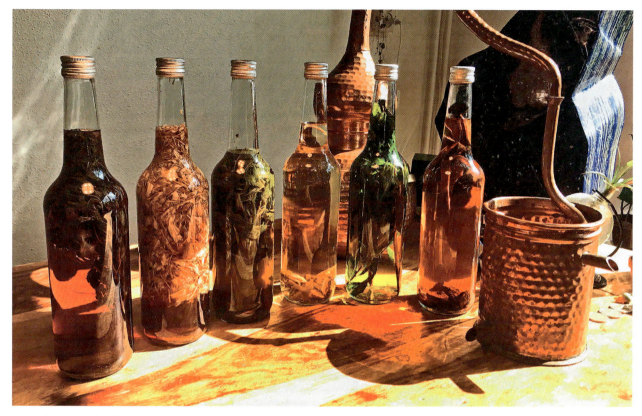

Extractions: cannabis, blue lotus, coca with kola, ginseng, gale, and chaga with reishi (from left to right)

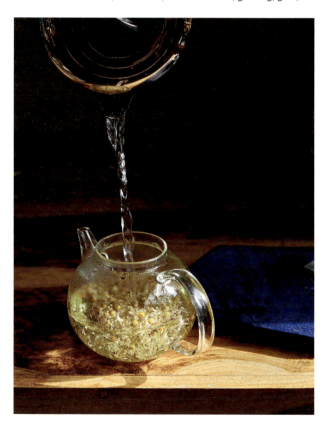

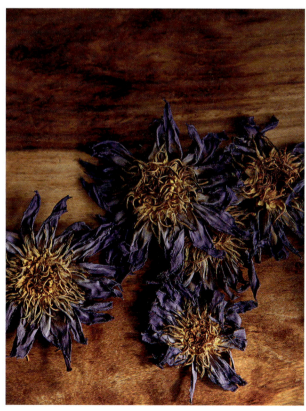

Example: *Making a Medicinal Cannabis Extract*

To take just one example, by making medicinal cannabis extract from its leaves (and buds), you experience what it is like to be a pharmacist. Collect dried leaves from the plant (perhaps including the buds), and crumble them by hand or in a food processor (10 grams/0.35 ounces of dried leaves yield approximately 0.9 grams/00.3 ounces of extract).

Place the ground leaves and buds in a nylon stocking or pantyhose (which functions as a very fine sieve) and tie it with a knot. Immerse the stocking in a bowl of 96 percent alcohol and leave for 1 hour. Remove the stocking from the alcohol, and wring it out thoroughly over the bowl wearing latex or cleaning gloves. This is important, because if you do not use gloves, you will get extremely high, because the psychoactive substances are absorbed through your skin, which we do not want. According to experts, the phytochemicals present in raw cannabis differ greatly from those in the smoke when you smoke cannabis. The medicinal effects of our cannabis extract is stronger if you do not heat the cannabis beforehand; this is great, because then you have a more potent plant medicine that does not make you high.

Leave the remaining green alcohol to evaporate in a pan with water or in a distillation device (if you want to recover the alcohol). If you have used 96 percent alcohol, the strongest available form is the last 4 percent of the substance remaining in your distiller or pan of water together with the cannabinoids. When making the extract in your pan, make sure that everything remains liquid and does not burn! The quickest way to evaporate alcohol is simply on a low heat. For safety reasons, the last part is best evaporated in a *bain-marie*, which is done by placing a heat-resistant bowl in a pan containing a layer of gently boiling water. You then pour the last remaining alcohol you want to evaporate into the heat-resistant bowl.

If necessary, use a kitchen thermometer to ensure that the extract does not get so hot that the THC-A is converted into THC. Some experts would say that THC-A does not produce a psychotropic effect. If you consistently expose THC-A and CBD-A to a temperature of 110 °C (230°F) for 30–45 minutes, it will be converted into CBD and THC, but that is not our goal here.)

Pour the extract into a sterile jar or bottle. The cannabis extract has a maximum shelf life of 1 year, after that, a psychotropic effect will still occur. Mix the extract with olive oil in a ratio of 1:10. Take a maximum of 1–2 drops per day. Use a dropper to drip the dose under your tongue.

This may come as a surprise but THC and all the other cannabinoids are lipids and are stored in your body fat. You can also cook the leaves in butter, causing the THC to bind itself to the fat in the butter. You can bake cakes with this. For the right proportions, see Wernard Bruining's *Weedology Handbook (Wietologisch Handboek)* from 1990, for example.

Hot Water Infusion (Tea)

As a rule of thumb, you can use 3 grams/0.10 ounces of dried leaves to 250 milliliters/8 ounces (1 cup) of hot water. Put the leaves in a tea bag or tea egg, and pour hot water over it. Cover the cup or pan with a lid, and let the infusion brew for a while, so that the medicinal substances work their way into your tea.

Cold-Water Extraction

Some plants need to be extracted in cold water in order to preserve the active substances, or because hot water extraction may extract toxins. Traditionally, valerian root and kava root are always prepared using cold-water extraction. Dry the roots or the other plant material and pound into powder. Scoop the powder into a piece of cheesecloth, which functions like a tea bag. Let it steep for a few minutes in cold water, and thoroughly wring out the cloth. Store the cold-water extraction in a sterile jar or bottle in the refrigerator.

Vinegar

Technically speaking, vinegar is an acidic liquid that is created by fermentation of alcohol. The fermentation into vinegar is carried out by *Acetobacter*, the acetic acid bacterium. If you want to make vinegar, you need this bacterium, in the same way that you do for kombucha or sourdough. You can use a little raw, unfiltered apple cider vinegar. If you want to make it regularly, you can also cultivate a so-called "mother," which you will see appear as a cloudy sediment at the bottom of your first bottle of vinegar.

You can make your own vinegar by pouring wine into a bowl, giving this a good stir to oxygenate it and adding in a splash of raw, unfiltered apple cider vinegar. That will start the process. Leave the bowl or jar in the dark at room temperature for a month. Cover the bowl with a tea towel or cheesecloth. After a few weeks, you will begin to smell the vinegar, and this means that it is ready. Also try enriching the vinegar by infusing it with flavorings (do not use garlic cloves; there is a risk of botulism).

Ointments

You can make beautiful ointments from olive oil by mixing 9 parts olive oil to 1 part beeswax using the *bain-marie* method. This involves suspending a bowl over a steaming pan so that the contents of the bowl do not make direct contact with the heat source.

If you want to make something really special, you can fill a jar to the brim with dried marigold petals (*Calendula officinalis*), add olive oil, seal the jar and let them steep for two months, allowing the medicinal substances to be transferred into the oil. Pour the petal and olive oil mix through a sieve or cheesecloth. With this calendula macerate, you can create a wound-healing ointment.

The oil has a regenerative and soothing effect on the skin and allows wounds to heal much faster. Adding beeswax turns it into an ointment. Allow it to solidify in small jars.

To make an even more potent ointment, you can also infuse a jar of finely chopped fresh turmeric root in oil in the same way as you did with the dried calendula flowers. Note that turmeric is a strong yellow dye. When making a facial ointment, do not add too much, and test it first on the skin of the back of your hand to see the effect. If you want to make a slightly thicker ointment or lip balm, you can change the ratio. For a balm, use 50 percent oil and 50 percent beeswax which, again, you mix in a *bain-marie*.

Experiment! I often make ointment from comfrey (*Symphytum officinale*), which is effective against bruising, sprains, back pain, and osteoarthritis. For this, use 10 grams (0.35 ounces) of beeswax, 20 grams (0.7 ounces) of coconut oil and 90 milliliters (3 fluid ounces) of comfrey oil, and prepare in the same way as the calendula maceration. Mix in a *bain-marie* again. To add fragrance, you can also add 30 drops of frankincense or lavender essential oil to your liking.

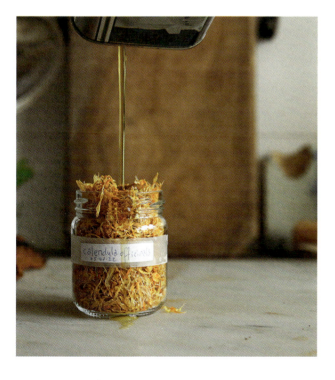
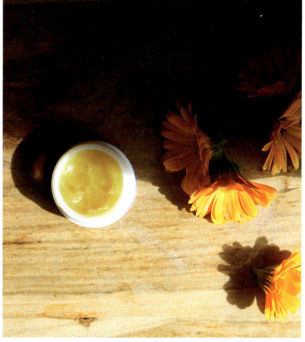

MUSHROOMS

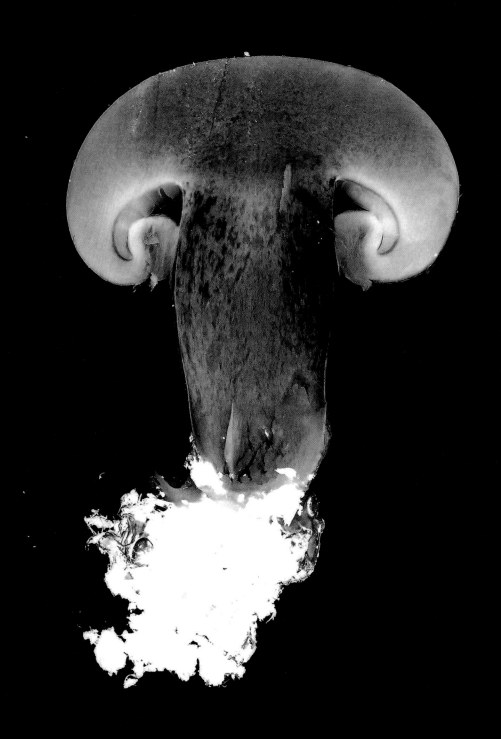

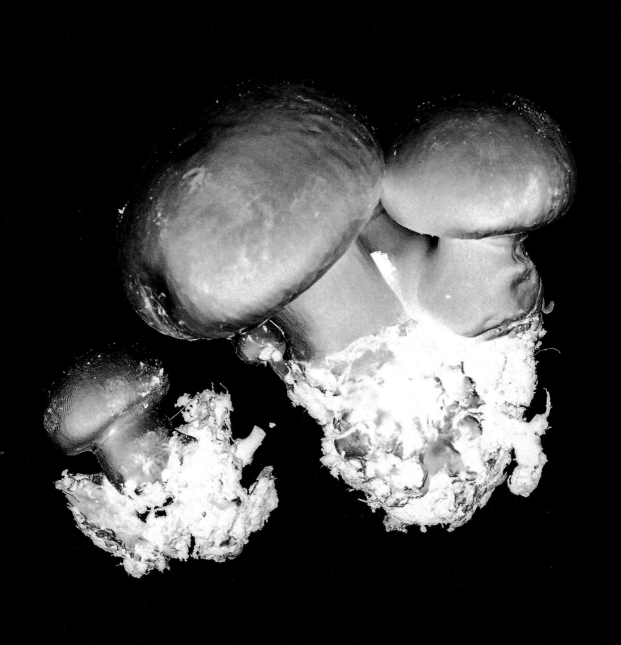

WOUTER "The first memories I have of mushrooms date back to my childhood, when I would go mushroom-picking with our father in the Belgian Ardennes. Our Christmas tree was always adorned with ornaments shaped like red mushrooms with white dots. At home, there was always a delicately crafted Chinese wooden statue of Zen teacher Bodhidharma with a large mushroom on his back. Do you remember how we used to go looking for mushrooms?"

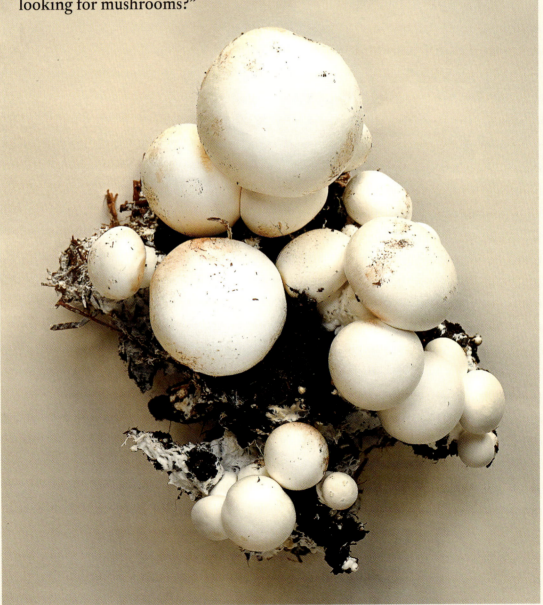

"Absolutely, I instantly picture our Belgian farm and the surrounding forest where we used to go every weekend. Chanterelles grew at the bottom of the mountain; there were pine boletes, porcini, and field mushrooms galore. After picking, we would fry our haul in butter and sprinkle it with pepper, salt, and parsley. It was so simple and delicious, a pleasure to remember. We really only picked the species we recognized, the rest we did not touch. Mushrooms add a rich and full flavor to dishes. They're almost like a kind of meat, if you ask me."

W "Some mushrooms contain quite a lot of protein and are very nutritious. I find them quite remarkable. Some astromycologists (scientists who study fungi in the universe) even believe they originate from space. Fungi were among the first inhabitants of the earth and can be found in nearly every bit of soil under our feet. They are capable of converting inorganic material into organic material on which plants can grow, in some cases producing mushrooms. These can be very tasty, but there are also many mushrooms that have strong medicinal effects, or are rather toxic or can even be deadly, such as the green death cap. That's why I always advise everyone not just to go picking, but to go out first with an experienced mushroom forager. Which mushrooms do you often use in the kitchen? And were the mushrooms featured in this book a challenge to come up with recipes for?"

J "In my restaurants, mushrooms are almost always on the menu. I like to cut mushrooms into raw slices, although I know you advise not to eat too much of this. But it has a really nice texture and adds freshness to a dish. I also love morels, ceps, and chanterelles. I didn't know all of the mushrooms you described so that was a great challenge. Chaga and reishi, for example, were completely new to me. I knew of lion's mane, but it was always hard to come by, until I met a lady who gave us two beautiful boxfuls of them.

You told me that lion's mane is good for the brain, and that's what I thought they looked like in terms of texture, and it also looked structurally like brains to me; that's why I prepared them the way I would have done with actual brains. How can it be that eating mushrooms are good for our brains?"

W "There are many similarities between the animal and plant kingdom. Fungi often live in symbiosis with plants. Through the mycelium, the network of fungal filaments, they exchange nutrients such as sugars and minerals with the plant kingdom. The mycelium also helps plants communicate with each other. From plant to plant, park to park, forest to forest—all across the entire planet there are connections between fungi and plants. We call this the "world wood web," the Internet *avant la lettre*, if you like. The below-ground mycelial system branches out and forms according to the same natural manifestation of electrically charged lightning. We find similar kinds of connections and branching in our own nervous system, brains, and brain cells. On a macro level, you can see this same pattern in the expansion of the universe in a network of galaxies; essentially a graphic representation of the world wide web, the data network of computers we know as the Internet. Thanks to the "wood wide web," plants can cooperate and communicate with each other. So, everything is connected on both micro and macro level. Not only in theory, but also in practice. Scientists from the University of Singapore have shown that consuming two servings of edible mushrooms per week significantly improves brain function. The study found that it did not matter which type of edible mushrooms were consumed."

CHAGA

INONOTUS OBLIQUUS

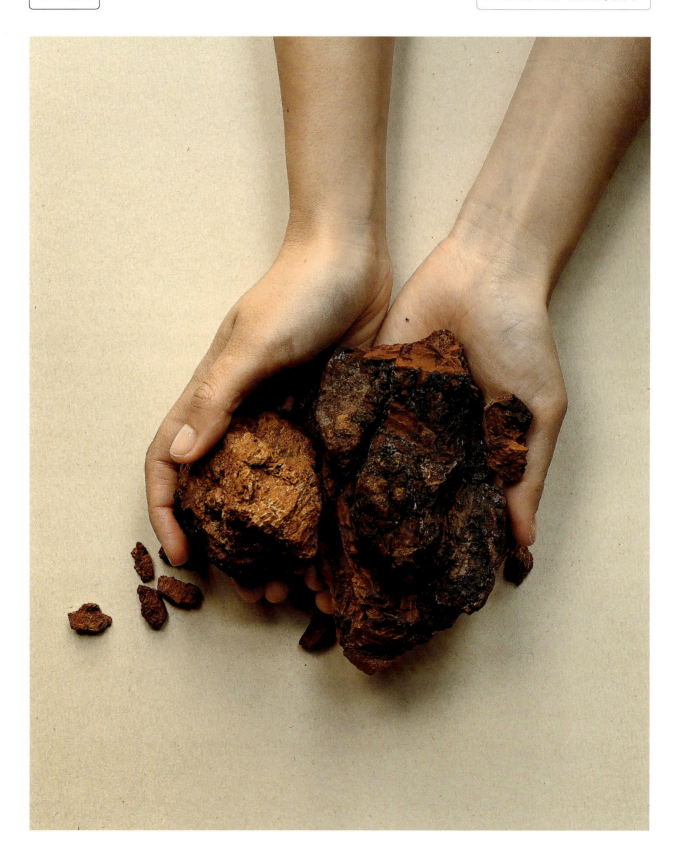

Healing Mushroom

The chaga mushroom grows around the Arctic Circle and is, rarely, found in the Netherlands, too. The name is derived from *czaga*, the Russian word for "mushroom." It is commonly known in the West as chaga. In Finland, where I first encountered these mushrooms, it is called *pakurikääpä*. I was invited by acquaintances to put on a magic show. By car and on foot, we traveled over 1,000 kilometers, all the way to the northernmost tip of Lapland. I had read about the medicinal properties of the chaga mushroom that grows on birch trees there and was eagerly hoping to find one.

In Lemmenjoki National Park, I spoke with Nils Aslak Näkkäläjärvi. He belongs to the Sámi people, one of Lapland's original Indigenous inhabitants. He sang a *joik* for us, an ancient song with magical sounds that celebrates the soul of natural phenomena such as trees. Traditional Sámi believe that all natural objects have a soul. During a joik, contact is made with the souls of nature. Afterwards, he told me about the chaga, which the Sámi use to combat flu, colds, and to strengthen their immune system. After a long search, we found a chaga mushroom. Since the beginning of our trip, I had been scanning just about every birch tree, but without luck. Nils's stories made me even more convinced of the powers of chaga, and I have been using it daily ever since in the form of teas or extracts.

Use

Chaga has been used for centuries to improve resistance. Scientific research indicates that the fungus can have a strong positive effect on the immune system and may help against the harmful effects of radiation. It appears that, in the suburbs of Moscow, there used to be much less cancer in the past, even though the living conditions there were worse than in the city center, with more pollution and greater poverty. People often did not even have enough money to buy tea, so residents in the suburbs made tea from chaga. Chaga was brewed in hot water in Russian kettles, known as *samovars*. Drinking it seemed to counter tumor growth, and it contained a substance that increased the absorption and elimination of, among other things, toxic heavy metals. The mushroom contains betulin, a substance that is now being extensively researched in connection with anti-cancer drugs.

Appearance

Chaga only occurs in the wild and, like bilberries (see page 88), requires really old, mature forests. Fortunately, there are plenty of those in Finland where 78 percent of the country is covered in forest. The fungus grows on the trunks of about one in 10,000 birch trees. The visible part of the fungus is not its fruiting body but a compact mass of mycelial threads. It looks like a sort of black, ridged clump. Inside, it is cork-like and brown. The mass tends to be rock hard and can only be removed from the tree with an axe or sturdy piece of wood.

PROPERTIES

- Antioxidant
- Antiviral
- Immune booster
- Helps remove toxins from your body

SOURCING

In countries around the Arctic Circle, you can go and forage for chaga yourself, but there are plenty of extracts and ground chaga available at health food stores and through online shops.

CAUTION

In very rare cases, chaga can cause an allergic reaction that manifests itself as breathing problems. Patients with kidney problems should avoid chaga. Excessive use of chaga can be harmful to your kidneys due to its high oxalate content.

Extracting and Dosing

Traditionally, dried chaga is extracted in two ways: in hot water and in alcohol. In Finland, the black outer part of the fungus is extracted in alcohol, and the brown inner part in hot water. In order to utilize the active substances effectively, it is best to grind the dried mushroom in a coffee grinder. Add the powder to water in a pan, and let it simmer gently for two hours. Filter the extract by pouring the liquid through a coffee filter. I will describe both the dosages that I use below.

Mushrooms

Hot-Water Extraction

Use 2 grams (0.07 ounces) of ground chaga powder per 1 liter (34 ounces) of water. I recommend making several liters at a time. Boil and filter as described above. The reservoir now contains the extract: chaga tea. The residue remains in the filter. You can drink the tea; the leftover residue can be dried and reused when you make your next batch. If you work in a hygienic way, this residue will last a long time.

Alcohol Macerate

Fill two-thirds of a sterilized small glass (preserving) jar with ground chaga. Pour vodka over this, or better still, safe-to-consume 96 percent alcohol, so that it just covers the chaga. Leave the sealed jar in a dark, cool place, and shake it once a week for 4–8 weeks. Label the jar with the date. When ready, filter the extract, and pour some of it into a dropper bottle with a pipette. Start with a few drops each day to see how you get on. You can also consume the extract in combination with the water extract.

As a maintenance dosage, and thus as a preventive against disease—prevention is better than cure— you can drink two glasses of chaga tea a week. Most people drink it as a substitute for coffee.

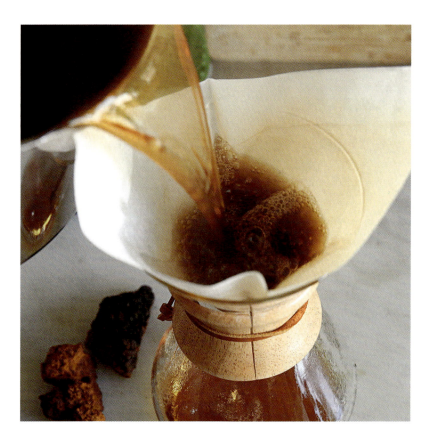

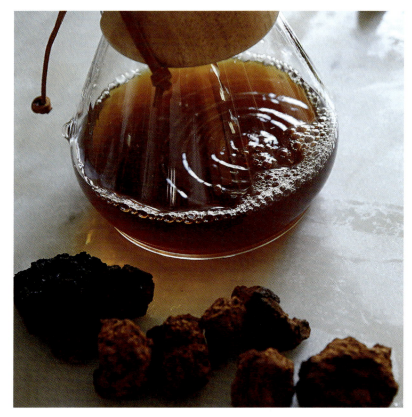

CHAGAKOMBUCHA

■ **FOR 1 LITER (34 FLUID OUNCES)**
- 1 L/34 fl oz water
- 30 g/1 oz (2 T) organic chaga powder (bought or ground yourself)
- 150 g/5 oz granulated sugar
- 50 ml/1.7 fl oz apple cider vinegar
- 1 kombucha mushroom (SCOBY, health food store or online)

■ **EQUIPMENT**
- coffee grinder for grinding (optional)
- sterilized glass jar with about 1L (34 fl oz) capacity
- cheesecloth or finely woven tea towel
- elastic band

method

Bring the water to a boil in a saucepan. Turn off the heat, and add the chaga powder and sugar while stirring.

Cover the pan with the lid, and leave for 6 hours.

Pour the liquid into a sterilized glass jar. Add the vinegar and the kombucha mushroom.

Cover the jar with a clean piece of (cheese) cloth, and secure with an elastic band.

Store the jar in a dark place at room temperature. Leave for 7–14 days. After that, store in the refrigerator.

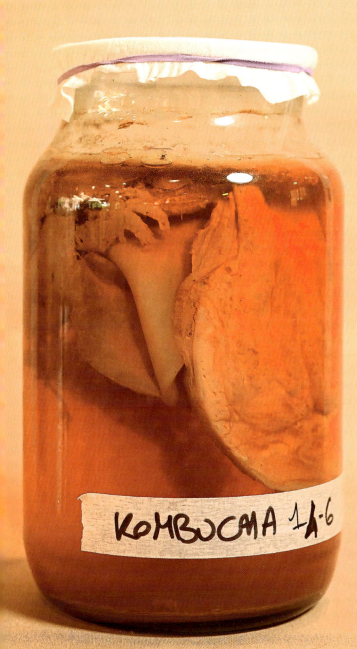

Mushrooms

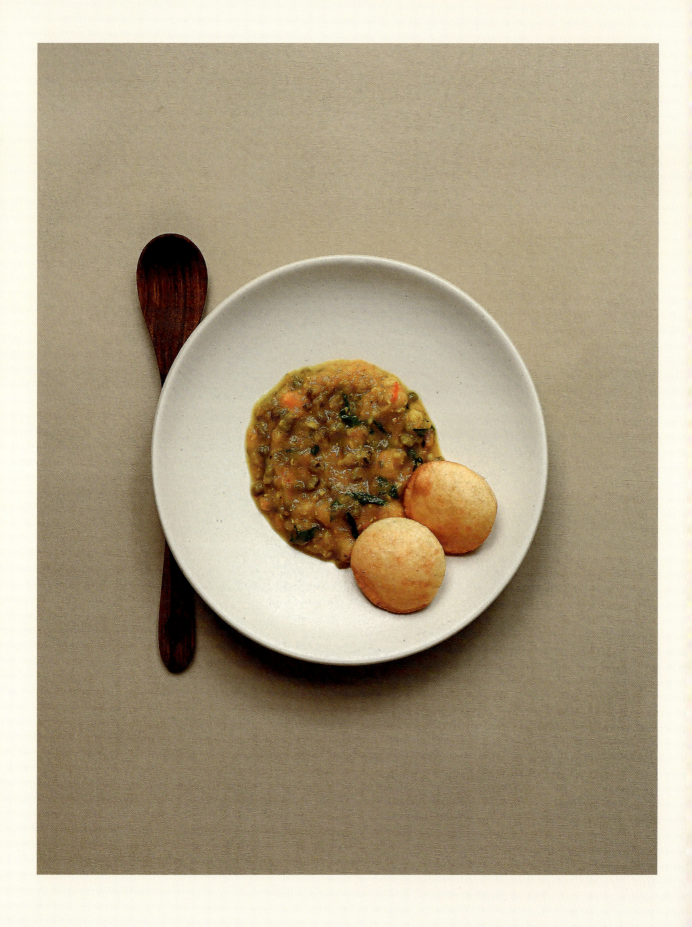

MUNG BEAN SOUP WITH CHAGA AND SOUFFLÉD NAAN

serves 4 people

■ **FOR THE SOUP**
- 100 g/3.5 oz mung beans
- 800 ml/27 fl oz water
- 4 x 1-cm/⅓-inch pieces chaga or 57 g/2 oz (4 T) ground chaga
- 8-cm/3-in strip kombu (Asian supermarket)
- 5 g/0.18 oz (1 tsp) cumin seeds
- 5 g/0.18 oz (1 tsp) turmeric powder
- 15 g/0.54 oz (3 tsp) coconut oil for frying
- 5 g/0.18 oz (1 tsp) coriander seeds
- 5 g/0.18 oz (1 tsp) fennel seeds
- 5 g/0.18 oz (1 tsp) fenugreek leaf
- 5 g/0.18 oz (1 tsp) mustard seed
- 3 cm/1-in piece ginger, grated
- ½ red chili pepper, seeds removed, and finely chopped
- pinch of fine sea salt
- 5 g/0.18 oz (1 tsp) freshly ground black pepper
- handful (about 20 g/0.7 oz) cilantro, finely chopped
- juice of 1 lemon

■ **FOR THE NAAN SOUFFLÉ**
- 40 ml/1.35 oz of water
- 6 g/0.2 oz dried yeast
- 100 g/3.5 oz flour
- pinch of fine sea salt
- 15 g/0.5 oz (1 T) plain yogurt
- 2 cloves garlic, grated or pressed (optional)

■ **EQUIPMENT**
- kitchen thermometer

method

Soak the mung beans for 6–12 hours in a pan with plenty of water, then drain.

Preheat the oven to 160°C (320°F).

Heat the water for the naan to about 38°C (100°F) in a bowl, and dissolve the yeast. Wait for the yeast to become active and then sift the flour into the bowl. Add the salt and yogurt, and knead into a dough. Leave to rest for 1 hour.

Meanwhile, place the water, chaga, kombu, cumin seeds, and turmeric powder in the saucepan along with the mung beans. Bring to a boil, then simmer for about 40 minutes.

Pour the oil into a frying pan, and fry the coriander and fennel seed, fenugreek leaf, and mustard seed until fragrant. Add the ginger and chili pepper, and sauté for 1 minute.

Remove the kombu and chaga from the soup, then add the contents of the frying pan and simmer gently for 10 minutes. Season the soup with salt and pepper.

While the soup is cooking, make 8 small balls of the dough, and roll them out flat into 2-millimeter- (0.07-inch-) thick discs about 4 centimeters (1.5 inches) in diameter. Place the dough discs on a baking tray lined with baking paper, and bake in the oven for 6 minutes. The dough soufflés in the oven into fluffy pads. Rub with garlic immediately afterwards to taste.

Ladle the soup into deep bowls, garnish with the cilantro and a squeeze of lemon juice. Serve with the souffléd naan.

Mushrooms

BUTTON MUSHROOM | AGARICUS BISPORUS

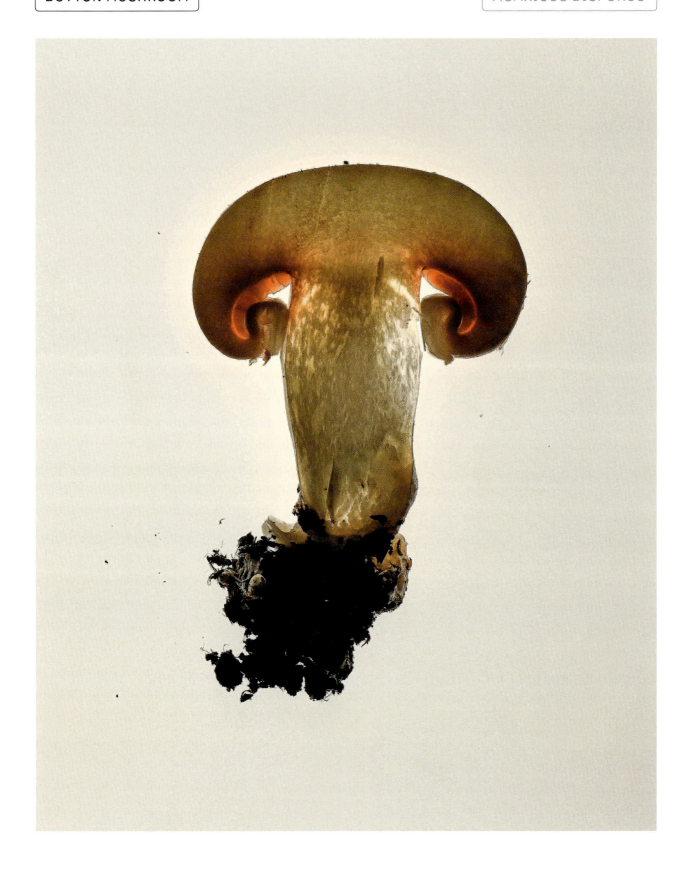

Omnipresent Fungus

Mushrooms were once regarded as enigmatic, mystical entities associated with witches and wizards, including what we know as "magic mushrooms." In the Netherlands and Belgium, mushroom consumption is mainly limited to white and chestnut mushrooms. About 260 million kilograms (573,201,882 pounds) of mushrooms are cultivated in the Netherlands each year, mainly for export. Mushrooms were not always so abundant. My father told me that, in his youth, mushrooms were a rare delicacy that you might be able to pick up occasionally, if you were lucky.

Use

The common mushroom contains a huge number of antioxidants and has anti-inflammatory properties. It is rich in copper, which is beneficial for your connective tissue, cartilage, and skin; vitamin B2 (riboflavin), which is essential for energy production; vitamin B3 (niacin), which is essential for a healthy nervous system and the production of sex hormones; and vitamin C, a powerful antioxidant and immune booster.[17]

Many people eat mushrooms as a meat substitute. Just like other fungi, button mushrooms contain proteins, but these are not the essential proteins found in, for example, meat or the alga spirulina. I eat mushrooms several times per week as a side dish, because I enjoy their taste and nutrients, but also because of a recent study by the University of Singapore, which showed that eating 100 grams (3.5 ounces) of any mushroom three times a week (regardless of the type) improves brain function (see reference list).

When eating mushrooms, it is important to chew them well, otherwise they are barely digested and the medicinal and other nutrients are not properly absorbed. It also helps digestibility to chop the mushrooms into small pieces and heat them before baking, frying, or incorporating them into a dish. Heating leads to the loss of some vitamins, but that is a trade-off you will have to accept. Breastfeeding mothers will be interested to learn that eating fresh mushrooms regularly can increase milk production.

According to the Chinese encyclopedic work *Icons of Medicinal Fungi from China* (Jiantze/Mao, 1987), mushrooms contain the substance tyrosinase, which has a blood pressure–lowering effect and can thus be used to reduce hypertension. The substance ergothioneine, which can also be found in mushrooms, is believed to have a positive effect on our bodies, due to its antioxidants.

Appearance

Button mushrooms look like white or light brown half-spheres. They are smooth and have a short stem when harvested. The fungus from which the fruiting body emerges lives underground, so no daylight is needed to grow mushrooms. They reach a height of 4–10 centimeters (1.6–3.9 inches) and are cultivated in special spaces in a specifically mixed growing medium that contains horse manure and topsoil.

Extracting and Dosing

It is recommended to incorporate mushrooms into dishes several times a week.

PROPERTIES
- Lowers blood pressure
- Source of antioxidants
- Increases milk production
- Protects our DNA
- Anti-inflammatory
- Source of vitamins
- Good for connective tissue, skin, and cartilage

SOURCING

Mushrooms are readily available from any greengrocer, farmers' market, or supermarket.

CAUTION

In my view, it is not wise to eat mushrooms raw, because they contain agaritine, which could have toxic effects. In large quantities, agaritine has been shown to cause damage in tests on mice and to increase the risk of bladder cancer in these rodents. This substance dissipates when you cook or bake mushrooms. You do not need to worry about occasionally consuming a few slices of raw mushrooms, as in Joris's recipe.

Mushrooms

MILLEFEUILLE OF RAW BUTTON MUSHROOM, COCOA, APPLE, AND AVOCADO

serves 4 people

■ FOR THE LEMON CREAM
(about 125 g/4.4 oz)
- 100 g/3.5 oz organic lemons (about 3)
- 500 ml/17 fl oz water
- 400 g/14 oz granulated sugar

■ FOR THE FEUILLES DE BRICK
- 4 sheets North-African brick dough (feuilles de brick); filo pastry may be substituted
- 10 g/0.3 oz butter
- 5 g/0.18 oz (1 tsp) honey

■ AS WELL AS
- 250 g/8.8 oz medium-sized button mushrooms, as fresh as possible with their stalks removed
- 2 avocados
- 2 green apples, such as Granny Smith
- pinch of cocoa powder

■ EQUIPMENT
- small bowl
- skimmer
- plate or approx. 20 cm/7.9 inch cake (cutter) ring
- mandolin

method

Start with the lemon cream. Cut a small piece off the top and bottom of each lemon and then cut them lengthwise into quarters and those quarters again into slices as thin as possible. Remove any seeds. Put the lemon slices in a stainless steel, glass, ceramic, or plastic bowl or container—acidic foods like lemons can discolor aluminum, copper, and iron bowls or trays, and make them taste metallic. Add the water, cover with a lid or tea towel, and leave the lemons on the counter overnight.

Put the lemons and the water in a saucepan and bring to a boil on a medium-high heat.

Simmer gently for about 45 minutes, or until the lemon peel is soft and tender. The time may vary depending on the variety of the lemon and the thickness of the slices.

Add the sugar, and cook on a low heat for about 20 minutes, until a thick marmalade forms. Skim off the foam that rises to the surface during the reduction process. Take 1 teaspoon (5 g/0.16 oz) of the marmalade and spoon onto a plate that has been chilled in the refrigerator. If the marmalade is firm, then it is ready. If it is still runny, then boil a little longer until further reduced.

If you want a smooth cream, then blend with a hand blender in the pan. Sealed airtight in a sterilized jar, the marmalade can be kept in the refrigerator for 4 weeks.

Preheat the oven to 80°C (176°F). Place a sheet of *feuilles de brick* or filo pastry on a cutting board and, using the plate or cake ring, cut or press 2 circles [out of the sheet]. Meanwhile, melt the butter with the honey in a small saucepan. Brush the *feuilles de brick* sheets with the butter-honey mixture, and stack them on top of each other.

Place the stack of *feuilles de brick* or filo dough sheets between 2 sheets of baking paper, and rest a weight on this, such as a heavy pan or an oven tray. Bake in the oven for 10 minutes until golden brown. Let it cool with the weight on top.

Slice the caps of the mushrooms horizontally over the mandolin, creating round slices. Do the same with the avocado and apple.

Place the cooled *feuilles de brick* or filo dough stack on a large plate, layer the slices of mushroom, then the apple and finally the avocado on top. Repeat until everything has been used up, finishing with a layer of mushrooms.

Sprinkle the cocoa powder on top. Cut into wedges, and serve with a spoonful of the lemon cream.

Mushrooms

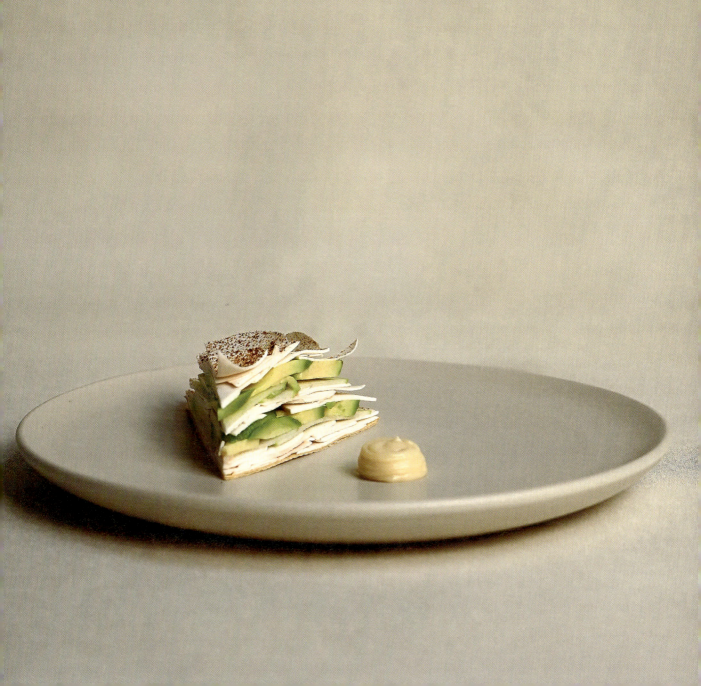

CHAMPIGNON Á LA GRECQUE WITH ARTICHOKE AND FENNEL SEEDS

serves 4 people

■ INGREDIENTS

- 300 g/10.6 oz button mushrooms, halved
- 400 ml/13.5 fl oz vegetable stock
- 100 ml/3.4 fl oz white wine
- ½ onion, cut into thin strips
- zest of 1 organic lemon, cut into thin strips
- 45 ml/1.5 fl oz (3 T) olive oil
- 30 ml/1 fl oz (2 T) apple cider vinegar
- 5 g/0.18 oz (1 tsp) fennel seeds
- 5 g/0.18 oz (1 tsp) coriander seeds, finely crushed
- 1 bay leaf
- 2 cloves garlic, grated
- 60 ml/ 2 fl oz (4 T) tomato paste
- 5 thyme sprigs, freshly picked
- fine sea salt and freshly ground black pepper
- 4 violet artichokes, cooked and cleaned

method

Put all the ingredients, except the artichokes, in a large saucepan and bring to a boil.

Simmer gently for 10 minutes, add the artichoke and simmer gently for another 5 minutes.

Using a skimmer, scoop all the vegetables out of the pan and place in bowls.

Boil the stock a little longer to strengthen flavor. Pour the hot stock around the vegetables on the plates.

Mushrooms

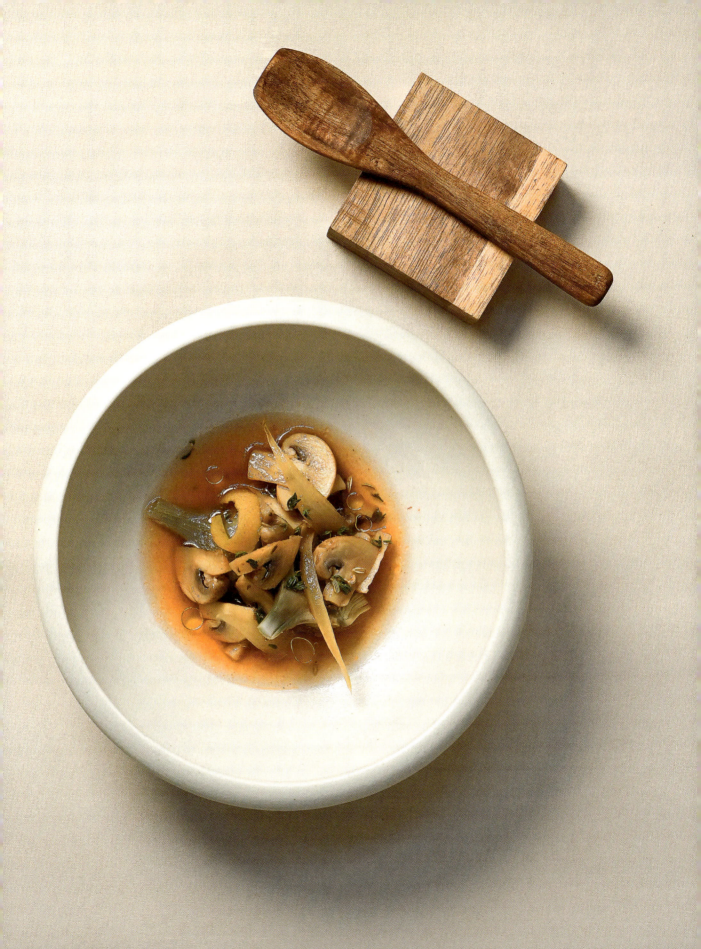

| INK CAP | | COPRINUS COMATUS |

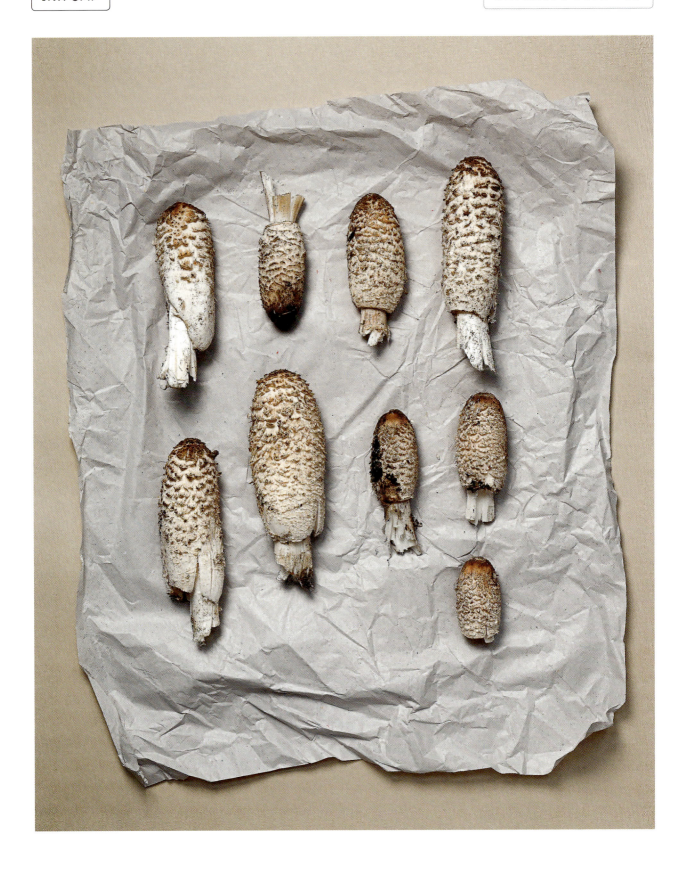

Blood Sugar-Reducing Delicacy

According to old reference books, ink cap mushrooms were actually used to make ink. This ink essentially consists of millions of mushroom spores.

My first memories of mushrooms stem from early childhood. My brothers and I were taught by our father how to recognize and pick young ink cap in the Belgian Ardennes. We baked them golden-brown as soon as we got home and ate them on a slice of buttered bread. They are delicious and taste a bit like asparagus.

The ink cap is not only extremely tasty but also has numerous medicinal properties and contains a host of vitamins and minerals. Ink caps grow in abundance all over the Netherlands and Belgium, as well as the rest of Europe and North America. In Asian countries, understanding about medicinal mushrooms is much more advanced—much knowledge was lost in Europe as a result of the witch hunts—but the great thing about the ink cap is that its medicinal recognition has a European origin. It really belongs to European culture and has been traditionally used as a medicine and eaten as a delicacy. The mushroom is also used in traditional Chinese medicine.

Use

Ink cap is rich in protein and contains all eight essential amino acids, vitamins A, C, D, and E, and the mineral zinc. In addition, it contains vanadium, a special mineral that helps regulate insulin production. The ink cap further helps fight off parasites by killing them.

Appearance

Ink caps look like folded umbrellas. They are egg or bell-shaped, white in color, with a light brown, smooth-centered cap with curled scales running down the side. The cap eventually opens out, collapses, and turns black. Its hollow stem stretches to 10–20 centimeters (3.9–7.8 inches). They can be found from May to October, usually in grass or lawns on sandy soil. Ink caps often grow along roads, on dikes, and in city parks.

Extracting and Dosing

To prepare ink caps, scrape the hat of the fungus clean with the blade of a knife. I only eat the bright white part. If you want to use the ink cap for therapeutic purposes, consult with a mycotherapist and your primary care physician. As a medicinal delicacy, you will probably only eat it a few times each season and no side effects are known about ingesting it in this quantity. It is helpful to know, however, that all edible (medicinal) mushrooms have a detoxifying effect: when first taken, they can cause a slight headache or nausea in some people.

To make ink, take around 10 already blackened ink caps. Put them in a pan with 2 cloves, and simmer for about 5 minutes. Strain into a bowl, and store in a sterilized airtight jar. Due to the cloves' preservative effect, the ink can be kept for years. Also, the cloves give the ink a pleasant fragrance, rather than smelling of rotten mushrooms.

PROPERTIES
- Immunomodulatory
- Antiviral
- Antiparasitic
- Antioxidant
- Promotes insulin production
- Contains all eight essential amino acids
- Source of vitamins and minerals

SOURCING

When in season, pick young, pointy ink caps in your neighborhood. Note: always pick with respect for nature, making sure the mushroom can carry on growing (cut them at soil level; don't pull them out), and always leave more than 75 percent of the mushrooms in place!

CAUTION

Avoid alcohol when eating ink caps. It will give you an unpleasant feeling inside. Only young ink caps are edible. Prepare ink caps as soon as possible, at least within a few hours of picking them, as they wilt quickly. Be sure you are eating the right kind of ink cap; join an experienced forager for a mushroom-picking session first.

Mushrooms

TOAST WITH FRIED INK CAPS AND PARSLEY BUTTER

serves 4 people

■ INGREDIENTS

- 10 ink caps
- 50 ml/1.7 fl oz sunflower oil
- 50 g/1.7 oz butter
- 1 shallot, cut into rings
- 1 bunch (approx. 40 g/1.4 oz) of leaf parsley
- 1 garlic clove
- 4 slices of sourdough bread, toasted
- fine sea salt and freshly ground black pepper

■ EQUIPMENT

- mortar

method

After the ink caps have been picked, you need to act quickly. Scrape the outside of the mushrooms with a small knife. This way, you will know for sure that you have removed the sand. Pull or cut the cap into strips.

Heat the sunflower oil in a skillet on medium heat, and fry the ink-cap strips until golden-brown.

Add half the butter, then the shallot, and sauté for a moment in the sizzling butter. Pick the parsley leaves from their stalks, and add half to the pan.

Meanwhile, crush the remaining parsley leaves and the garlic in a mortar, and mix with the remaining butter. Spread this onto the slices of sourdough bread. Season the mushrooms with salt and pepper, and divide them over the slices of bread with the parsley butter.

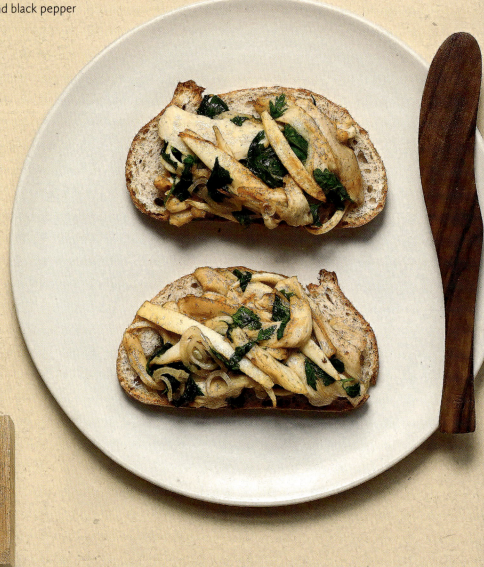

Mushrooms

VEGETARIAN PASTA CARBONARA WITH INK CAP AND REMEKER CHEESE

serves 4 people

■ INGREDIENTS

- 400 g/14 oz spaghetti
- 3 egg yolks
- 1 whole egg
- 100 g/3.5 oz Remeker cheese, grated (a raw Gouda-style cheese)
- 200 g/7 oz ink caps
- 15 ml/0.5 fl oz (1 T) olive oil
- fine sea salt and freshly ground black pepper

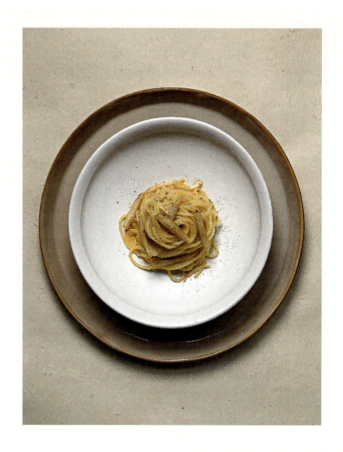

method

Make this dish as soon as possible after you have picked the mushrooms, as they only last a short time. Cook the spaghetti according to the package instructions in a pan with plenty of salted water. Meanwhile, whisk the egg yolks, the whole egg, and the grated Remeker cheese in a bowl.

Scrape the outside of the mushrooms with a small knife. This way, you will know for sure that you have removed the sand. Pull or cut the cap into strips.

Heat the olive oil in a skillet on medium heat, and fry the ink-cap strips until golden-brown. Turn off the heat.

Drain the spaghetti, but save a cup of pasta water. Add the spaghetti to the pan containing the ink caps, and pour in half the saved pasta water.

Roll around the pan, and add the egg mixture. Stir and roll around until the spaghetti is evenly coated with the sauce. Work quickly to prevent the eggs from congealing. If necessary, add the remaining saved pasta water. Season with salt and pepper.

| REISHI | | GANODERMA LUCIDUM |

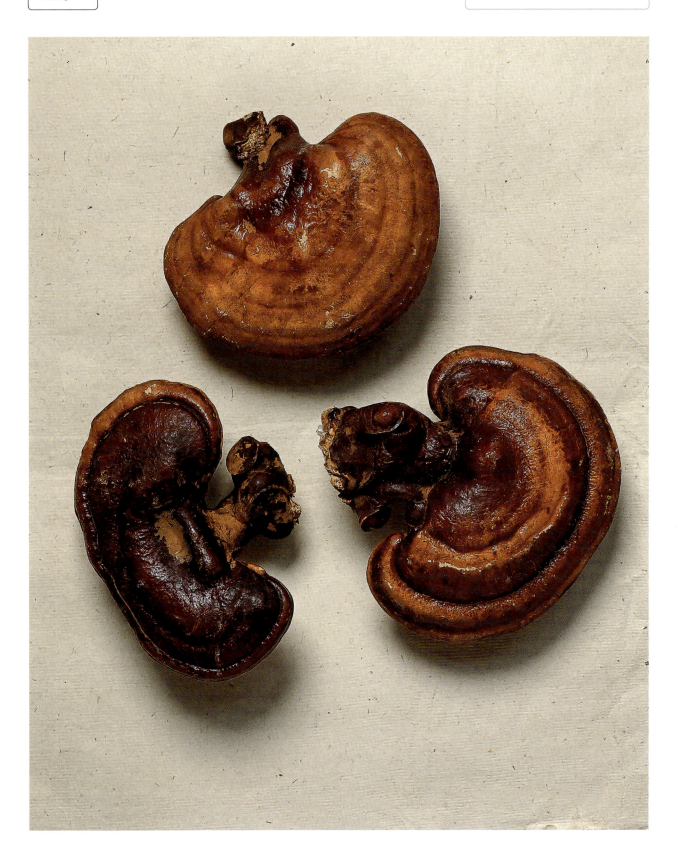

Mushroom of Immortality

Reishi has various medicinal properties. In traditional Chinese medicine, reishi is regarded as fortifying, detoxifying, and warming, and is one of the life-extending medicines.[18] The mushroom has a beneficial effect on the immune system and is used therapeutically for liver disorders. Reishi is officially recognized by the Japanese and Russian governments as an efficacious mushroom against certain types of cancer, as research has shown that reishi significantly interferes with the formation of new blood vessels in cancerous tissue, preventing those tissues from growing and spreading. Several scientific studies have shown that reishi has antitumor properties.[19] The book *Icons of Medicinal Fungi* from China asserts that reishi render mice resistant to radioactivity.

Reishi additionally acts against nervous weakness and forgetfulness. The mushroom is also prescribed to reduce stress and is used as an antidote to poisonings caused by toxic mushrooms.

The mushroom contains many bioactive substances such as polysaccharides, vitamins, and minerals and trace elements such as chromium, copper, selenium, boron, and germanium. Germanium is involved in stabilizing the immune system. Germanium is also found in garlic and ginseng.[20] Reishi is beneficial for respiration, as it improves oxygen uptake via the lungs, and therefore, like ginseng and coca, has a beneficial effect on endurance. Finally, the fungus has strong antiviral and antibacterial properties.

Appearance

When the mushroom is wet on top it looks almost lacquered; the cap then has a beautiful woody-brown color, which is why it is called "Japanese lacquer mushroom" in Dutch. It is native to several places, from the Amazon to the southern states of North America and many countries in Asia, but the mushroom is rare in the wild. The fungus tends to grow on logs of wood. Holes are drilled in the sides of fresh logs. Rods of wood-infused mycelium spawn are then inserted into those holes. After about a year, reddish-brown reishi mushrooms grow from the logs.

Extracting and Dosing

Reishi extracts can be used preventively on a daily basis. If you can get it in powder form, ½ a teaspoon (2.5g/0.07oz) of extract is sufficient. Swallow it with some water, or mix it with food or drink; for example a smoothie. *The Pharmacopoeia of the People's Republic China* recommends 6–12 grams (0.2–0.4 ounces) of reishi extract daily.[21]

Fungotherapists can prescribe and use very strong medicinal active extracts from often wild or specially grown fungi. If you really want to cure something, I highly recommend you to work with a well-trained fungotherapist like Aurora Grigorjeva, for example.

PROPERTIES
- Improves breathing and endurance
- Antiviral
- Antibacterial
- Anti-stress
- Antitumor
- Enhances mental strength
- Boosts the immune system
- Helps detoxify the body
- Appears to be life-extending
- Combats forgetfulness

SOURCING

Reishi extracts are available in powder and capsule from health food stores, better specialty drugstores, and online.

CAUTION

Reishi could affect other medicines. According to Dr. Geert Verhelst, it has a blood-thinning effect and, in theory, could interact with blood-thinning medication; therefore, do not use reishi before or after surgery and in cases of active bleeding, such as stomach ulcers.

Mushrooms

TIRAMISU WITH REISHI COFFEE

serves 4 people

■ **FOR THE PASTRY CREAM**
- 200 ml/6.8 fl oz whole milk
- 50 g/1.7 oz granulated sugar
- ½ vanilla pod
- 15 g/0.5 oz custard powder
- pinch of fine sea salt
- 1 egg yolk

■ **FOR THE TIRAMISU**
- 100 g/3.5 oz mascarpone
- 100 g/3.5 oz whipped cream
- 20 lady's finger cookies
- pinch of cocoa powder

■ **FOR THE COFFEE SYRUP**
- 40 g/1.4 oz granulated sugar
- 5 g/0.17 oz (1 tsp) reishi powder
- 200 ml/6.6 fl oz hot espresso

■ **EQUIPMENT**
- fine sieve

method

For the pastry cream, in a saucepan, gently bring the milk to a boil, along with 40 grams (1.4 ounces) of the sugar and the vanilla, including the scraped-out pod. Do not let the milk boil over.

Meanwhile, in a bowl, mix the custard powder with the salt and the rest of the sugar. Add the egg yolk, and stir to form a lump-free paste.

While stirring, pour a ladleful of hot vanilla milk into the custard paste. Mix well—this way the mixture warms up a little, which will set in motion the thickening process. While stirring, add the paste to the pan of hot milk, and bring gently to a boil. Keep stirring. Remove the vanilla pod.

Gently simmer the pastry cream for 2 minutes, until it has the thickness of custard. Turn off the heat, and pour the cream into a bowl. Cover with plastic wrap (clingfilm). Really press the plastic wrap onto the cream so there is no air between it and the cream, otherwise a skin will appear. Allow to cool.

In a bowl, mix together 100 grams (3.5 ounces) of cooled pastry cream into the mascarpone until there are no more lumps. Beat the whipping cream until thick, and gently fold into the mascarpone cream.

Make the coffee syrup by dissolving the sugar and reishi powder in the hot espresso. Dip the lady's fingers in this espresso mixture. If you like the cookies a little harder, dip for 1 second. If you prefer them softer, dip them for longer.

Build the tiramisu by covering the bottom of a glass or bowl with the dipped lady's fingers. Spoon a layer of mascarpone cream on top of that. Repeat, so that there are two layers of cookies and two layers of mascarpone. Just before serving, sprinkle a thin layer of cocoa powder through a sieve on top.

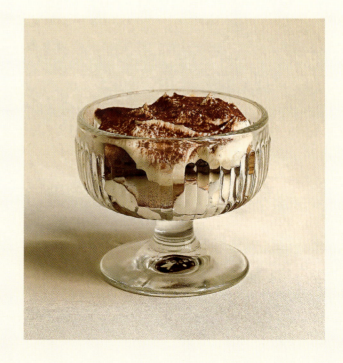

REISHI CHAI LATTE

serves 4 people

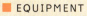
INGREDIENTS
- 500 ml/17 fl oz water
- 15 g/0.5 oz (1 T) reishi powder
- 1 cinnamon stick
- grated zest of ½ organic orange
- 4 cardamom pods
- 8 black peppercorns
- 4 star anise
- 4 cloves
- 1 thumb-sized piece of ginger, sliced
- 1 vanilla pod, halved
- 400 ml/13.5 oz whole milk

EQUIPMENT
- milk frother

method

In a saucepan, bring the water to a boil. Turn off the heat and, while stirring, add all other ingredients except the milk. Put the lid on the pan, and leave to soak for 30 minutes.

Pour the contents of the pan through a sieve into a bowl. Pour the collected liquid back into the pan, and bring to a boil again.

Meanwhile, in a saucepan, heat the milk, and froth up using a milk frother.

Fill glasses halfway with the frothed milk, and top up with the reishi chai.

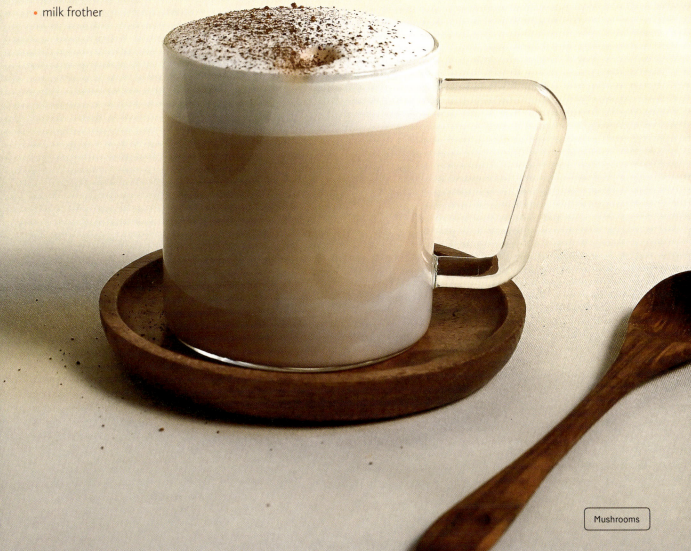

Mushrooms

SHIITAKE | LENTINULA EDODES

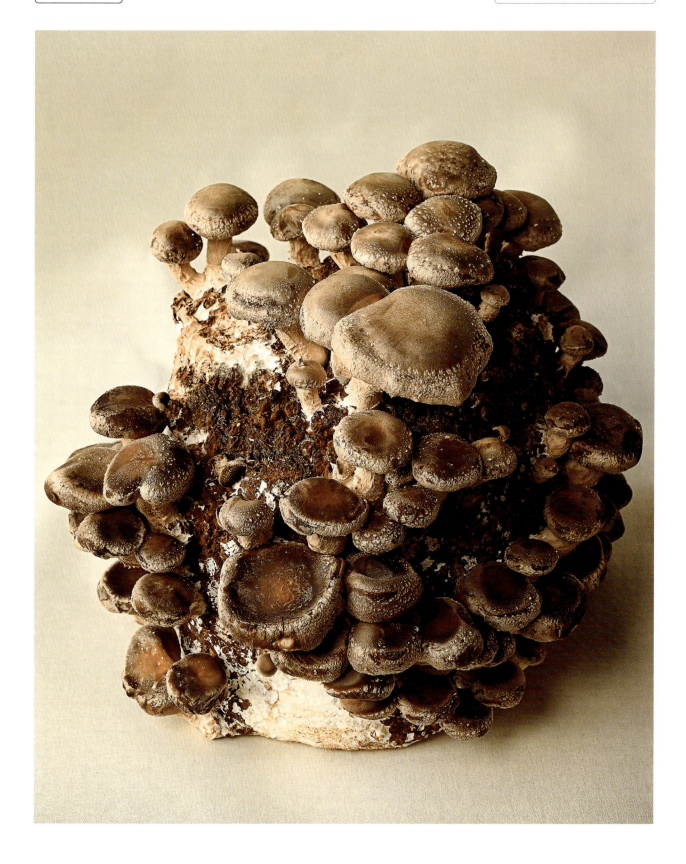

Mushroom of Eternal Youth

After button mushrooms, log-grown shiitake is one of the most popular edible mushrooms in the world. A quarter of all mushrooms consumed globally are shiitake. They are a traditional delicacy in Japan, China, and Korea. The name shiitake comes from the Japanese word for a particular species of chestnut tree, *shiia*, and the Japanese word for mushroom, *take*.[22] Its Latin name is derived from the word *lentus*, meaning "pliable," a reference to its pliable stalks, and *edodes*, meaning "edible," a specific reference to its cap. In Asia, the fungus has also been called "elixir of life" because of its life-enhancing qualities.

During the 1990s, I would occasionally buy dried shiitake with my Chinese Wing-Chun kung-fu teacher on the Geldersekade in Amsterdam. After training, he would often cook a delicious Chinese meal. In Flanders, the Netherlands, and elsewhere in the world, shiitake mushrooms are now also available in every supermarket's fresh food section. They were introduced to us by the macrobiotic scene and by Asian influences and have now become mainstream.

Compared to the common button mushroom, shiitake contain a great deal of protein, as much as 13 grams (0.4 ounces) per 100 grams (3.5 ounces), whereas button mushrooms contain 2.7 grams (0.09 ounces) of protein per 100 grams (3.5 ounces). The protein content of meat is around 20 grams (0.7 ounces) per 100 grams (3.5 ounces). Spirulina leads the way as far as protein is concerned: almost 70 percent of this alga consists of protein. Combined with shiitake and nuts, this makes it a good vegetarian protein substitute.

Aside from the fact that shiitake have numerous health-promoting properties, they are also delicious, with a so-called umami flavor. Dried shiitake develop an even stronger umami flavor. To prepare these, soak them in water for 1 hour. The soaking liquid can then form the basis of a potent stock.

Use

Shiitake are very rich in trace elements and minerals (calcium, potassium, magnesium, manganese, selenium, zinc, copper, iron, and phosphorus), and other compounds including vitamins A, B2, B3, B6, B12, C, D2, and E. As a result, they are an important support for muscles, tendons, and nerves. They also contain a wide variety of antioxidants. These active compounds are known to detect and neutralize free radicals before they can cause chronic disease, premature aging, and mental problems. Shiitakes contain all the essential amino acids that are important for humans.

Shiitake promote blood flow and counteracts calcification on the cell walls of veins.[23] Shiitake also have an interesting and powerful antiviral quality and inhibit the development of a number of viruses, such as the herpes simplex virus.[24]

PROPERTIES
- Immunopotentiating
- Virus-inhibiting
- Anticarcinogenic (reduces the risk of cancer)
- Anti-inflammatory
- Reduces cholesterol
- Reduces blood pressure
- Rich source of vitamins, minerals, and trace elements
- Contains all eight essential amino acids

SOURCING
Fresh and dried shiitake can be bought in specialty Asian markets, supermarkets, and at greengrocers. Extracts are available from drugstores and health food stores. Mushroom growers sell mycelium-infected wood plugs that you can insert into logs with drilled holes. Keep the fresh logs (3 weeks old) moist and in the shade. Once the logs have been inoculated, they will produce fruiting bodies after about 6 months. If you use solid hardwood such as oak, the logs will continue to produce mushrooms for up to 6 years.

CAUTION
A very small group of people might be allergic to shiitake. This manifests itself through sensitivity to light on the skin.

Mushrooms

Shiitake are also used to reduce cholesterol and blood pressure. In traditional Chinese medicine, shiitake are consumed to counter inflammation and arthritis and rheumatic diseases, as well as colds, flu, and cardiovascular diseases.[25]

According to American mycologist Paul Stamets, shiitake appear to activate killer- and helper T cells so that they could potentially be deployed to treat some cancers.[26] In addition to lentinan, a well-known substance that is used in hospitals in Japan as a complementary agent in cancer therapy, it has become clear that shiitake, like a number of other medicinal mushrooms, contain antitumor compounds.

Over the past few years, more than 100 scientific studies have been published in which the health-promoting properties of shiitake have been set out. As a preventive measure, to support nutrition and in consultation with my doctor, I would definitely continue to eat mushrooms or consume mushroom extracts alongside regular forms of treatment.

Appearance

The caps grow 5–25 centimeters (approx. 2–10 inches) wide. They are dark brown to black in color at first and become lighter as they mature or dry. When young, they are somewhat spherical, flattening out as they continue to grow. The stems are fibrous and sturdy. They grow on dead (oak) logs, and these days also in mushroom farms on a substrate of bags of sterilized sawdust.

Extracting and Dosing

Add shiitake to your diet a few times a month. Eat them fresh, make a stock from dried shiitake, or use extracts.

Mushrooms

AVOCADO WITH FERMENTED SHIITAKE POWDER

serves 4 people

■ **INGREDIENTS**
- 1 kg/2.2 lbs shiitake
- about 20 g/0.7 oz salt (2% of the weight of the shiitake)
- 1 avocado

■ **EQUIPMENT**
- large, sterilized jar with lid

method

Cut the shiitake into equal pieces and, in a bowl, mix them thoroughly with the salt. Leave for 5 minutes, then mix well again. The shiitake should now start to give off some juices.

Fill the jar with the shiitake, and press down well into the bottom of the jar. There should be as little air in the jar as possible. Leave approximately 1 centimeter (0.4 inch) below the rim of the jar. Close the jar. The juice should just cover the shiitake. Leave the jar in a dark place at room temperature for 5–7 days. Small bubbles will form.

Once the shiitakes are fermented, they can be dried. Preheat the oven to 60°C (140°F).

Spread the shiitakes in a single layer on a parchment-lined baking tray, and leave to dry in a warm oven for at least 8 hours. The shiitakes should be bone dry—no more juice should come out when you squeeze them. Put the dried shiitakes in a food processor, and grind to a powder.

Cut the avocado lengthways into 4 equal segments. Remove the kernel, and peel. Sprinkle the flesh with the fermented shiitake powder.

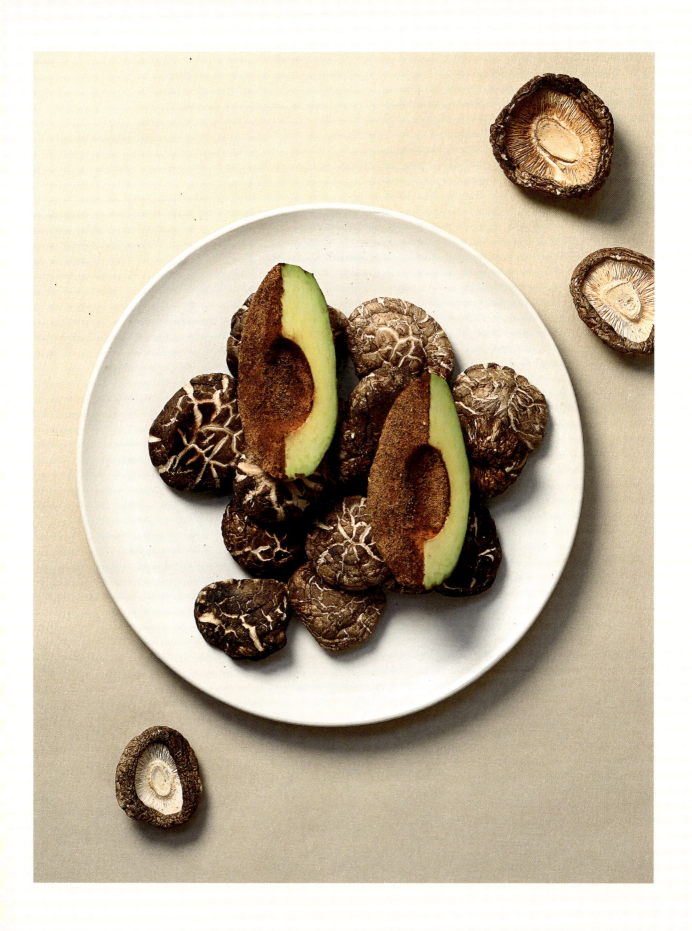

SHIITAKE DASHI WITH FURIKAKE EGGS

serves 4 people

■ FOR THE SHIITAKE DASHI
- 1 pointed cabbage
- 1 green cabbage
- 1 white onion
- ½ kombu leaf (Asian and other supermarkets)
- 50 g/1.8 oz dried shiitake (Asian and other supermarkets)
- 2 L/68 fl oz water
- 50 ml/1.7 fl oz ponzu (Asian and other supermarkets)

■ FOR THE EGGS WITH FURIKAKE
- 4 eggs
- 10 g/3.5 oz wasabi sesame seeds (Asian supermarket)
- 50 g/1.8 oz white sesame seeds
- 15 g/0.5 oz poppy seeds
- 5 nori sheets (Asian supermarket)
- 4 g/0.14 oz sushi vinegar powder (Asian supermarket)
- 5.7 g/0.17 oz (1 tsp) onion powder

■ AS WELL AS
- 1 white radish (approx. 450 g/1 lb, Asian supermarket), peeled
- 25 g/0.9 oz fresh shiitake, in pieces
- 100 g/3.5 oz enoki (Asian supermarket), separated
- 1 nori sheet (Asian supermarket), cut into 4 strips

■ EQUIPMENT
- spiral cutter
- barbecue

method

Start with the *dashi*. Fire up the barbecue. Cut both cabbages into quarters and halve the onion, then char-grill both vegetables on the barbecue until they are blackened on all sides. This takes about 30 minutes.

Put the blackened pieces of cabbage and onion in a large pan, and cover with the water. Add the kombu and shiitakes. Bring to a boil, then simmer for 2 hours. Turn off the heat, put the lid on the pan, and set aside for a while.

Strain the stock through a fine sieve or cloth into a large bowl, and stir in the ponzu.

Save the uncharred insides of one section of pointed cabbage for later; cut into pieces.

Soft-boil the eggs, about 5–6 minutes. Meanwhile, mix the rest of the ingredients for the *furikake* in a flat bowl. Plunge the boiled eggs in cold water, and peel. Roll the peeled eggs through the furikake, and cut each into four wedges.

Cut the white radish with the spiral slicer so that you have a kind of spaghetti.

In each bowl, place 4 wedges of egg, followed by some sliced radishes, fresh shiitake and enoki, a strip of nori sheet, and the inside of the pointed cabbage. Pour the hot dashi over this.

Mushrooms

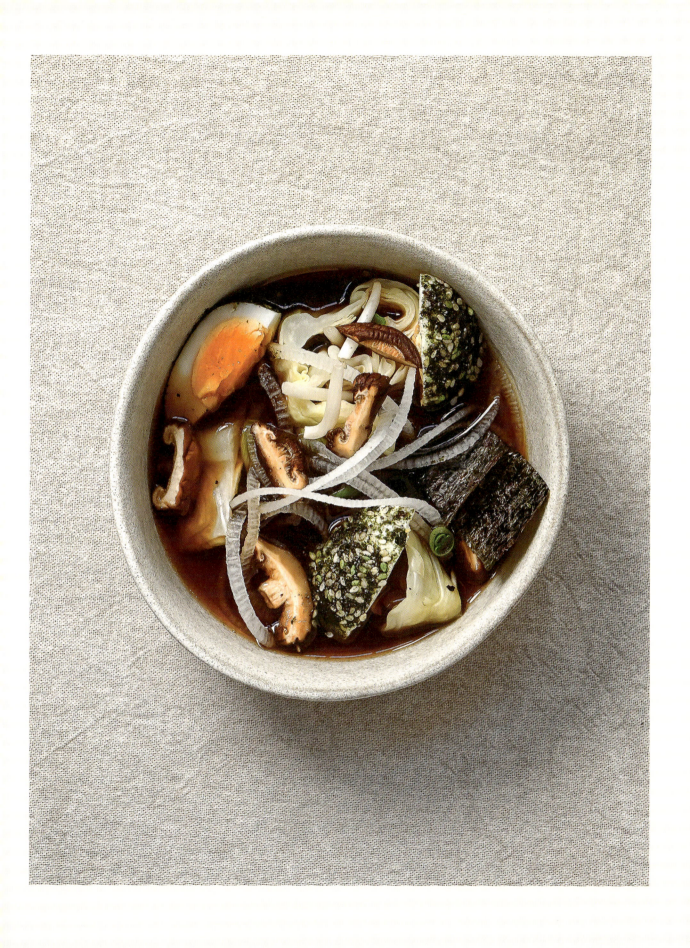

LION'S MANE | HERICIUM ERINACEUS

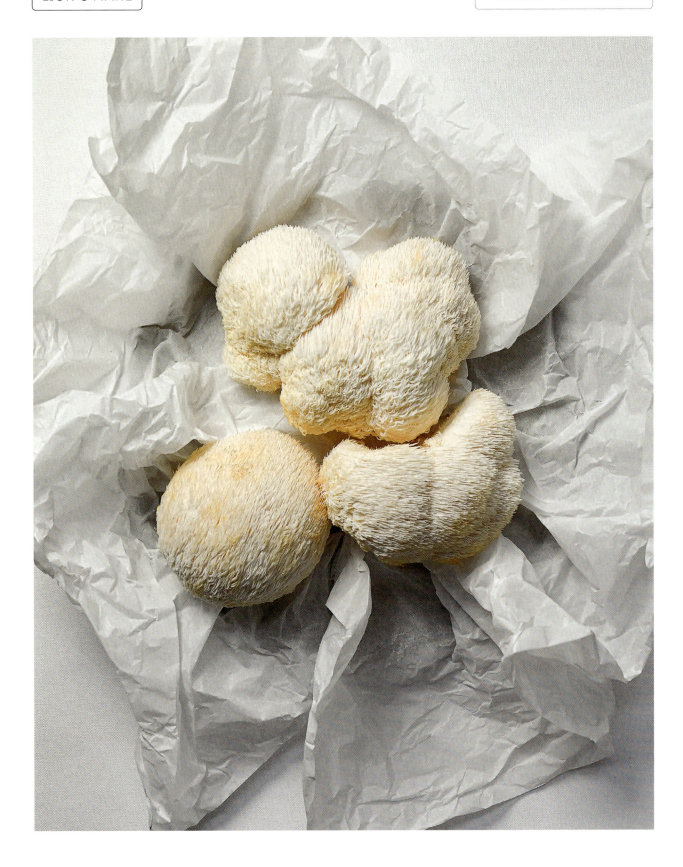

Mushroom of Neurogenesis

I initially consumed lion's mane mushroom as an extract in capsule form, and later discovered herbalist Aldo Hakman's outstanding extracts. I noticed a significant improvement in my ability to think. In Amsterdam, I first came across the fresh mushroom at a mushroom stand at the Zuidermarkt (South Market). I cooked the fungus, and just one hour after eating it, I felt much brighter and sharper. My mother works as a volunteer at the organic fruit and vegetable stand at this market every week. Thanks to her, I became aware of the power of organic food at a very young age. She taught me about health and how to stay healthy.

Lion's mane grow in the wild on deciduous trees and in cavities and crevices, as well as on dead stumps of wood. It is native to Europe, Asia, and North America, and has long been used in Asia as a delicacy and as medicine.

Use

Like many other medicinal mushrooms, this fungus has been used in traditional Chinese medicine for a long time. Lion's mane is used for stress, emotional issues, gastrointestinal problems, and for the prevention of gastrointestinal cancer. This antitumor effect has been confirmed in a Japanese study by Dr. Mizuno from 1995.[27] Lion's mane additionally has a positive and strengthening effect on the immune system. The most interesting thing about this mushroom is that it helps regenerate nerve cells. It stimulates nerve growth factor (NGF). That is why I believe this species of mushroom is very important for the prevention and cure of Alzheimer's disease and dementia. It can contribute to improved thinking and everything you do with your brain.

Lion's mane is known for its anti-inflammatory and cognitive supporting properties. It also has a beneficial effect on the cardiovascular system. The fungus is rich in minerals, such as zinc, potassium, phosphorus, and selenium, as well as in essential amino acids. When combined with a microdose of psilocybin mushrooms (see page 67), special results can be achieved. To achieve these, at your own risk, follow the protocol that mycologist Paul Stamets describes in his books and online video. Numerous scientific studies in recent years have substantiated these results.

Appearance

Lion's mane resembles a large white wig, or to some people, a lion's mane. The white spherical fungus looks somewhat fluffy and appears to be composed of thin threads that have grown together. The fungus is usually white in color with the occasional pale-yellow tone.

Extracting and Dosing

Take 2 capsules of dried mushroom 1–3 times daily, or consume 5–20 grams (0.18–0.7 ounces) of fresh mushroom per day. If you have a potent extract, you can do a course twice a year, by taking one-third of a dropper bottle of extract 3 times per day for a maximum of 20 days.

PROPERTIES
- Neuroregenerative
- Strengthens the immune system
- Anti-inflammatory
- Beneficial effect on the cardiovascular system
- Contains numerous minerals and essential amino acids

SOURCING

You can find lion's mane online and in some health food stores, but you can also grow your own. You do this by ordering from an (online) trader mycelium-inoculated wood dowels that you a tap into drilled-out holes in a tree stump. The freshly cut stump should be 3 weeks old. The wood is then sufficiently decayed and has not yet been infected by other fungi. Lion's mane likes to grow on oak, beech, birch, and horse chestnut stumps. After a few months, you can harvest lion's mane you have cultivated yourself. In the Netherlands and other countries, including some US states, lion's mane is an endangered species, so do not pick the fungus in the wild.

CAUTION

Lion's mane may interact with certain psychiatric medications.

TEMPURA OF LION'S MANE WITH GARLIC POWDER AND PARSLEY AIOLI

serves 4 people

■ FOR THE PARSLEY AIOLI
- ½ bunch (approx. 40 g/1.4 oz) curly parsley
- 250 ml/8.5 fl oz sunflower oil
- 1 egg white
- 25 ml/0.8 fl oz sushi vinegar

■ FOR THE TEMPURA
- 3 egg yolks
- 200 ml/7 fl oz ice-cold sparkling water
- 80 g/28 oz flour, plus extra
- 4 tangerine-sized lion's mane mushrooms
- about 1.5 L/51 fl oz sunflower oil
- pinch of fine sea salt

■ AS WELL AS
- 15 g/0.5 oz (1 T) garlic powder
- 15 g/0.5 oz (1 T) onion powder

■ EQUIPMENT
- pan for deep frying
- kitchen thermometer
- skimmer
- fine sieve

method

Pick the leaves off the parsley. Put in a blender together with the sunflower oil, and whizz until smooth. Strain into a bowl through a fine sieve or cloth. Put the egg white with the sushi vinegar in the blender, blend well and then, with the machine still running, slowly add the parsley oil until you have an *aioli* (garlic mayonnaise). Set aside in the refrigerator until you need it.

Make the tempura batter by whisking the egg yolks, the ice-cold sparkling water, and flour in a bowl. A few lumps of flour are not a disaster, but it is better if you do not have too many. Meanwhile, heat the sunflower oil in a high-sided, thick-bottomed pan to 180°C (350°F).

If necessary, clean the lion's mane by brushing off any sand or soil. Cut the mushroom in half. Sprinkle some flour on a plate, and dip the mushroom's "hairy" side into this and then into the tempura batter. Carefully place the mushroom in the hot oil.

To achieve a good result, it is important that the lion's mane mushroom is dry, the oil remains hot, and the tempura batter very cold.

After about 3 minutes, remove the golden-brown and crispy lion's mane from the oil, and drain on paper towels or a wire rack. Sprinkle with a little salt afterwards. Repeat with the rest.

Spoon a generous tablespoon of parsley aioli onto each plate, and place 2 halves of lion's mane on top. Mix the garlic and onion powder in a small bowl, and sprinkle over the mushrooms through a fine sieve.

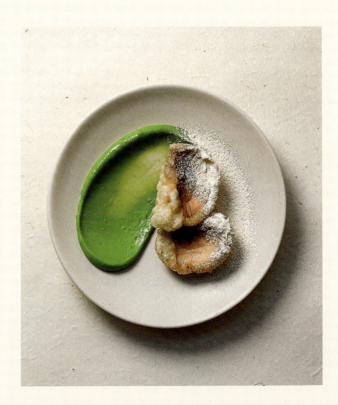

Mushrooms

POACHED POM POM BLANC WITH PONZU AND GINGER

serves 4 people

■ **FOR THE JAPANESE SWEET AND SOUR PONZU STOCK**

- 30 ml/1 fl oz rice vinegar (Asian and other supermarkets)
- 120 ml/4 fl oz mirin (sweet rice wine, Asian and other supermarkets)
- 30 g/1 oz kombu (Asian supermarket)
- 120 ml/4 fl oz yuzu juice (Asian supermarket; lime juice will do as well)
- 120 ml/4 fl oz light soy sauce (Asian and other supermarkets)

■ **FOR THE SPRING ONION OIL**

- 5 spring onions with lots of green
- 100 ml/3.4 fl oz sunflower oil

■ **AS WELL AS**

- 500 g/17 oz lion's mane, which may be 1 or 2 large, or about 8 small ones
- 2 thumb-sized pieces of ginger, peeled
- 2 spring onions, just the green
- 15 ml/0.5 fl oz (1 T) spring onion oil

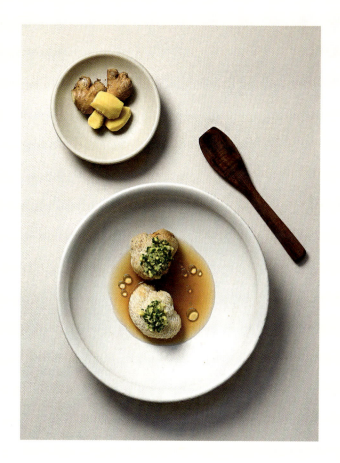

method

Start with the ponzu stock. Put the rice vinegar, mirin (rice wine), and kombu in a saucepan, and bring to a boil. Put the lid on the pan, and simmer for 10 minutes. Turn off the heat, and let the stock cool completely with the kombu still in it. When the stock has cooled down, stir in the yuzu juice and soy sauce. (You can also buy ready-made ponzu, but make sure that this is not shoyu ponzu, which is made with dark soy sauce.)

For the spring onion oil, finely chop the green tops of the spring onions. Put the chopped leaves in a stainless steel or other fireproof bowl; be sure to use a deep bowl, because there will be some splattering when you make this dish. Heat the sunflower oil in a pan to about 185°C (365°F). Ladle the hot oil, drop by drop, onto the spring onion leaves. Wait for it to stop splashing before adding the next drop. Allow the spring onion to cool down completely.

Put the lion's mane in a generously sized pot. Add the ponzu stock. Bring to a boil, put the lid on the pot, and simmer for 15 minutes.

Meanwhile, peel the ginger, and remove the green tops from the spring onions. Mince the ginger and spring onions, and mix in a small bowl with the spring onion oil.

Divide the braised lion's mane into 4 portions, and place in bowls. Pour a layer of the ponzu stock into each bowl, then arrange the spring onion and ginger mixture on top of each mushroom. Drizzle a small amount of spring onion oil into the stock.

Mushrooms

FURTHER PLANT JOURNEYS

FLY AGARIC

Amanita muscaria

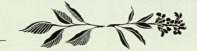

The Magic Mushroom

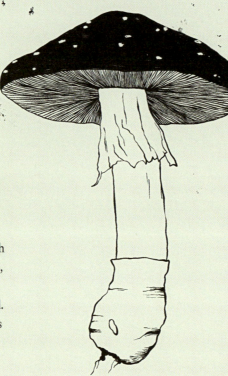

Fly agaric is one of the most evocative mushrooms in the world. Known from the forest and through fairytales, the red-capped mushroom with its white dots is associated with magic, witchcraft, strength, and power. Since the Stone Age, fly agaric has been used by shamans as a consciousness-expanding agent. In ancient times, people were amazed by its way of growing without seed. After birth from an egg (a womb with a fetus), the fungus resembles a penis, which is erect, just like the human male organ when sexually stimulated. Every description of the mushroom's existence was loaded with sexual associations.[28]

The mushroom has also numerous medicinal properties, as demonstrated in *Microdosing with Amanita Muscaria: Creativity, Healing, and Recovery with the Sacred Mushroom* (Masha, 2022) by the Russian physician Baba Masha. For example, fly agaric seems to help against psoriasis and Alzheimer's disease, and the mushroom improved stamina, creativity, and was effective against a number of allergic diseases. In her book, Masha says that she first thought that the fly agaric was a dangerous mushroom because of all the warnings in various mushroom guides she came across, but she now believes that fly agaric can be used medicinally. She even quotes from *Les Misérables* by Victor Hugo to underline her findings: "No army can withstand the power of an idea for which the time is ripe."

The mushroom has been associated nearly worldwide with thunder, lightning, and rain, as it emerges from the earth after a rainstorm. In Iran, fly agaric is called *banat-al-ra'd*, which means "daughters of thunder."[29]

In Lapland and Siberia, fly agaric is common, and it was once equal in value to a whole reindeer. I was told by ethnobotanist Aldo Hakman that some reindeer eat fresh fly agaric. A Scandinavian shaman-to-be bonded with a reindeer, and when that bond of trust was realized, drank the animal's urine for one lunar cycle. The animal was subsequently killed and its heart eaten raw. A magic drum was fashioned from its skin. The budding shaman then went into the forest alone to work with the magic mushroom—only then was he strong enough to consume the dried mushroom in undiluted form. Fly agaric was usually used in combination with chaga (see page 34), with chaga seen as the king and fly agaric as the jester, as they keep each other in check.

The Vikings and Vedic Aryans used fly agaric to increase their prowess and fighting spirit. In 1736, Swedish colonel P.J. von Strahlenberg, who spent 12 years in Siberia as a prisoner of war, wrote about the fungus. He described the Koryaks tribe, who collected large supplies of the mushroom for winter use. On festive occasions, they made tea from these fungi to get pleasantly drunk.[30]

I myself have regularly, out of ethnobotanical interest, tried dried fly agaric mushrooms and extracts. In the words of artist Jesse Faber, it felt like "having drunk an intelligent cup of coffee" and becoming a kind of Ferrari: I did everything faster and in a more focused way.

Mushrooms

FURTHER PLANT JOURNEYS

FLY AGARIC

Amanita muscaria

At somewhat higher doses, I could perceive color more sharply and had creative thoughts. I have never eaten large quantities of the fungus myself. Hakman told me of his experience that the fungus made him use his primitive (reptilian) primal brain more, and that other functions of consciousness began to operate more in the background, as if he was more in touch with his primal intuition.

In Europe, fly agaric was presented as something diabolical. This was partly due to the Inquisition, with its witch burnings, because the fungus induced a visionary state of consciousness that was seen as a threat to the power of the Church; thus, the popular and widely appreciated mushroom was shown no mercy and banned.

This is unusual because, according to John Allegro, who taught Old Testament Studies at the University of Manchester, Christianity is not an original religion, but rather, emerged from the pagan fertility rite surrounding fly agaric.

Allegro was part of the team that examined the Dead Sea Scrolls. His conclusion came after years of comparing the original Hebrew Bible texts with words from the Sumerian and other ancient languages of the Middle East. Allegro described his conclusion in his book *The Sacred Mushroom and the Cross*. The title refers to one of the ancient Hebrew words for mushroom, "small cross." Allegro believes that the secret meanings and uses of fly agaric in sacred texts such as the Bible were hidden in codes. Another way was to hide the information in magic formulas or special names in a document that seemingly dealt with an entirely different matter.[31] Allegro's book has been criticized, but there are nonetheless many people who support his theories.

According to other researchers, even the Pope's habit refers to Christianity's primal origins: a white robe with a short red cloak over his shoulders and the miter supposedly referring to an opening mushroom. The fungus also appears in numerous stained-glass windows in churches and cathedrals, including those in Chartres. The Roman Mithras cult, which was linked to the ancient Persian magical cult of sacred fire, centered on the use of *Amanita muscaria*. Among the Persians, the divine drink of immortality was called *haoma*. In the *Rig Veda*, a sacred Hindu scripture, its name was *soma*.

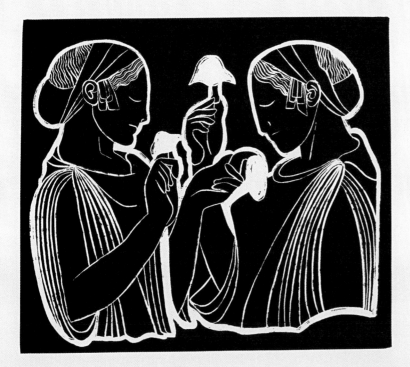

DEMETER AND PERSEPHONE – Psychedelic mushrooms were central to the mystery cult of the temple of Eleusis. The mystery cult revolved around a beatific vision-inducing potion consumed by adepts after a nine-day initiation period. The temple was dedicated to the Greek goddess Demeter, goddess of the earth, agriculture, grain, and *pharmaka*, and her daughter Persephone, goddess of the underworld. In the image left, they share sacred mushrooms. This image of the original stone is displayed in the Louvre opposite the Mona Lisa.

Mushrooms

FLY AGARIC

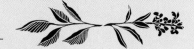

Amanita muscaria

The fact that the followers of Darius, the king of ancient Persia at the time, drank his urine is all the more evidence for Carl Ruck, a professor of classical studies, that fly agaric was part of the haoma sacrament. This is something we also see among Sámi shamans in Lapland and Siberia. Fly agaric was consumed as a sacrament in Mithraic banquets. These took place in closed rooms without windows. The mushroom was consumed in several ways; for instance, through drinking blood and eating the meat of a bull that had been fed fly agaric. Religious animal sacrifices in antiquity were first fed *pharmaka*, or entheogens. The mystical symbolism of bull sacrifice is still found in Spanish bullfighting and the sacrificial Muslim feast of Eid al-Adha.

As was true during the time of the Eleusian Mysteries, when the Ancient Greek potion *kykeon* made with true ergot fungus (*Claviceps purpurea*) was drunk, initiates of other rituals were deified by consuming fly agaric. The god Mithras is usually depicted dressed in red with white polka dots and wearing a kind of distinctive forward-flopping Santa hat. This cap represents fly agaric and is called the Phrygian cap. Ruck believes fly agaric is the drug that civilized Europe and formed the basis of our civilization. For hundreds of years, Mithraism was one of the Roman Empire's two state religions.

Many elements from this religion were adopted by the first Christians, such as the consumption of the (consciousness-altering) Eucharist. According to various traditions, the First Supper was actually the eating of the Tree of Knowledge by Adam and Eve in the Garden of Eden. Graham Hancock considers this to be the first psychedelic crackdown of our people.

The Last Supper is the consumption of the psychedelic Eucharist that was still brewing in the first Christian house churches and in the catacombs located beneath the Vatican. Now that the Eucharist is consumed as a placebo in church, it lacks the proper chemical composition and works for some people by suggesting other things. Plato called the transcendental state of consciousness induced by the holy *kykeon* at Eleusis "the holiest of holiest." The second psychedelic crackdown was the prohibition on the use of these sacraments, followed by the War on Drugs, first against peyote (see page 212) and later Mexican marijuana. The question now is, what is the next Supper? Many of the most significant developments in Western culture were inspired by a central spiritual, ecstatic impulse, often but not always induced by entheogens. Freemasonry also adopted elements of these cults. The 1789 French Declaration of Human Rights has, in at its center, a red mushroom with white dots as a Phrygian cap (symbol of the *Amanita Muscaria*).

As explained by professor Carl Ruck, the top of the declaration is adorned with the incorporeal eye, which refers to visions.

According to entheogenic theories, the origins of religions such as Christianity are said to lie in the use of psychoactive plants and mushrooms that induced a visionary state of consciousness. Entheogenic basically means "derived from the god within ourselves," or "something that generates the divine within ourselves." Donald Teeter, author of the 2005 ebook *Amanita Muscaria: Herb of Immortality* thinks that the Christian holy grail was in fact a clay bowl in which vision-inducing fly mycelium was grown. The word "grail" in our language is Celtic in origin and means "brew of inspiration." [32] The grail therefore probably contained a magical potion based on fly agaric.

So who knows, we may owe more to fly agaric than we previously thought. In ancient Europe, during the Yule feast celebrated on December 21 (winter solstice), fly agaric mushrooms were eaten that had previously been dried on the Christmas tree. During this fertility festival, people blackened their faces with soot and celebrated the return of light. Bringing a Christmas tree into the house at this time is a remnant of the ancient European tree cult. Coincidentally, the Christmas tree is one of the trees that fly agaric lives in symbiosis with.

Mushrooms

FURTHER PLANT JOURNEYS

PSILOCYBIN

incl. *Psilocybe semilanceata*
and *Psilocybe cyanescens*

Sons of the Gods

During the 1960s, mushrooms containing psilocybin became known through hippies as "magic mushrooms." But magic mushrooms have been used for centuries as sacraments in a range of cultures. People have been ingesting them for at least 7,000 years and probably much longer. Psilocybin mushrooms are believed to have played an important role in the evolution of human consciousness. Researchers at Johns Hopkins University have used psilocybin to explore the nature of our consciousness, among other things. "Human consciousness ... is a function of the ebb and flow of neural impulses in different parts of the brain—the substrate on which drugs such as psilocybin act," says Charles Schuster, former director of the U.S. National Institute on Drug Abuse (NIDA). "Understanding what makes these effects happen falls clearly in the domain of neuroscience and warrants research."

American ethnobotanist Terrence McKenna believed that psilocybin mushrooms were the "evolutionary catalyst" from which our language, projective imagination, art, religion, philosophy, science, and in fact our entire human culture emerged. McKenna's hypothesis is known as the "stoned ape theory."[33]

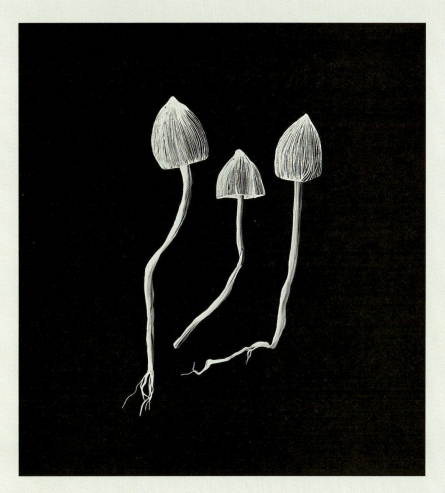

The oldest artistic expressions to clearly show that mushrooms have been used by man for magical purposes in ritual setting have been found carved into a cave on the Tassili plateau in present-day southern Algeria. The petroglyph was made 7,000 years ago. The human figure has the head of a bee, a body with mushrooms growing from it, and holds several large mushrooms in each hand. There are indications of psilocybin mushrooms in Egyptian hieroglyphics and some Egyptologists believe Osiris's crown is a mushroom. Likewise, in Mexico and Guatemala, multiple images and artistic expressions of enchanting mushrooms can be found in ancient Mayan temples. This is also where mushroom stones originate, which were used for crushing the sacrament for consumption. In Aztec, the psilocybin mushroom is called *teonanacatl*, which means "god's flesh." Psilocybin is an "Einstein drug," which means it is supposed to make you a smarter and better human.

67

Mushrooms

FURTHER PLANT JOURNEYS

PSILOCYBIN

incl. *Psilocybe semilanceata* and *Psilocybe cyanescens*

These allies of humanity have helped many people overcome traumas and regenerate their brains and nervous systems. Shamans and witches have known for millennia that one of their holy sacraments (psilocybin mushrooms) can induce predictions about the future.

Much has already been written about spiritual and mystical experiences with magic mushrooms and, as we know, they have been used for millennia all over the globe, including in Europe. Both Plato and Socrates participated in religious ceremonies in which magic mushrooms (*Claviceps purpurea*) were consumed.[34] I have also experimented with psilocybin mushrooms. They give you visions that are said to be similar to what you might experience with LSD. I cannot compare it myself because I have never tried LSD. An expert in such experiences told me that you should see LSD as a master—if you do not follow him, you will have a bad trip; whereas, mushrooms are a friend not a master—they go along with you.

In California's Silicon Valley in the United States, LSD and psilocybin mushrooms are commonly taken therapeutically in microdoses. Under the influence of LSD, biochemist Kary Mullis, like Steve Jobs, had visions and special insights. He won the 1993 Nobel Prize for Chemistry for the invention of PCR, a method by which you can show the tiniest amount of DNA in a material. He said: "Would I have invented PCR if I hadn't taken LSD? I seriously doubt it. I could sit on a DNA molecule and watch the polymers go by. I learned that partly on psychedelic drugs."[35]

Microdosing does not lead to tripping, only improvement in certain brain functions. Studies have shown that after microdosing psilocybin mushrooms for six weeks, brain connections improved significantly and had multiplied. You might even say there had been a case of neurogenesis or neuroregeneration; nerve cells were being renewed and restored.

Psilocybin has enormous potential for getting rid of anxiety and depression with positive long-term effects. Many people have banished their depression for good through one single good mushroom trip. Presently, several universities are conducting scientific studies into the microdosing of psilocybin mushrooms. More and more outcomes appear to be positive and are being published.

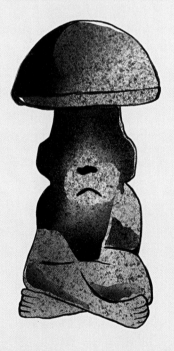 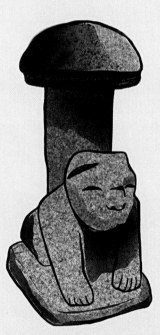

MUSHROOM STONES – After Europe had been for the most part stripped of psychedelic-sacramental use, Catholic missionaries in the Americas tried to eliminate humanity's deepest primal tradition. Some 200 mushroom stones from Mexico and Guatemala (the oldest found dates from 3000 BCE) have survived their destruction. These stones were used to pulverize the dried magical sacrament into powder for consumption. Western civilization is the only civilization on Earth in which, following the killing of the wise herbalists and their beer-brewing daughters ("witches"), for the past 500 years, the use of sacraments has been prohibited, gone underground, and become taboo.

Mushrooms

FURTHER PLANT JOURNEYS

PSILOCYBIN

incl. Psilocybe semilanceata and Psilocybe cyanescens

In the United States, 40 studies into microdosing and the therapeutic use of psilocybin are currently underway at leading institutions, and in Europe some 20 studies. So it is a global phenomenon. There is even talk of a psychedelic renaissance.

The beautiful thing about psilocybin mushrooms is that they are cheap, especially compared with the conventional drugs generally used for depression. It is a completely natural remedy, a true natural medicine. With this ally, people regain their original and independent power. Physicians are also working increasingly more often with patients who would like to try it, for example so that they can stop taking antidepressants.

In addition, psilocybin has proved to be a promising remedy for alleviating pain from cluster headaches. In a 2006 study, 22 out of 26 patients mentioned a favorable result after using psilocybin in order to prevent a pain attack, and 18 out of 19 psilocybin users reported longer seizure-free periods. People who are terminally ill, likewise, tend to benefit from the mystical experience psilocybin mushrooms can generate. As a result, they are better able to cope with death, as has also been demonstrated in studies at John Hopkins University.[36] They teach us that the world as we see it normally is, in fact, not normal, and that many different realities exist, which become observable with the help of these small friends.

How you see the world is in large part determined by the state of your consciousness. As a result of the spiritual experience and of feeling part of something bigger, people obtain an inner peace that makes it easier for them to accept death. Psilocybin, especially in combination with lion's mane, is strongly neurogenic.

TASSILI ROCK SHAMAN – This ancient rock painting (8000-6000 BCE) of a costumed or supernatural figure was found on the Tassili plateau in eastern Algeria and appears to represent a prehistoric bee medicine man. The rock shaman is one of the first surviving images of what looks like psychedelic mushroom use.

The protocol formulated by Paul Stamets and other mycologists and scientists, such as Dr. James Fadiman, can be easily found online. Neurogenetics and synaptogenetics are possible and borne out by research.

These small mushrooms appear in the autumn, when the weather starts to get wetter—in meadows (*Psilocybe semilanceata*) and on wood chips in parks (*Psilocybe cyanescens*).

Mushrooms

FRUIT AND NUTS

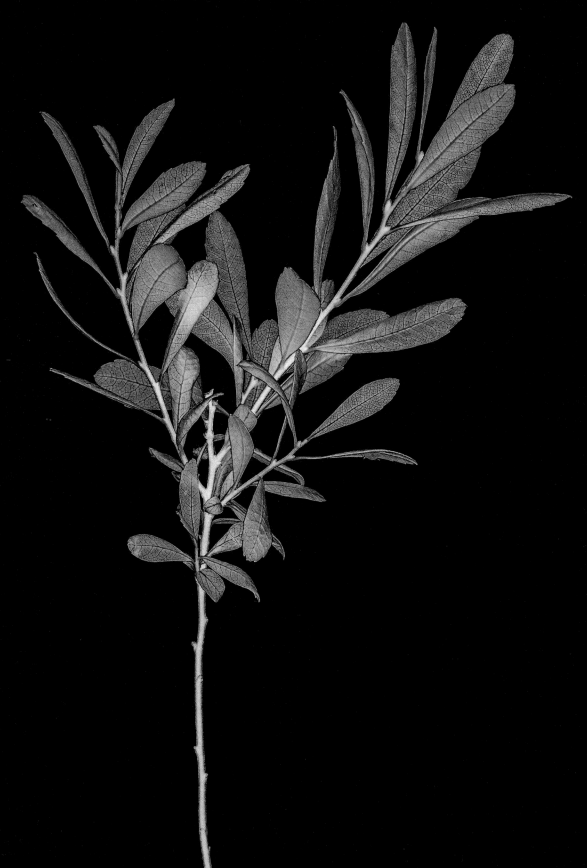

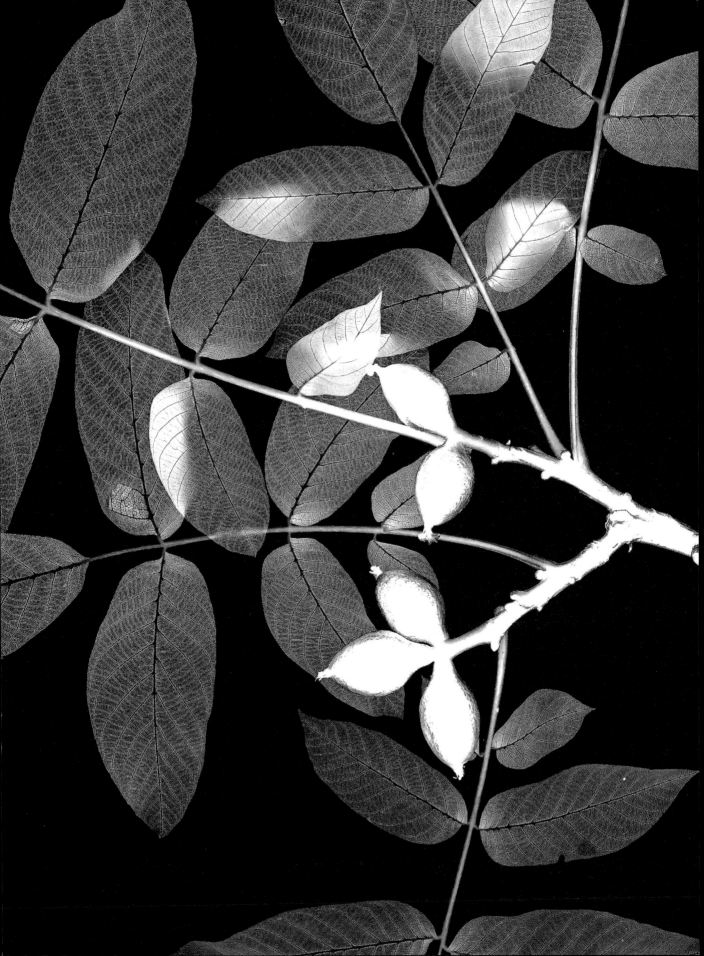

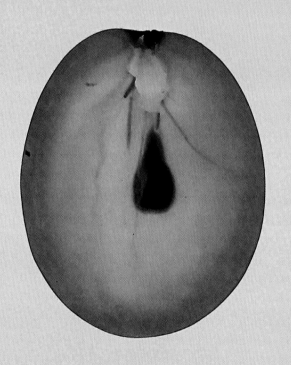

WOUTER "Just about everyone knows that fruits and vegetables should be a regular part of a varied diet, so that you get as many vitamins, minerals, and other plant ingredients as possible. Many fruits and vegetables should be eaten immediately to ensure maximum flavor and quality. Just compare the head of lettuce we freshly pulled from the vegetable garden with the one cut two days ago. The spark of life has gone, and with it much of its nutritional value. You can hardly ever say that about nuts and seeds, which retain their potency. Their life force is sometimes preserved for centuries. I eat fruit mostly unprocessed. Do you actually use it in your cooking?"

"When I worked at Le Jardin des Sens restaurant in France, I learned from the chef, Laurent Pourcel, how refreshing it can be to incorporate fruit in our cooking. Tomato and raspberry salad, slices of ripe peach alongside roast duck, red wine, and passion fruit sauce to accompany roast beef—it works. I use nuts in my cooking for their savory notes and umami flavor when roasted. By the way, the difference in taste between a fresh and dried nut is huge. *Ajo blanco* (white gazpacho) soup is not the same if you use toasted almonds instead of fresh ones straight from their green husk, which is like eating vegetable caviar. So the point at which you eat may not affect nutritional value, but it does affect the taste.

Remember when we used to go bilberry picking in the Ardennes? In season, bakeries would sell all kinds of delicious bilberry cakes and confectionery. We also used to turn them into *crème de cassis*. That is the beauty of nature and the seasons. For quite a long time, something is not there. Then when they do appear, there are masses and masses but for a short time only. To my mind, those bilberries always really perked me up. I guess you know what lies behind that?"

W "You can read a detailed explanation later in the book, but it is indeed well known that eating lots of fruits and vegetables reduces cardiovascular disease, cataracts, and cancer risk. Bilberries are good for your intestinal flora, among other things, and partly because of this have a beneficial effect on our immune system. They also have a beneficial effect on our brain and eyes, strong antioxidant properties, and are rich in vitamins. Alarmingly, people with the lowest fruit and vegetables intake are twice as likely to develop several types of cancer than those who eat more of them. How do you think we can help people become more aware of eating fresh fruit instead of candy from the supermarket?"

J "We learned this by always helping out on our vegetable plot and by watching how everything grows. In the process, you develop a kind of appreciation and love for delicious fresh fruits and vegetables.

That's why I am such a fan of school gardens. In our school garden at RIJKS, we also have a walnut tree. For me, fat is a very important flavoring. Are the fats from nuts and seeds in any way good for you?"

W "When we think of fat, we immediately think of toxic trans-fatty acids that are created by fats in food going rancid, or by deep-frying and industrial hardening of fats for the food industry. Those fats contribute to cardiovascular disease. Many other fats, which you find in nuts and seeds, are actually essential for our health; for example, the omega-3 fatty acids in walnuts are good for brain function. You do not just use healthy fats in the kitchen, I assume?"

J "Without realizing it, we use liters of fat every day in the restaurant kitchen. In my kitchens, fat represents flavor but also gives the right structure to dishes. Think of mayonnaise. The fats we use can be animal-based, and I'm talking about lard or goose fat, for example, but also butter of course. But the fatty substances we most use are oils. In some cases, we need a neutral oil. For example, if we want to give the oil itself a flavor. That's the beauty of oil; it's a kind of flavor chameleon. Whizz oil with a bunch of parsley in a blender or food processor, and it turns green and pops with flavor. It's a technique we use on a daily basis, and it never ceases to surprise me. And don't forget the all-purpose olive oil! With a good olive oil, basically everything becomes tasty."

PAPAYA CARICA PAPAYA

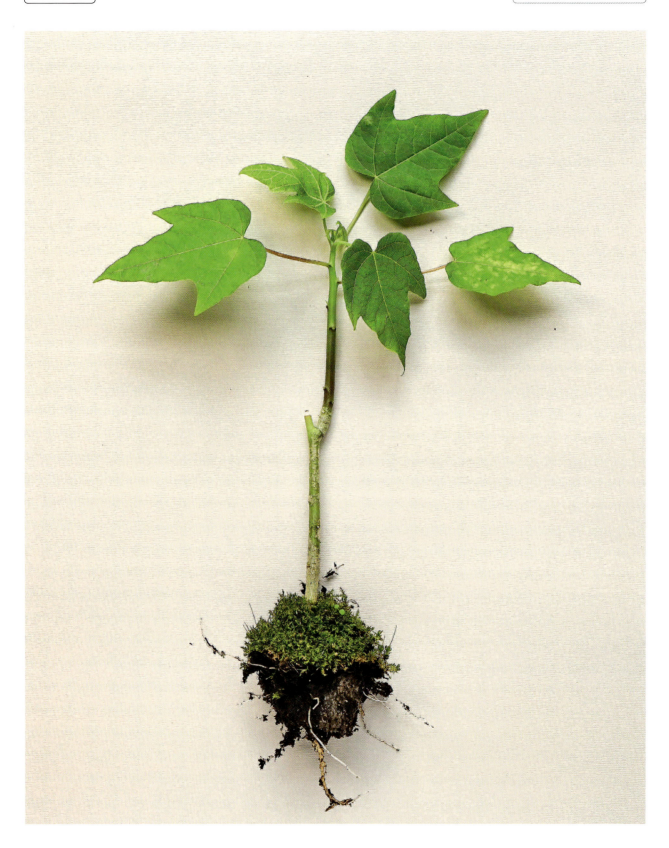

Fruit of Angels

Sweet papaya originates in South and Central America and the Caribbean Islands. From there, starting in the 16th century, it was spread by the Spanish to almost all the tropical regions on the planet. According to some accounts, papaya was said to have been the favorite fruit of the explorer Christopher Columbus. After he and his men arrived in the Americas, on an island in the Bahamas, the local food made them ill. Local Carib Indians fed them papaya, after which they recovered and regained their strength. The Carib called the fruit *ababi*, which means "fruit of angels." The entire tree, including its fruit and the seeds, is used medicinally throughout the world. Some people in the tropics regard papaya as mystical, because the plant, like the human embryo, takes nine months to develop.

The most interesting thing about the papaya tree is perhaps that its seeds, when ingested, render some men temporarily infertile. The fact that incidental infertility occurs after consuming the seeds is no guarantee that it would work as a 100-percent-effective contraceptive. Because it has a strong effect on male reproductive cells only when used, it might well form part of a future contraceptive.

Appearance

The fruits grow directly on the tree trunk; the tree's wood is very soft. Most papayas we eat come from a hermaphrodite tree. According to biologist Ray Ming, it's likely that the hermaphrodite variant came into being because Mayan people from the Yucatan Peninsula of Mexico cultivated and improved the tree. The Mayans, Aztecs, and Olmecs of Mexico were known for their great horticultural knowledge. Thanks to them, we are also familiar with tomatoes and cocoa, for example. One of the reasons the papaya was important to them was because it was among the fruit used as an offering on their annual November Day of the Dead altars (*ofrendas*).

Use

The fruit contains beta-carotene and other carotenoids. As pro-vitamin A, beta-carotene contributes to a strong immunity. Papaya also contains vitamin C and vitamins B1, B2, and B3. In addition, the fruit contains calcium, phosphorus, iron, calcium, and sodium.

Papaya leaf is used as a worm repellent. After use, large amounts of papaya fruit are also often eaten for their laxative effect, flushing out the parasite's eggs as well. Even without worms, papaya leaf likewise cleanses the intestines of heavy food and old embedded food particles. Do not eat papaya at the same time as a meal, but in between.

Some people say that eating papaya leaf twice a week keeps malaria at bay. The leaves are quite bitter. Almost all bitter substances from nature are used against malaria and stimulate digestion.

PROPERTIES
- Counters constipation
- Improves digestion
- Intestinal cleansing (both the fruit and the leaf)
- Anti-candida properties
- Immune-strengthening
- Anti-inflammatory
- Rich source of various vitamins and minerals
- Papaya tenderizes meat when cooking

SOURCING

Papaya can be purchased in tropical stores, farmers' markets, greengrocers, and many supermarkets.

CAUTION

Papaya seeds may make some men temporarily infertile. Carpaine in the seeds can slow the heart rate. This substance also occurs in the leaves of the tree, and is therefore not allowed to be used in dietary supplements. If you rub papaya onto your skin, do not leave it there for too long. When exposed to light, dark orange skin spots will appear that remain in place for three days

The enzyme papain in papaya leaf and the fruit gives it its protein-digesting properties. Everyone in the tropics knows that you can wrap tough meat in papaya leaf to tenderize it. In the meat industry, papain is injected into meat to make it more tender.

Fruit and Nuts

Papain also has a cosmetic action: it removes dead skin cells in the epidermis. Enzymes from papaya affect our macrophages, so eating papaya can help boost our immune system naturally.

In Suriname, the fruit is eaten as fruit, but is also recommended for high blood pressure, stomach pain, constipation (*tranga bere*), bloating, and hemorrhoids. The fruit (or the juice) is believed to "keep your belly cool" and encourage lactation in breast-feeding women. However, it is said that eating a lot of papaya makes your body watery (*yu watra a skin*),[37] causing other herbal medicines to "dilute" and thus reduce their effectiveness. According to a Creole woman from Amsterdam, papaya leaf tea is supposed to "bring out hidden diseases."

In the wild, there are two other types of papaya, the so-called male and female forest papaya, both of which are used for medicinal purposes. Their leaves have several medicinal applications, so it is useful to find out whether you are dealing with the cultivated or wild papaya. In their book *Medicinal and Ritual Plants of Suriname*, scientists Tinde van Andel and Sofie Ruysschaert note that the leaves of the domesticated variety form part of the ingredients for a herbal bath for getting rid of a spirit tormentor. At funerals, people tap papaya leaves on the coffin to offer peace to the deceased's spirit and to make sure that it does not start to wander.

Extracting and Dosing

For medicinal purposes, occasionally eat a few pieces of papaya for 3–4 days.

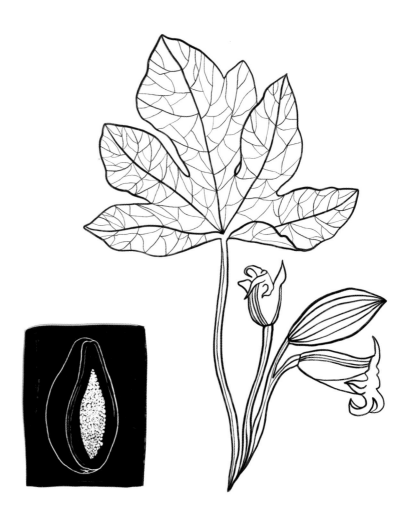

Fruit and Nuts

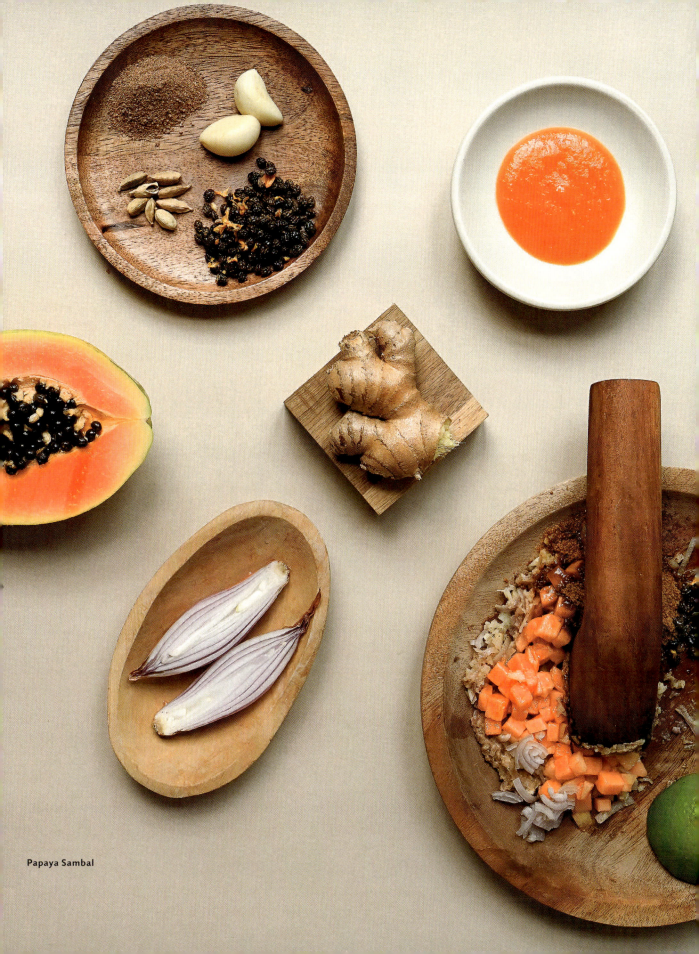

Papaya Sambal

PAPAYA SAMBAL

for 1 jam jar

■ INGREDIENTS
- 1 small ripe papaya (approx. 500 g/17.6 oz)
- 1 shallot
- 3-cm/1-inch ginger, peeled
- 2 Madame Jeanette hot chili peppers, de-seeded; Habanero or Scotch Bonnet peppers may be substituted
- 5 cardamom pods
- 3 garlic cloves
- pinch of nutmeg
- 50 g/1.8 oz soft brown sugar
- pinch of fine sea salt
- 100 ml/3.4 fl oz white wine vinegar
- juice of 1 lime

■ EQUIPMENT
- mortar
- sterilized jam jar with lid

method

Peel the papaya, cut it in half, and scrape out the seeds with a spoon. Cut the flesh into cubes. Cut the shallot, ginger, and Madame Jeanette/Scotch Bonnet/Habanero chilis as finely as possible. Crush the cardamom pods, and remove the seeds. Discard the pods.

Pulverize the papaya, shallot, ginger, pepper, cardamom seed, garlic, nutmeg, sugar, and salt in a mortar with a pestle until it is a smooth paste. Add the vinegar and lime juice. Mix well, and spoon into the clean, sterilized jam jar. This sambal is quite runny. In an airtight jar, it can be kept in the refrigerator for at least 2 weeks.

You could dry the papaya's scooped-out black seeds separately on kitchen paper. Once dried, the seeds start to taste peppery, a little like nasturtiums. Use them as you would use pepper.

GREEN PAPAYA SALAD

serves 4 people

■ INGREDIENTS
- 350 g/12 oz green papaya
- 3 garlic cloves
- 1 Madame Jeanette hot chili pepper, de-seeded; Scotch Bonnet or Habanero may be substituted
- 14 g/0.5 oz (1 T) palm sugar
- 16 cherry tomatoes, halved
- 3 sprigs of cilantro including stems, coarsely chopped
- 1 spring onion, cut into thin rings
- 1 shallot, cut into rings
- 30 ml/1 fl oz (2 T) fish sauce
- 45 ml/1.5 fl oz (3 T) lime juice

■ EQUIPMENT
- serrated peeler, mandolin, or box grater (optional)
- large mortar or bowl

method

Peel the green papaya. There are special peelers you can use for grating into slivers, but you can also do that with a mandolin with a julienne blade, a box grater, or by just cutting them into thin slices first and then julienning into neat strips.

You need a large mortar and pestle for this recipe so that you can pound firmly, but otherwise a solid bowl will work just as well. While preparing, crush the ingredients with the one hand and, with the other, run a spoon or spatula along the edge of the mortar or bowl to make sure nothing gets stuck. Everything should be really well mixed.

Pulverize the garlic, chili pepper, and sugar into a paste in the mortar using a pestle. Add the papaya and tomatoes and pound until the papaya is soft. Everything should be well mixed. Add the cilantro, spring onion, shallot, fish sauce, and lime juice. You can play with the amounts of sugar, lime juice, and fish sauce to taste.

Mix well again, and serve the salad immediately.

Fruit and Nuts

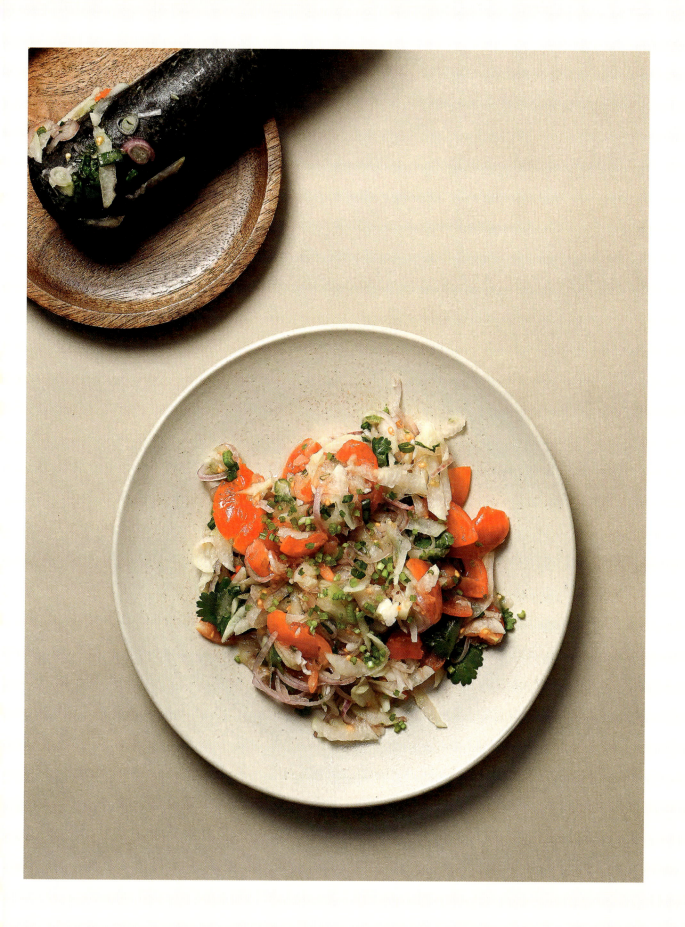

GRAPE

VITIS VINIFERA

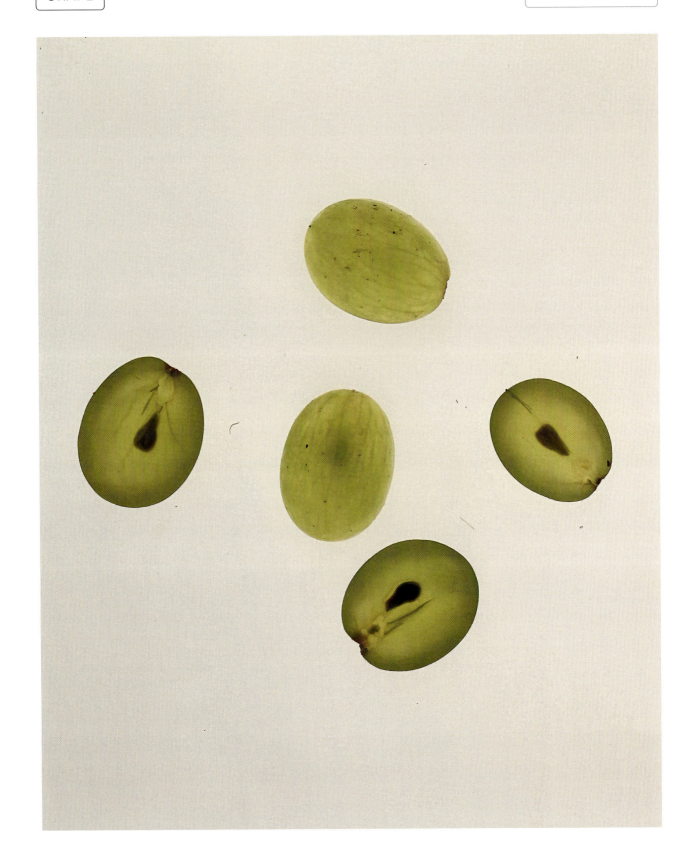

Pupils of the Eyes of Horus

In ancient times, practically every herbalist used the vine liana, wine, and grapes as a medicine. The symbolic meaning of grapes features in all cultures where vines were grown.[38] The metamorphosis of grape juice into intoxicating firewater has always enthralled people. Wine was reputed to sharpen predictions, generate magical powers, and transport people into heavenly ecstasy.[39] It occupies an important place in the culture, religion, and rituals of Europe and the Middle East.

The ancient Egyptians, Sumerians, and Persians had a rich wine culture as far back as 3,000 BCE. In the ancient Egyptian religious texts, grapes are referred to as the Pupils of the Eyes of Horus, with wine considered its "tears." The Egyptians carefully recorded the soil and the year in which the wine was grown on the labels of their wine jars. The Roman writer Pliny the Elder (AD 23–79), who is considered to be the founder of botany, described a great many types of wine in his *Naturalis historia*. He mentions no fewer than 150 different wines.[40] Archaeologists have found the oldest traces of wine making in Georgia and Armenia, to the east of present-day Turkey, where wine was made from crushed grapes as far back as 8,000 years ago. The humid and temperate climate there provide excellent conditions for viniculture. Around 600 BCE, Greek settlers introduced wine growing to present-day France. The French learned the art of wine making from the Greeks. France has since become one of the most influential winegrower countries in the world.

Wine has been associated with religion and cults for a long time. The ancient Greek calendar followed the year of the winegrower. The Greek god of nature, wine, fertility, and ecstasy Dionysus (Bacchus) was charged with watching over the harvest, thus putting an end to worries and misery. In the cult surrounding Dionysus, followers attained religious ecstasy through wine, pharmaka, music, and dance. The god of the followers of Jesus Christ displayed similarities with Dionysus. Both gods offer redemption, and their supporters drink their god's blood, symbolized by wine. Both spiritual movements arose from a fertility cult, and in both movements, pharmaka were consumed.

The Maenads (Bacchantes), who worshipped and accompanied Dionysus, used a *thyros*, or "staff," to collect the mind-altering herbs that were incorporated into the wine. According to Professor Carl Ruck, the wand—still used by some conjurers and magicians—was originally a staff with which the nymphs accompanying Dionysus collected narcotics by pricking the point of this staff into the narcotic leaves. This is probably where our idea of the magic wand comes from.[41]

PROPERTIES

- Tonic for blood vessels and counteracts arteriosclerosis
- Improves blood flow to the eyes
- Delays skin aging
- In small doses, wine appears to help prevent cardiovascular disease
- Antioxidant effect
- Cardioprotective effect
- Protective effect for the nervous system
- A limited gut course (cleanse) for the intestines and gallbladder
- Helps remove toxins from the body
- Tonic for capillaries and vessel walls

SOURCING

Wine and vinegar can be found in supermarkets, liquor stores, and specialist wine stores. Ambrosia wines can be bought in beekeeping stores and from beekeeping associations. Grapeseed oil can be purchased in many food stores and delicatessens. In season, you can buy grapes at farmers' markets, greengrocers, or supermarkets. Grapes are also sold in their dried form. Currants and raisins feature in numerous dishes and offer the advantage of a long shelf life and are therefore a useful provision when traveling.

CAUTION

Beware of alcohol addiction. Do not drink alcohol when pregnant or breastfeeding.

Fruit and Nuts

The symbol of the staff surrounded by the double helix of two snakes wrapped around it, known as the caduceus, is also the symbol of medicine in many parts of the world.

Use

The fact that the French tend to eat large amounts of saturated fats but have little cardiovascular disease is called the French Paradox. This is said to be due to a trio of compounds found in red wine: procyanidin, resveratrol, and alcohol. Drinking moderate quantities of wine every day (no more than two glasses) is believed to have a beneficial effect on the prevention of cardiovascular diseases. Doctors recommend that you not drink alcohol for a minimum 2–3 days a week to let the liver regenerate. Alcohol can be dangerous and carcinogenic. It's the dose that can make it harmful or medicinal.

Wine was, and is, an excellent medium in which to dissolve medicinal plant ingredients. The first surgical interventions in Egypt were done by priests. They dissolved mandrake, blue lotus (see page 208), and opium in wine and used this as an anesthetic during surgery. Beekeepers have been making a somewhat milder but nevertheless medicinal wine for centuries. Medicinal ambrosia wine made with honey, propolis, and herbs works as a heart tonic, stimulates the blood flow, and has anti-inflammatory and immunity-building properties. Ambrosia means "food of the gods" and brought the gods immortality and eternal youth.

The pharmaceutical industry turns grape seeds into a purified and standardized extract, *oligomeric proanthocyanidin*. This convoluted term stands for a specific group of flavonoids, in other words antioxidants; in this case, the blue dye found in plants, and especially in their kernels and peel. Procyanidin has a positive effect on blood vessels and counteracts arteriosclerosis.[42] This substance can also pass through the blood–brain barrier and thus also affects the veins in your brain. It is an excellent brain medicine in combination with *Ginkgo biloba* (see page 174) and gotu kola. Procyanidin also improves the blood supply to the eye.

Due to its high concentration of strong antioxidants, grape seed oil slows down our natural aging process. You can incorporate it into salads or use it in other culinary ways, as well as applying it to your skin. The oil contains many omega-6 fatty acids that help your body attract oxygen and ensure that oxygen can penetrate the cell walls. It works well against skin blemishes, wrinkles, and crow's feet.

Many of the ingredients in this oil act as an antimicrobial for both plants and humans. Grapevines produce the antibody resveratrol in their grapes. This substance has a large number of beneficial health effects on our bodies: it has an antioxidant effect and cardioprotective benefits.[43] In addition, it has a protective effect on our nervous system and anticarcinogenic and anti-inflammatory qualities.

Wine is also turned into vinegar, see pages 28 and 84. In this process, the alcohol present in wine is converted into acetic acid, along with oxygen from the air. Acetic acid is an efficient disinfectant and detergent: it kills bacteria and removes mineral lime deposits. You can therefore also use it to descale your kettle. In many northern countries, gherkins and onions are pickled in vinegar in jars to preserve them.

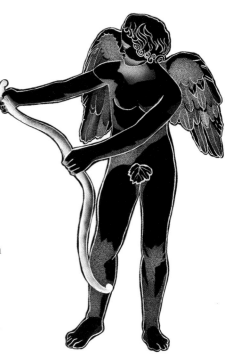

EROS – The god of love with a grape leaf. Eros is the son of Kronos (personification of time) and Gaia (the goddess of the earth). (After a drawing from Mythology Pictures, Pepin Press, 2006.)

Fruit and Nuts

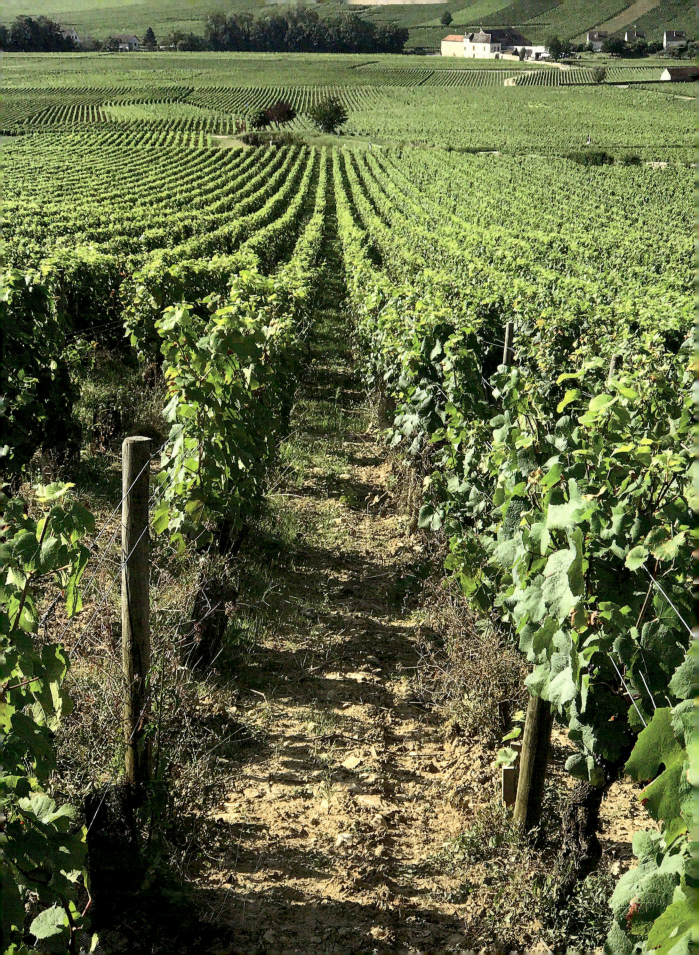

The sour taste is sometimes camouflaged by adding large amounts of sugar to the vinegar. Vinegar is also used as the basic ingredient of mustard. You can use vinegar in the kitchen to add flavor contrast to your dishes and make them more interesting to eat.

Vinegar can be used for culinary purposes, but also has medicinal uses. It can help against nettle stings and some jellyfish bites if you dab it on the area that has been stung. It dissolves the lime in the stinging hairs causing them to detach themselves. Vinegar also ensures that the glycemic index drops and your blood sugar levels do not rise too much. It is therefore a good idea to have a small salad with vinaigrette dressing made from 4 tablespoons oil, 1 tablespoon vinegar, 1 teaspoon mustard, salt, and pepper at the start of a meal.

Fresh grapes are therapeutically used to cleanse the intestines and gallbladder. Fasting for a few days on grapes is said to cleanse the entire body of toxins. Grape leaves are also eaten and are a tonic for the capillaries and vascular walls. Many people know grape leaves as the casing around the Greek dish of *dolmades*, cooked rice wrapped in pickled grape leaf.

Appearance

In the wild, forest-dwelling vines climb from branch to branch across the trees. The plant can reach a height of 35 meters (115 feet) with vines as thick as your upper arm. Bunches of wild grapes measure 50 centimeters (nearly 20 inches) and contain grapes the size of ping-pong balls. Cultivated grape plants (canes) are perennial, shrubby plants characterized by vines and a twisted trunk. They are pruned regularly to grow no taller than approximately 1 meter (about 3 feet). The trunk has peeling bark, and leaves are three to five lobed, palmate, incised, and coarsely serrate. The green leaves turn red in the fall. In summer, it has pale yellow flowers that form into bunches of oval-shaped or round green to dark purple berries. The shape and the color may vary depending on the variety. Normally, all grapes contain seeds.

Extracting and Dosing

You can make your own vinegar by pouring wine into a bowl, stirring well to oxygenate it, and then adding a splash of unfiltered apple cider vinegar. This will start up the process. Cover the bowl or jar and leave for a month in a dark place at

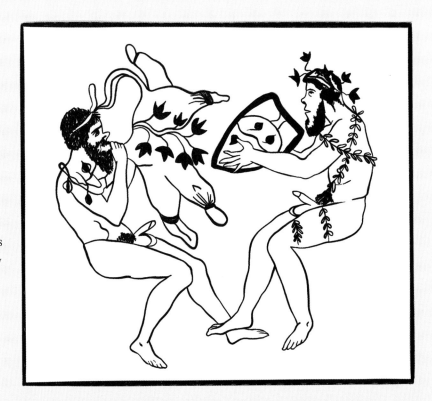

DIONYSUS AND SATYR – The cheerful forest creature and fertility spirit Satyr (the companion of Pan, god of the wilderness) and Dionysus (the Greek god of fertility, psychedelic wine, and fun) play the bagpipes and drink. (After a drawing from Mythology Pictures, Pepin Press, 2006.)

Fruit and Nuts

room temperature. After a few weeks, you will begin to smell the vinegar.

Drink no more than 2 small glasses of wine a day. Choose organic or natural wine preferably, so that you do not have to ingest chemical pesticides.

A few times a week, I like to stir a tablespoon of cold grapeseed oil into my yogurt with muesli. I soak my muesli in the yogurt the night before in the traditional way, making it easier to digest.

When following a grape diet, you can eat 1–1.5 kilograms (2–3 pounds) of organically grown grapes every day, spread over several grape meals. After about three days, the body will have been greatly cleansed and your bowels will be almost completely empty. It is sensible to stop the course after three days and slowly resume your regular diet. During the course, you only drink water, so it is in fact a kind of grape fast.

From the grape leaf, you can also make a mother tincture (see page 26). The dosage is 40 drops three times daily for 12 weeks.

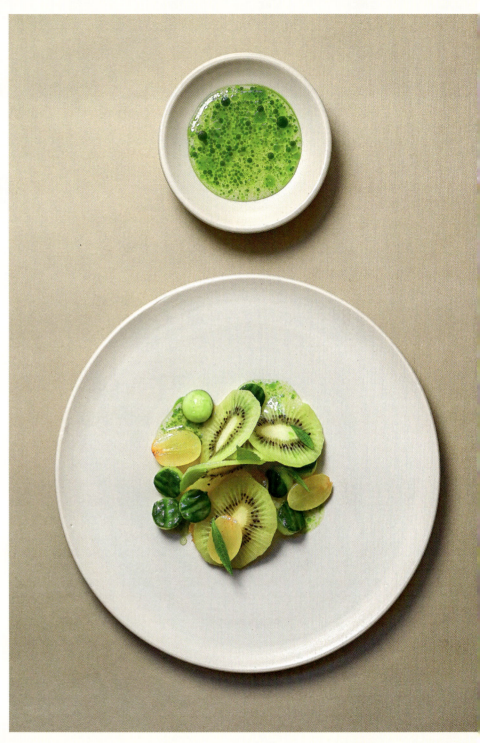

Kiwi, Cucumber, Verbena, and Fried Grapes Salad

Fruit and Nuts

KIWI, CUCUMBER, VERBENA, AND FRIED GRAPES SALAD

serves 4 people

■ **FOR THE SALAD**
- 1 kiwi
- 1 cucumber
- 12 (lemon) verbena leaves
- 30 g/1 oz butter
- 12 grapes

■ **FOR THE GREEN OIL**
- handful (approx. 20 g/0.7 oz of each) of leaf parsley and verbena leaves
- 100 ml/3.4 fl oz grapeseed oil

■ **FOR THE VINAIGRETTE**
- 3 T grape juice
- 1 T white wine vinegar
- 1 T green oil (see above)

■ **EQUIPMENT**
- melon baller (optional)
- fine sieve

method

Peel the kiwi, and cut into thin slices. Wash the cucumber and, using a melon baller, cut out small balls including skin (or cut the cucumber into cubes if you do not have a melon baller). Put the kiwi, cucumber, and verbena leaves in a bowl. Heat the butter in a skillet on medium-high heat, and fry the grapes in the bubbling butter until their outsides have browned slightly. Cut the fried grapes in half, and add them to the bowl. Make the green oil. Blend the herbs and grapeseed oil into a green, smooth liquid using a hand blender in the blender's beaker. Strain into a bowl through as fine a sieve as possible. In a small bowl, whisk the ingredients for the vinaigrette until you have beautiful green pearls. This happens naturally because the oil does not form an emulsion with the moisture. Dress the salad with the vinaigrette, and arrange everything attractively in the center of a serving plate. The green oil can be kept in the refrigerator for at least 1 week and can be used in all your other salads.

AJO BLANCO WITH MELON

serves 4 people

■ **FOR THE AJO BLANCO (WHITE GAZPACHO)**
- 100 g/3.5 oz white almonds
- 2 slices of white bread, crusts removed
- 100 g/3.5 oz white seedless grapes
- ½ Granny Smith apple, peeled and cored
- 1 garlic clove, peeled
- 250 ml/8.5 fl oz water
- 35 ml/1.2 fl oz sushi vinegar
- 35 ml/1.2 fl oz apple cider vinegar
- 50 ml/1.75 fl oz olive oil

■ **AS WELL AS**
- 1 cantaloupe melon
- 100 g/3.5 oz white grapes
- 100 g/3.5 oz almond flakes

■ **EQUIPMENT**
- mandolin (optional)

method

Put all the ingredients for the *ajo blanco* in a blender, except for the olive oil, and blend. Add the olive oil little by little, and blend until you have a smooth soup. Set aside in the refrigerator for at least 1 hour until it is ice cold.

Preheat the oven to 180°C (350°F).

Cut the melon into quarters, scoop out the seeds and peel. Cut the melon quarters into thin slices using the mandolin or a sharp knife.

Halve the grapes lengthwise.

Toast the almond flakes for about 5 minutes in the oven until golden-brown.

Arrange the melon along the side of a deep bowl. Arrange the grapes on top, and sprinkle with the almond flakes. Pour the ice-cold *ajo blanco* on the other side of the plate, next to the melon and grape mix.

Fruit and Nuts

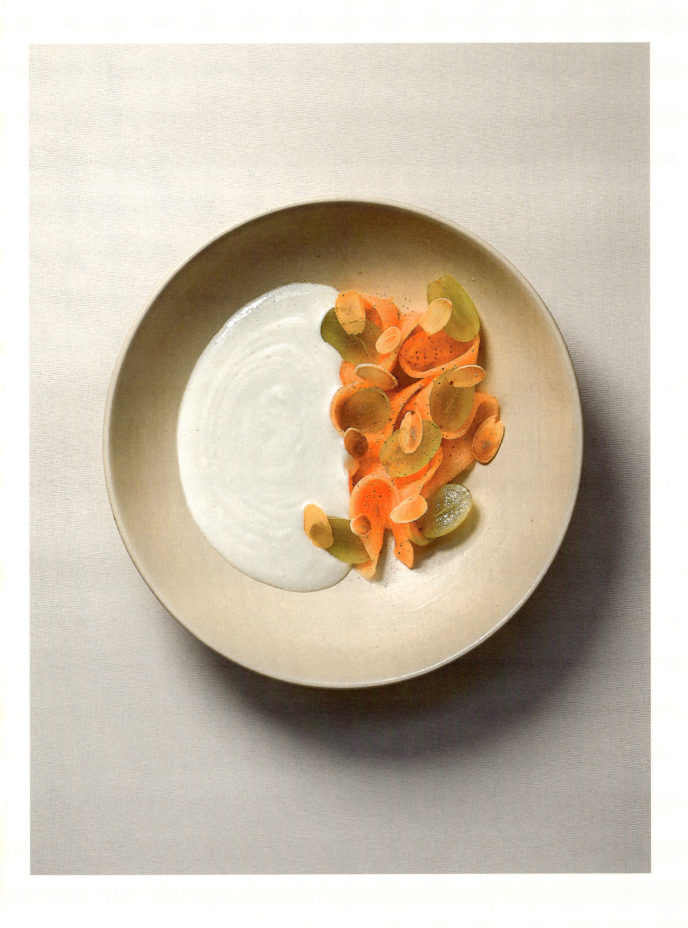

BILBERRY

VACCINIUM MYRTILLUS

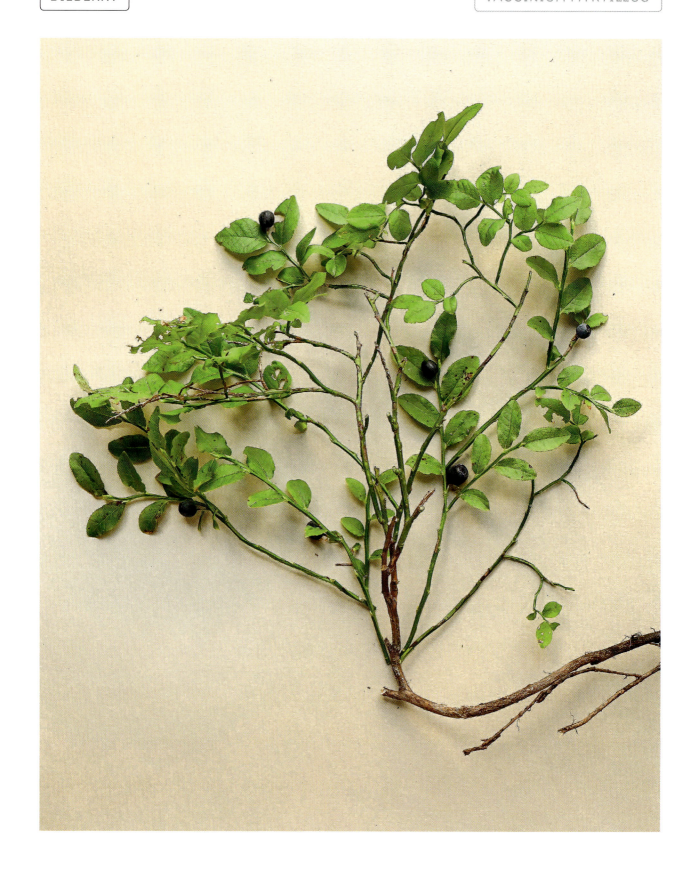

DNA and Eye Tonic

The bilberry or wild blueberry is native to many places in Europe and elsewhere in the world. The berries thrive in Scandinavia, and around 20 percent of Sweden is covered in bilberry plants. The Belgian Ardennes is another region in Europe where you will find a great many bilberry bushes. Near our (vacation) home in the Ardennes town of Vielsalm, known as "the bilberry capital," the annual blueberry festival is celebrated on 21 July with a parade including so-called Macralles, witch-type creatures named after the legendary witch Gustine Maka (1836–1915), who lived in the valley of the Salm. When we were children, this celebration was the highlight of the year in Belgium.

Elsewhere, bilberries are also collected traditionally in the third week of July. During the Irish-Celtic festival of Lughnasadh, they are gathered on the last Sunday of July, the first traditional harvest festival of the year. According to this tradition, the quality and quantity of the bilberry harvest is an indication of how good the crop will be the rest of the year. Bilberries tended to be picked by children, who would sing bilberry rhymes, some of which are still well known. The first three berries were always placed on a stone as an offering to the forest spirits. This was a way to guarantee a good harvest.[44]

The berry has been used for centuries for its medicinal properties. As far back as the 16th century, apothecary Michel Nostradamus wrote:

"Whoever wants to give his eyes a beautiful radiant shine should eat bilberries as often as possible." In the 12th century, Hildegard of Bingen is believed to have written about the medicinal properties of the bilberry. Contemporary scientific studies have now also shown that these berries have special properties.

Use

I grew up with these berries. You end up with bright blue fingers if you pick them yourself. We were crazy about them. I later found out that the blue pigment (anthocyanin) is a strong antioxidant with antibacterial and anti-inflammatory properties, and that it improves insulin secretion and can thus help with diabetes.[45] In the Ardennes, many people keep bilberries in their freezer as a remedy for gastrointestinal symptoms and flu.

While traveling in Finland, my friend Jani Asikainen told me that, before flying, Swedish F16 pilots eat up to 1 kilogram (2 pounds) of bilberries, because the phytonutrients in them was said to have a beneficial effect on their eyes. I later read that, during the Second World War, English pilots ate bilberry jam in order to see better. I then found out in scientific studies that there is actual evidence that bilberries have a beneficial effect on the eye.[46]

A study from Tufts University in the United States showed that the berries had a rejuvenating effect. They did an experiment with rats in which

PROPERTIES
- Eye tonic
- Strengthens vessel walls and improves (micro-vessel) blood circulation
- Blood-thinning
- Antioxidant
- Anti-inflammatory
- Antibacterial
- Improves insulin secretion
- Has a positive effect on the gastrointestinal system
- Improves intestinal flora
- Stimulates the appetite
- Mild laxative (mild stool softener)
- For flu support

SOURCING

When in season, gather the berries yourself in the forest, or buy them frozen from better health food stores and some supermarkets or greengrocers. The berries are also sold in dried form or as jam. Ensure that these are the real bilberries and not the larger blueberries.

CAUTION

The berry has a blood-thinning effect, and eating them is not recommended before you have to undergo (dental) surgery. Potential interactions may occur with drugs and plants that also have blood-thinning effects. Excessive use may cause diarrhea.

Fruit and Nuts

some had been given bilberries as additional nutrition for eight months and the control groups spinach and strawberries. The brain activity of the rats that had eaten berries was chemically younger than before the study.

Appearance

The bilberry grows in acid soils in partial shade in spring and summer (sometimes into autumn). The plants are very slow-growing and reach a height of 15–50 centimeters (about 6–20 inches). The berries, 5–9 millimeters (0.2 –0.35 inch) in diameter, are deep purple-blue, almost black, with a dull gray waxy coating. The bilberry is not the same berry as the American blueberry, which is easy to grow. The American version is much larger and is the most common variety on our supermarket shelves. This is a shame, because through cultivation, many of the berries' beneficial properties have been lost. The bilberry, the real blueberry, is not commercially grown because it does not produce a large crop and is, therefore, not attractive financially. For commercial purposes, the species is only collected in the wild where, fortunately, it is easy to find.

Extracting and Dosing

The berries can be eaten just as they are, in cream or yogurt, or as jam. For constipation and diarrhea, eat 100–300g (3.5 –10.5 oz) of fresh berries three times daily. This sounds contradictory but really works in most cases.

To improve your eyes, you can eat a handful of bilberries three times a week, and take an astaxanthin supplement alongside this. In addition, you may also consider putting a few drops of Sananga (*Tabernaemontana undulata*) in your eyes. It has helped me get rid of a blur in my left eye. It comes from the Amazon, where it was taken by the Kaxinawá and the Yawanawá tribe before they went out on a hunt, in order to see more sharply. Sananga can be purchased from ethnobotanical suppliers, such as UK-based online supplier Katukina. If you are successfully managing to stop your eye tissue from degenerating, it is also important to continue using maintenance doses. In Belgium, pharmacies sell bilberry eye drops.

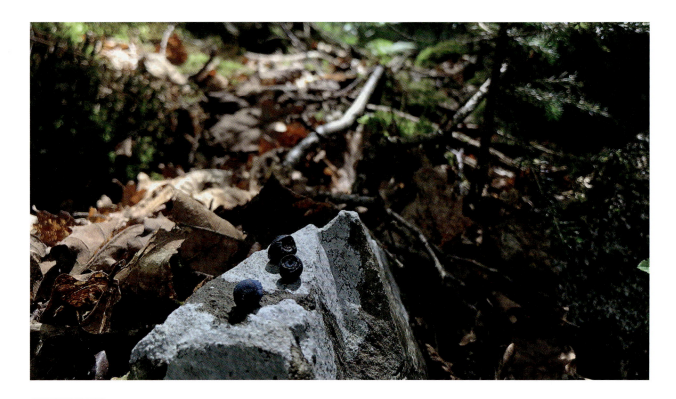

Fruit and Nuts

BILBERRY CANDY

makes about 15 pieces

■ INGREDIENTS
- 1 piece of licorice
- 125 ml/4.2 fl oz water, plus extra
- 125 g/4.4 oz bilberry or blueberry puree (health food store or puree the berries in a blender or food processor)
- 1 gelatin leaf
- 15 g/0.5 oz (3 tsp) soft brown sugar
- 5 g/0.18 oz (1 tsp) salty licorice powder (health food store or online)
- 42.5 g/1.5 oz (3 T) wheat flour

■ EQUIPMENT
- (silicone) molds of your choice

method

Cut the licorice into small pieces. Put them in a small saucepan with the water, and bring to a boil. Simmer for 5 minutes, then strain in a sieve into a second small pan. Add the bilberry puree to the strained liquid, and bring to a simmer again. Reduce by one-third.

Meanwhile, soak the gelatin leaf in a bowl of cold water.

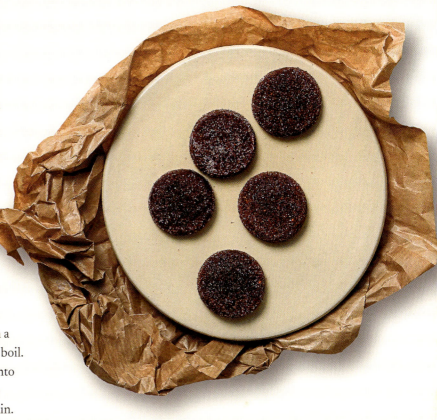

Add the sugar and salty licorice powder to the pan, reduce the heat further, and stir frequently.

In a bowl, make a paste of the flour with a small splash of water.

Squeeze out the gelatin, and add this to the pan, together with the flour mix. Keep stirring to stop any lumps from forming. When it is smooth and creamy, it is ready.

Pour the mixture into the molds, and leave to set for 24 hours.

Fruit and Nuts

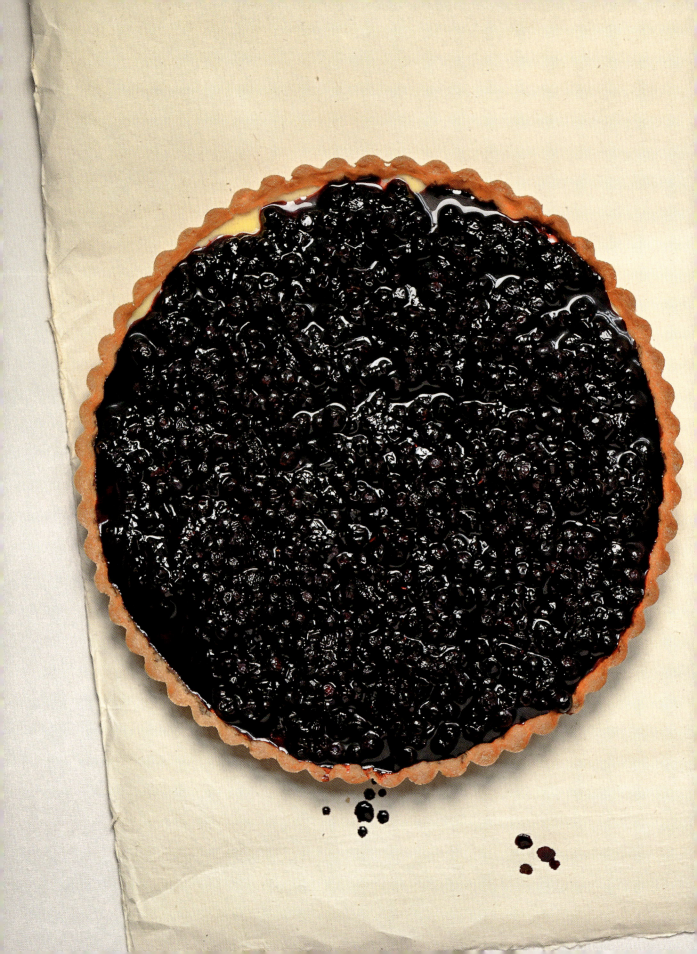

BILBERRY PIE

serves 8 people

■ **FOR THE PIE CRUST**
- 125 g/4.4 oz soft white sugar
- 2.5 g/0.09 oz (½ tsp) fine sea salt
- ½ egg, beaten
- 15 ml/0.5 fl oz (1 T) cold water
- 125 g/4.4 oz butter, at room temperature and cut into small cubes
- 250 g/8.8 oz flour, plus extra
- 5 g/0.18 oz baking powder
- butter for greasing

■ **FOR THE PASTRY CREAM**
- 250 ml/8.5 fl oz whole milk
- 60 g/2.1 oz granulated sugar
- ½ vanilla pod
- 20 g/0.7 oz custard powder (Bird's or similar)
- pinch of fine sea salt
- 2 egg yolks (approx. 40 g/1.4 oz)

■ **AS WELL AS**
- 500 g/17.6 oz bilberries or blueberries
- icing sugar

■ **EQUIPMENT**
- 26 cm diameter x 2.5 cm deep/10 in x 1 in pie dish or cake tin
- ceramic baking or dried beans or similar
- piping bag

method

Start with the pie crust. In a bowl, mix the sugar with the salt, egg, water, and butter. Add the flour and the baking powder, and knead into a smooth dough. Do not knead it for too long otherwise it will become tough.

Roll the pastry into a ball, and cover with plastic wrap (clingfilm). Allow to rest in the refrigerator for least 1 hour.

Preheat the oven to 180°C (350°F). Grease the cake tin or pie dish with some butter. Roll out the pastry, and line the tin or dish with it. Cover the pastry with a sheet of baking parchment, fill it with the ceramic baking beans or similar, and bake blind for 20 minutes. When the pastry has turned a nice golden-brown it can be removed from the oven. Remove the beans and baking parchment, and leave to cool.

For the pastry cream, in a saucepan, bring the milk to a gentle boil together with 50 grams (1.8 ounces) of sugar and the vanilla, including the scraped pod. Do not let the milk boil over.

Meanwhile, in a bowl, mix the custard powder with the salt and the rest of the sugar. Add the egg yolks, and stir into a lump-free paste.

While stirring, add a ladleful of hot vanilla milk to the custard mixture, and mix well. This allows the mixture to warm up a little, which will set in motion the thickening process. While stirring, add the paste to the saucepan of hot milk, and bring gently to a boil. Keep stirring. Remove the vanilla pod.

Gently simmer the pastry cream for 2 minutes, until it has the thickness of custard. Turn off the heat, and pour the cream into a bowl. Cover with plastic wrap, really pressing the film onto the cream so there is no air between it and the cream, otherwise a skin will appear. Allow to cool.

Reheat the oven to 180°C (350°F).

In a bowl, lightly whip the cooled cream to loosen it, and scoop it into a piping bag. Generously fill the baked pie crust with this to 5 millimeters (0.2 inches) below the edge. Smooth out the cream with a spoon or spatula.

Spread the bilberries over the pastry cream, and sprinkle with icing sugar. Bake the pie in the oven for another 25 minutes.

Fruit and Nuts

| OLIVE | | OLEA EUROPAEA |

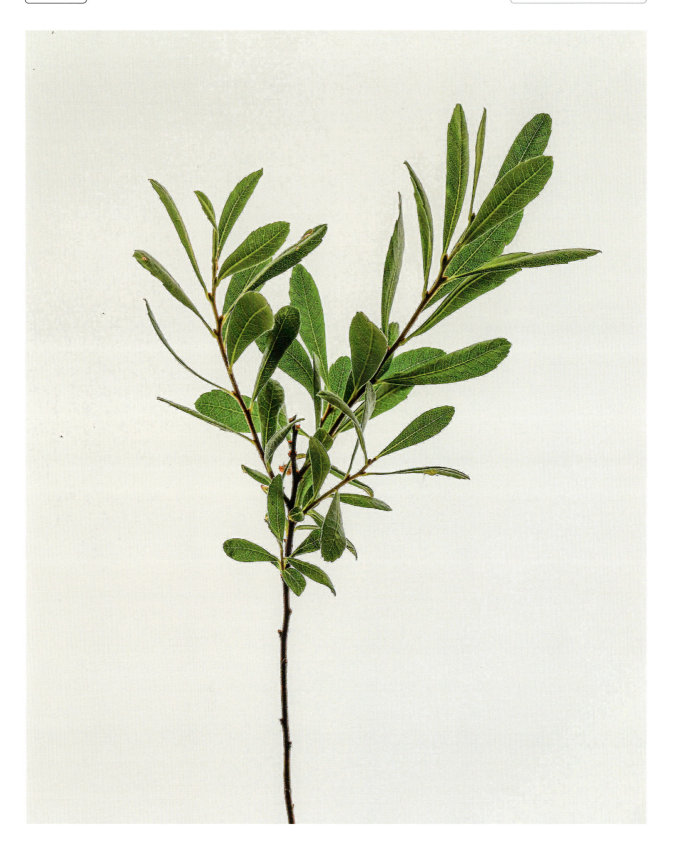

Honored Oil

I well remember, aged 16, stepping off the train in Delphi at the end of my first major train journey, from Amsterdam to Greece, how the silvery sea of olive trees in the mountains surrounding the ancient oracle temple made a huge impression. The olive tree was one of the first plants to be domesticated around the Mediterranean, and in all the countries surrounding it, olive (oil) use has been a feature.

It was used not only in the preparation of food; people also rubbed it into their skin and used it as a carrier oil for flower perfumes or as lamp oil. Olive branches were additionally used during ceremonies and sacrificial rites; in antiquity, the winner of the Olympics was given an olive wreath, for example. In the Bible, in the book of Genesis, the dove returns to Noah's ark with an olive branch in its beak. This image has become a global symbol of peace, goodwill, hope, and prosperity. In several faiths, the olive tree was regarded as a blessed tree. In Tutankhamun's tomb, three wreaths with olive branches were found. [47] The first written mention of olive oil was found on the pharmaceutical clay tablet texts from Ebla in present-day Syria. The texts date from 4,500 years ago.

Olive oil was a common remedy for diseases in Biblical times. It is a custom that originated with shepherds. Insects would nest in the wool fleece of their sheep. As a preventative remedy, they would rub sheep's heads with olive oil so that the insects were less able to reach the sheep's ears. Anointing thus became a symbol of strength and protection. In the story about the Good Samaritan, we read that he healed wounds by pouring wine and olive oil onto them and then dressing them. The miracle child from Bethlehem himself is called the Anointed One, the Christ. According to Professor Carl Ruck, the ointment in question contained cannabis and thus, as an entheogen, induced visions.

In ancient times, both objects and persons were dedicated to God by anointing them with fragrant olive oil. Anointing was a sign of connectedness and a sign of being chosen. If you were anointed, you were under the influence of God. Anointing with scented oil was also an important moment in the initiation rite of the early Christians, and later, that of priests and kings.

The Greek island of Crete has the highest consumption of olive oil and the lowest incidence of cardiovascular disease in the world.[48] The island is home to the world's oldest olive tree; more than 2,000 years old, it is still producing edible olives. These ancient trees that have accompanied civilizations have forged a direct link between mankind's oldest forms of culture and the present. Through their age, they connect us with antiquity in one direct living line. In Sarve-Abarqu in Iran stands an Italian cypress that is more than 4,000 years old. Gümeli on the Black Sea in Turkey has a yew tree with a similar life span. The oldest living tree known to us is an ancient bristlecone pine tree in the California White Mountains that is well over 5,000 years old. In the Netherlands, there is an old sacred oak tree in the Brabant village of Den Hout that is 600–800 years old; similarly, in the Dutch town of Oisterwijk, a 600-year-old summer lime tree graces De Lind behind the town hall. The Fortingall Yew in Perthshire is considered to be the oldest tree in the

PROPERTIES
- Prevents cardiovascular disease, age-related complaints, gallstones
- Laxative
- Lowers blood pressure
- Anti-inflammatory
- Neuroprotective

SOURCING

Available from stores specializing in Mediterranean food, supermarkets, health food stores, oil specialists, at farmers' markets, and sometimes direct from a local producer.

CAUTION

At least two effects have been proven with olive leaf, and it is therefore widely prescribed and applied by herbalists as a blood pressure–lowering remedy and to widen the walls of the coronary arteries, but little is known about any toxicity.[49]

Fruit and Nuts

United Kingdom, with an estimated age of at least 2,000–3,000 years, possibly much older.

Even though we eat (processed) olives almost everywhere in the world, it is primarily the oil from the fruit and kernel that we use for medicinal purposes. The oil is obtained by pressing and filtering the whole fruit and kernel together.

Use

Olive oil is an excellent carrier for substances from other medicinal plants. A large number of studies have confirmed the health-promoting effects of olive oil used as part of the Mediterranean diet, including prevention of neurodegenerative disorders and age-related diseases.

By regularly consuming extra virgin olive oil you will be ingesting healthy fats, as it contains omega 3, 6, and 9 oils. The oil is also rich in vitamin E and K and a protective antioxidant called eulorpein, which is known for its blood pressure–lowering, anti-inflammatory, cardioprotective, and neuroprotective properties.[50]

Seventy percent of olive oil consists of healthy, monounsaturated fats. These help balance the fat levels in your blood and counter high cholesterol and blood clots resulting from an excess of unhealthy fats and processed sugars.[51] The oil is also rich in many polyphenols, which help improve the immune system, cognition, and alertness.

In addition, olive oil is one of the safest laxatives. According to herbalist Mellie Uyldert, nothing works better for intestinal inflammation, cramp, or constipation than olive oil.[52]

The leaf of the olive tree is phyto-therapeutically applied as a blood pressure–lowering agent, as an antioxidant to protect the vessel walls, and to stabilize irregular heart rhythms.[53]

Eating an olive right off the tree is not very enjoyable; they are hard and bitter. So they are mostly processed in some form or other. In Greece, the olive is scored and then preserved in vinegar. In Crete, I was told that people swallow the occasional olive kernel. The kernel is said to be digested in your intestines and contain various antioxidants and other beneficial substances that are believed to benefit muscles and the cardiovascular system.

Traditionally, olive oil is taken in combination with lemon juice as a remedy for gallstones.[54]

Appearance

Olive trees can grow to a considerable girth with an ash-gray bark. The tree grows slowly and eventually is blessed with a thick, gnarled, short trunk and long roots. This is taken into account when it is planted. It only starts to bear fruit after 5–10 years. The branches have lanceolate, leathery, sage-green leaves. The oval fruits are green and measure 1–3½ centimeters (0.4–1.4 inches).

Olive trees grow best in sunny, dry regions with mild winters, such as around the Mediterranean Sea.

Extracting and Dosing

Eat at least 2 tablespoons (30 millileters/1 fluid ounce) of olive oil every day for the prevention of cardiovascular disease and age-related conditions.[55] Traditionally, olive oil is also used as a folk remedy in so-called oil pulling, whereby, after rising in the morning, you roll a hefty gulp of olive oil around in your mouth for 20 minutes; your body's toxins will be absorbed into the oil, and this is said to improve the hygiene of your teeth. You spit out the oil afterwards. (Coconut oil can also be used for this purpose.)
You can make beautiful ointments with olive oil; see page 29.

To make an olive leaf infusion, pour 150 milliliters (5 fluid ounces) of boiling water over 16 ounces/ 431 grams (2 cups) of finely chopped olive leaves. After 30 minutes, strain into a bowl. You can drink 3–4 small tea cups of the extract a day. Little is known about the safety of this treatment in terms of toxicity, but it has been proven to contain active components.

Make sure you use high-quality, first cold-pressed olive oil (extra virgin), preferably organic. Store the oil airtight in a dark place, otherwise it can quickly become rancid. It is best to consume the oil cold. Heated oil loses its medicinal properties.

Fruit and Nuts

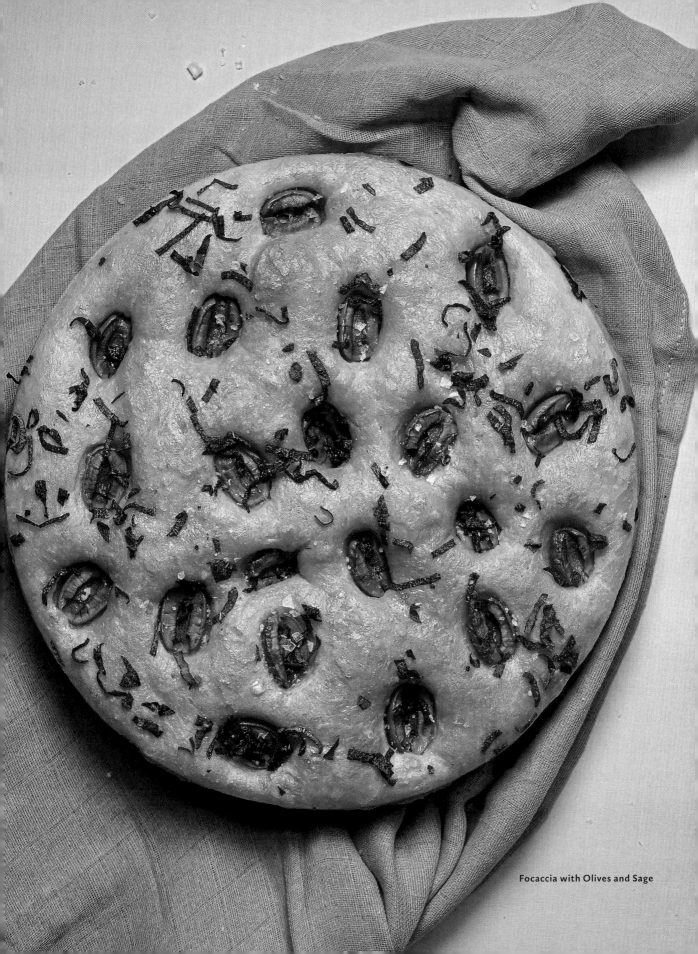

Focaccia with Olives and Sage

FOCACCIA WITH OLIVES AND SAGE

for 1 loaf

■ INGREDIENTS
- 7 g/0.25 oz dried fast-acting yeast
- 400 ml/13.5 fl oz lukewarm water
- 500 g/17.6 oz white bread flour, plus extra
- 10 g/0.3 oz (2 tsp) fine sea salt
- 75 ml/2.5 fl oz (5 T) olive oil, plus extra
- ½ bunch (approx. 40 g/1.4 oz) sage leaves, cut into fine strips
- 5 g/0.15 oz (1 tsp) fleur de sel
- 100 g /3.5 oz green olives, halved and pitted

■ EQUIPMENT
- round baking or springform tin measuring 24 centimeters (10 inches) in diameter.

method

Dissolve the dry yeast in the lukewarm water. Put the flour and fine salt in a bowl, and make a well in the center. Pour the water with the yeast along with 30 milliliters (1 fluid ounce, or 2 tablespoons) of olive oil into the well. Gently mix the flour into the liquid so that a dough is formed.

Dust the countertop with flour, and drop the dough onto it, scraping along the sides of the bowl so that everything comes out. Knead for about 10 minutes until your dough is soft and less sticky. Put the dough in a clean bowl, cover with a tea towel and leave to rise in a warm place for 1 hour until it has doubled in volume. Grease the baking tin with some olive oil and place the dough in it. Stretch to fill the tin. Cover with a tea towel, and leave to rise for another 45 minutes or so.

Meanwhile, preheat the oven to 220°C (425°F). Drizzle the dough with the remaining olive oil, sprinkle with the sage and fleur de sel. Press the olives about 1 centimeter (0.4 inch) into the dough.

Bake the focaccia for 20 minutes until cooked and golden-brown.

PASTA AGLIO E OLIO

serves 4 people

■ INGREDIENTS
- 400 g/0.8 lb spaghetti
- 150 ml/5 fl oz extra virgin olive oil
- 4 garlic cloves, finely chopped
- 1 red chili pepper, seeds and membrane removed and finely chopped
- ½ bunch (approx. 40 g/1.4 oz) leaf parsley, finely chopped
- fine sea salt and freshly ground black pepper

method

In a pan with plenty of salted water, cook the spaghetti for 1 minute less than the package instructions. Drain but save a cup of the pasta water.

Heat the olive oil in a large skillet on medium-high heat. Fry the garlic and red chili pepper for 30–60 seconds. Add the parsley, and roll the pan around to distribute the parsley and olive oil.

Turn down the heat, and add the spaghetti. Add a few tablespoons of pasta water, and roll around the pan again so that everything is well distributed and the oil sticks to the pasta. Season with salt and pepper, and serve immediately.

Fruit and Nuts

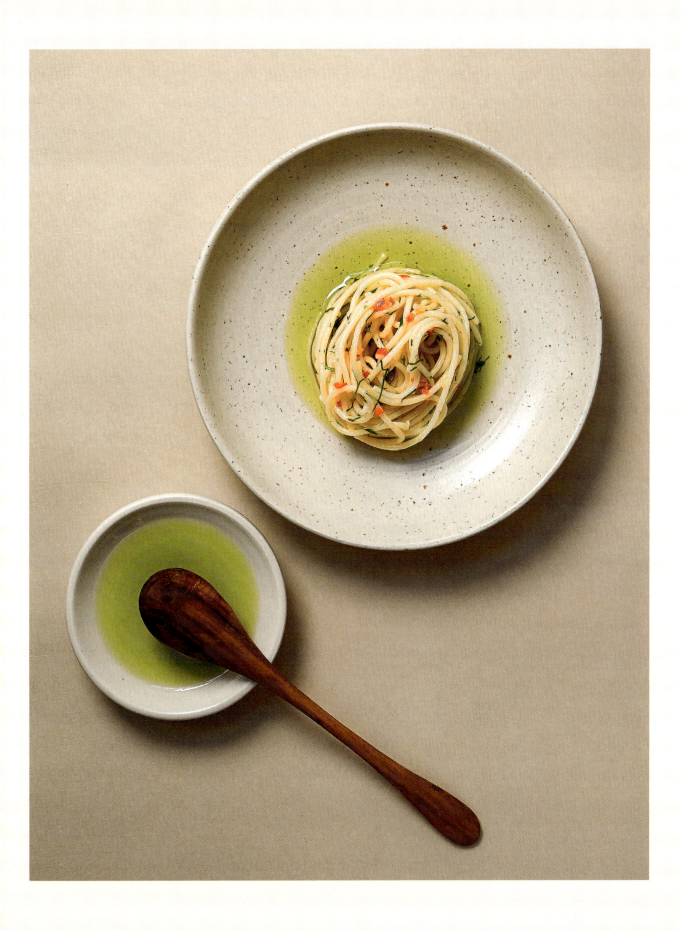

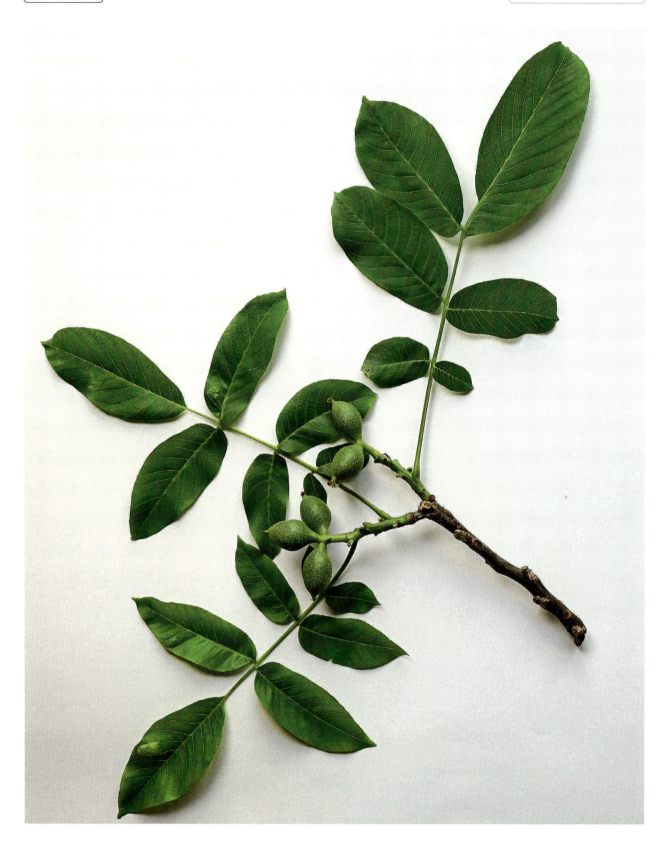

Provisions for the Brain

When I think of walnuts, I think of the brownies I bake every year on my birthday—and I immediately think of my favorite Persian dish, *fesenjān*, a delicious sweet and sour stew with walnuts and pomegranate juice. In English, the walnut is also called "Persian walnut." The English word walnut literally means "foreigner's nut." In antiquity, the walnut was brought from Persia to Greece and was then spread through Europe by the Greeks and Romans. Eastward, the walnut found its way into China via Afghanistan. This nut that is among humanity's oldest cultivated crops is now grown in many more places. France, Italy, and the United States are currently the largest producers of walnuts.

Among the Greeks and Romans, the walnut tree was dedicated to the supreme god Zeus (Jupiter). Walnuts were seen as the food of the gods. The sacred union between the tree and their supreme god is also found in its botanical name *Juglans regia*, meaning "royal acorn of Jupiter." The tree has always been associated with death and is widely planted in cemeteries, but the nut was also long used as a fertility symbol at weddings, when walnuts were sprinkled over young brides.

I learned from Belgian professor of ethnobotany Marcel de Cleene that, in Europe and the Latin-speaking countries, walnut trees were regarded the favorite haunt of witches. Witches would gather under the walnut tree on June 24, St. John's Day.[56] Brian Muraresku, author of the book *The Immortality Key*, also talks about the walnut tree as a gathering place of wise herbal women, later known as witches. The holiest witchcraft pilgrimage site in the world was the walnut tree of Benevento in Italy, where women gathered from all over Europe. "There they frolicked under the branches, which were sacred to the Greek goddess Artemis. And paid homage to a female divinity who bore many names: the Matromne, the Teacher, or the Wise Sibilla, the King of the Fairies and the Greek Mistress."

Like all sabbaths, the ritual at Benevento was an alternative mass with a different Eucharist in honor of an alternative deity.[57] The Eucharist used by the "witches" tended to be a psychoactive witches' salve. According to Muraresku and other historians, including Professor Carl Ruck, psychedelics served as a shortcut to enlightenment and formed the basis of Western civilization.

These historians have proven that the Vatican tried to ban the original (psychedelic) Eucharist—first in the mysteries of Eleusis, followed by the mysteries of Dionysus, then in the first Christians' domestic churches and in the catacombs of the Vatican, and later the witches who gathered under walnut trees—in order to deprive people of beatific visions.

PROPERTIES
- Source of omega-3 fatty acids
- Anti-inflammatory
- Antithrombotic (helps prevent heart and vascular diseases)
- Improves mood
- Source of antioxidants
- Fortifying

SOURCING

Walnuts and walnut oil can be bought at farmers' markets, greengrocers, and supermarkets.

CAUTION

Walnut oil can go rancid quickly. Store it in a dark, airtight bottle in a cool place.

They saw these changes of consciousness as one of the great dangers to their power. This prohibition was first implemented in Europe and then with Catholic colonization also in Africa, Asia and Latin America.

The Catholic faithful now receive a somewhat empty ritual and a placebo (a host and a sip of wine) every Sunday during mass instead of the original psychedelic sacrament. Currently, more and more people are finding out about this history, and we are in the midst of a psychedelic renaissance. We see a worldwide revival of one of humanity's deepest primal traditions of sacramental use dating back to Neolithic times. Who knows, we may be gathering under walnut trees again in Europe, reviving ancient rituals.

Fruit and Nuts

The walnut was considered an oracle tree in ancient Europe, and there were numerous ancient customs during which the nuts revealed prophecies about marriage and life.

In Belgium, it is customary to plant a walnut tree when a son is born. My mother planted a walnut tree in the garden of our farm in Wallonia even before I was born. The names Wallonia and Wales still refer to the word walnut. Walnut trees also used to be planted near farms, as the bitter substances and aromas of the leaves kept mosquitoes and flies at bay. Walnut leaves were also hung in cribs for that reason.

Walnuts are not actually nuts. This is because they do not meet the official definition of a nut: a nut is a fruit with one seed, the shell of which hardens, like a hazelnut. Walnuts are actually stone fruits. Yet we have simply come to call them nuts.

Use

According to traditional medicine, walnuts are used to strengthen kidneys, lungs, and intestines. They have warming properties, and therefore, a beneficial effect on the libido. In Chinese cuisine, the walnut is one of the most commonly used nuts. It is a rich source of protein and fats and is highly nutritious.

According to the ancient Doctrine of Signatures healing theory, plants that resemble body parts may be used for healing; thus, the walnut, which resembles a brain, is associated with cerebral health. As a result of its healthy essential omega-3 fatty acids, this nut is in fact good for the brain. "Essential" means that our bodies cannot make these fatty acids themselves, so we must consume foods that contain them. Our brain is made up of cell membranes that are themselves made up of fat. Omega-3 fatty acids have an anti-inflammatory effect and also help prevent numerous degenerative diseases such as Alzheimer's, cardiovascular disease, and arthritis. Walnuts contain the amino acid tryptophan, which, on consumption, is converted into the neurotransmitter serotonin. This "mind-boosting happiness hormone" is one of the primary brain chemicals responsible for maintaining a positive mood.

Walnuts are high in antioxidants and fiber. Vitamin E in walnuts helps prevent blood clots, among other things, and is thus important in preventing cardiovascular disease. It also supports proper reproductive function and helps prevent infertility and miscarriages.

A well-known home remedy for colds and digestive problems used to be young walnuts with their green husks soaked in brandy, often with cloves and cinnamon.

Appearance

The walnut tree has lanceolate, aromatic, oval leaves and produces nuts with a hard bivalve shell with leathery partitions. The shell is covered with a green smooth skin, which later turns black due to oxidation and falls away from the shell. The nut inside the shell resembles two brains grown together.

Extracting and Dosing

For most adults, the recommendation is to eat one handful (approx. 25 grams / 0.8 ounces) of unsalted nuts a day. Walnuts make you feel satiated for a long time, so you are less likely to get hungry. You can incorporate a good quality walnut oil into a vinaigrette or another salad dressing a few times a week.

Fruit and Nuts

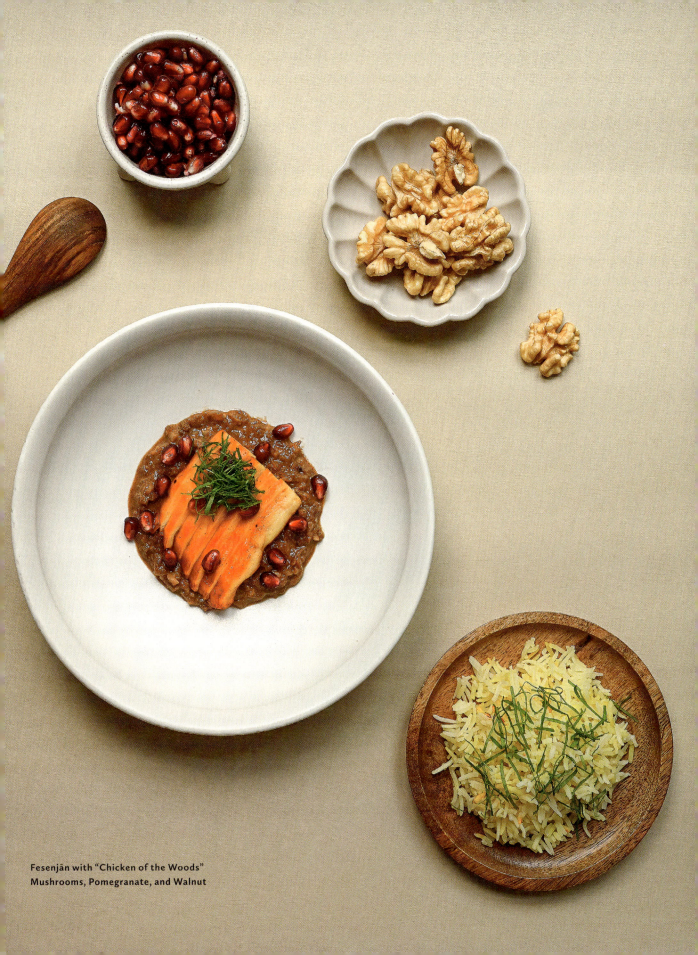

Fesenjān with "Chicken of the Woods" Mushrooms, Pomegranate, and Walnut

FESENJĀN WITH "CHICKEN OF THE WOODS" MUSHROOMS, POMEGRANATE, AND WALNUT

serves 4 people

■ INGREDIENTS

- 100 g/3.5 oz shelled walnuts
- 30 ml/1 fl oz (2 T) olive oil, plus extra
- 1 red onion, chopped
- 2 garlic cloves, finely chopped
- 7.5 g/0.25 oz (½ T) cinnamon powder
- 7.5 g/0.25 oz (½ T) cayenne pepper
- 200 g/7 oz cooked chickpeas
- 250 ml/8.5 fl oz vegetable stock
- 45 ml/1.5 fl oz (3 T) pomegranate syrup
- 15 ml/0.5 fl oz (1 T) maple syrup
- fine sea salt and freshly ground black pepper
- 400 g/1 lb "chicken of the woods" mushroom (health food store or greengrocer)
- seeds of ½ pomegranate
- rice as a side dish

method

Heat a dry large skillet over medium-high heat, and add the walnuts. Toast them a few minutes until golden brown. Briefly grind the walnuts in a food processor to a fine crumb.

In a tall, thick-bottomed pan, heat the olive oil on medium-high heat. Add the onion and garlic and sauté for about 5 minutes, until they begin to brown. Add the cinnamon powder and cayenne pepper, and sauté briefly. Add the nut crumbs, chickpeas, vegetable stock, pomegranate syrup, and maple syrup. Bring to the boil, and put the lid on the pan. Let it all simmer and thicken for about 10 minutes. Season to taste with pepper and salt.

Meanwhile, brush or rub clean the mushrooms. Heat a splash of olive oil in a skillet on high heat, and briefly fry the mushroom just *al dente*. Slice the mushrooms, and place them on top of the nut stew. Sprinkle with the pomegranate seeds. Serve with rice.

WOUTER'S BIRTHDAY BROWNIES

serves 20 people

■ INGREDIENTS

- 250 g/8 oz butter, plus extra
- 400 g/0.8 lb raw cane sugar
- 16 g/0.5 oz (2 sachets) vanilla sugar
- 35 g/1.2 oz cocoa powder
- grated zest of 1 organic lemon
- 4 eggs
- 190 g/6.7 oz wholewheat spelt flour
- 225 g/8 oz walnuts, coarsely chopped
- 100 g/3.5 oz dark chocolate

■ EQUIPMENT

- brownie tray measuring approximately 20 x 30 cm (approx. 8 x 12 in)

method

Melt the butter in a saucepan and allow to cool. Preheat the oven to 175°C (350°F).

In a bowl, mix the melted butter, both types of sugar, the cocoa powder, lemon zest, and eggs with a whisk or hand mixer. Add the spelt flour and the chopped walnuts, and mix well again. Line the baking tray with baking parchment, grease with some butter, and pour the batter into it. Bake for 40 minutes in the middle of the oven.

Insert a toothpick or the tip of a knife to see if the brownies are baked. If any batter sticks to it, they are not yet ready. If so, return to the oven for a few more minutes.

During the last minute, break the chocolate in pieces over the brownies, and allow to melt briefly in the oven. Remove the tray from the oven, and spread the melted chocolate over the top of the brownies with a spoon or spatula until it is smooth. Allow to cool completely, then cut into 20 pieces.

Fruit and Nuts

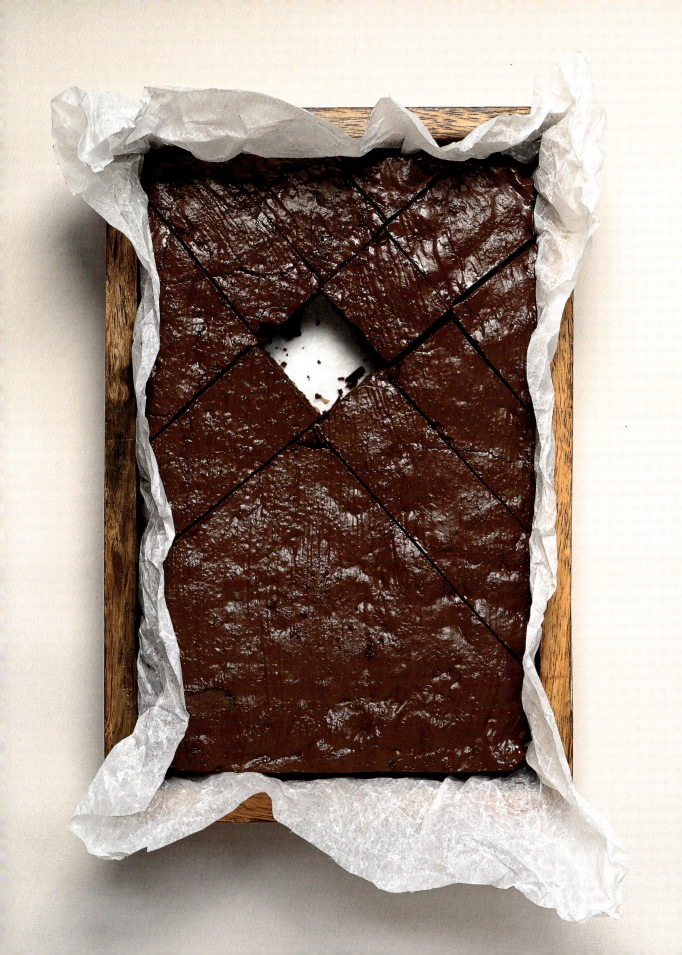

CLOUDBERRY | RUBUS CHAMAEMORUS

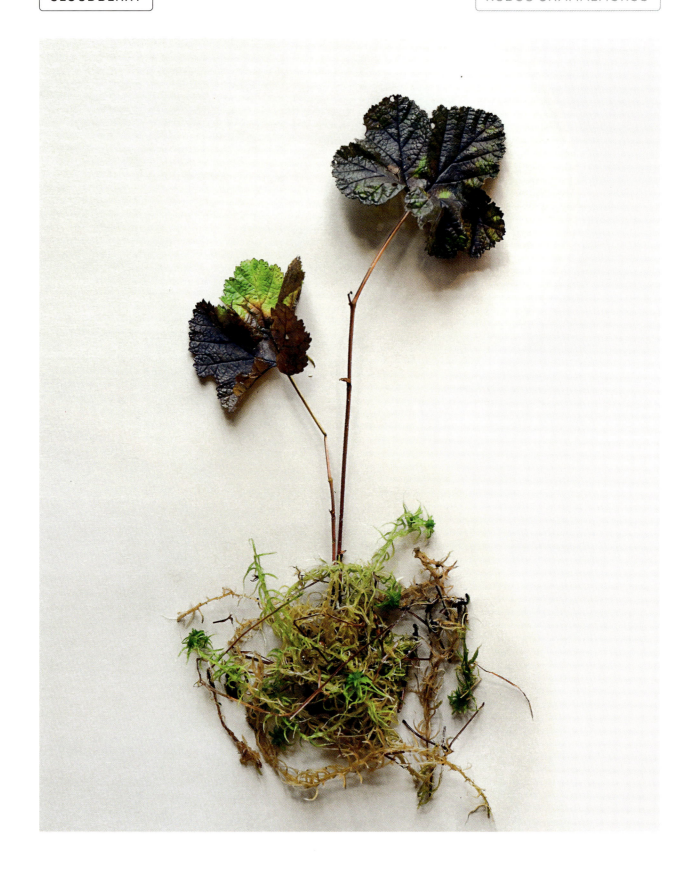

Immune Booster

Cloudberry typically grows above the Arctic Circle, between the latitudes of 78°N and 55°N, as well as scattered locations farther south. It grows in places where almost no other crop can grow and can take temperatures of minus 40 degrees Celsius (-40° Fahrenheit). The berry can be cultivated, but it usually only grows in the wild. In North America, it may be found in Canada and some locations in the northern US states of Alaska, New England, northern Minnesota, New Hampshire, Maine, and upstate New York.

It is not common in the Netherlands, but in countries such as Finland it is highly rated, where the berries are sold dried or as jam. The berry is even depicted on the Finnish 2-euro coin. It has been used for centuries in Nordic folk medicine for its powerful effect on our immune system.

Fresh cloudberries taste quite sharp, which is why the berry is mostly incorporated into dishes, confectionery, or jams before it is eaten. In Finland, cloudberries are eaten for breakfast on soft, buttered rye bread, or sometimes with *Leipäjuusto*, a Finnish flat oven-baked cheese; cloudberry jam is served as dessert mixed into yoghurt. The berry is regarded a delicacy in the country and also drunk as a liqueur during special celebrations. There, in Europe's most wooded country, this power berry is known as *lakka, hilla, valokki*, or *suomuurain*.

They are difficult to find and only in the wild in the boreal forests in the mountains, making the berries seem quite pricey to us. They are also known as "the gold of the Arctic."

Use

Cloudberry helps protect against cardiovascular disease as it is high in polyphenols, a category of plant compound that offers various health benefits, including anthocyanin, micronutrients, and fiber.[58] Cloudberries also help our bodies to detoxify and strengthen our immune system, partly because of the high concentration of vitamins A and C.

The berries are used to counter aging or to slow down the aging process. These berries have a positive effect on our eyes as they contain pro-vitamin A and A-carotene. In addition to being a rich source of vitamins and minerals, they also contain ellagic acid, which protects human skin cells from UV radiation damage and also binds to and eliminates carcinogenic substances. Due to the presence of ellagic acid, prepared foods made from these berries remain naturally preserved and are easy to store. If chilled, cloudberries can be kept in their own juices without added sugar.

Due to their positive effect on the skin, extracts from the berries are also incorporated into cosmetics such as shampoos, hand creams, and body lotions.

PROPERTIES
- Immune booster
- For the prevention of cardiovascular diseases
- Good for the heart because of omega-3 and -6 fatty acids
- Anti-aging
- Rich source of vitamins, minerals, and ellagic acid
- Protects against UV-radiation

SOURCING
In the Netherlands, you can buy the jam in The Finnish House store in Rotterdam or online. In Finland and other countries around the polar circle, the berry is also available as a dried powder, which is also available online elsewhere. In their habitat, they can also to be found in the wild in early fall.

CAUTION
There are no known side effects.

Extracting and Dosing

Stir in 1 tablespoon of dried berries into a smoothie or yogurt. In addition, use the jam on bread or stir into yogurt.

Fruit and Nuts

CLOUDBERRY JAM WITH COULOMMIERS CHEESE, HERB SALAD, AND CLOUDBERRY BREAD

serves 4 people

■ **FOR THE CLOUDBERRY JAM**
- 125 g/4.4 oz cloudberries
- 75 g/2.6 oz granulated sugar
- 75 g/2.6 oz preserving sugar

■ **FOR THE HERB SALAD**
- 1 bunch (approx. 80 g/2.8 oz) sweet cicely
- 1 bunch (approx. 80 g/2.8 oz) green sorrel
- 1 bunch (approx. 80 g/2.8 oz) red sorrel
- 50 g/1.8 oz mizuna
- 50 g/1.8 oz bronze fennel
- 25 g/0.9 oz cornflowers (bachelor buttons)

■ **AS WELL AS**
- Approx. 250 g/8.8 oz Coulommiers cheese, a soft raw cheese with a bloomy rind similar to brie, in 1 piece

method

Mix the cloudberries and the two kinds of sugar in a bowl, and leave in the refrigerator overnight. In the morning, transfer to a saucepan, and simmer over a low heat for 10 minutes. Remove the pan from the heat when the mixture has thickened a little and begins to resemble jam. Allow to cool.

Bake the cloudberry bread according to the recipe on the opposite page. Note that this takes some time because the dough needs to prove.

Make the herb salad by removing the stems from all the ingredients and roughly tearing the leaves. Mix in a bowl. If you like, you can add a dressing, but I find that the fresh herbs and flowers have enough flavor of their own.

Slice the cloudberry bread when it is as fresh as possible. Serve with the the Coulommiers cheese, cloudberry jam, and herb salad.

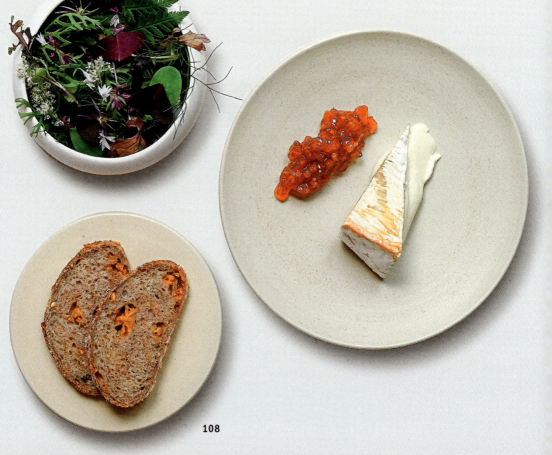

CLOUDBERRY BREAD

for 2 loaves

■ **FOR THE POOLISH (PRE-FERMENT OR YEAST STARTER)**
- 20 g/0.7 oz fresh yeast
- 60 ml/2 fl oz cold water
- 60 g/2.1 oz flour

■ **FOR THE DOUGH**
- 500 g/18 oz cloudberries
- 600 ml/21 fl oz water, plus 2 T (30 ml/1fl oz)
- 120 g/4.2 oz poolish
- 500 g/18 oz French white T65 (high-gluten) bread flour, plus extra
- 300 g/10.6 oz wholewheat flour
- 18 g/0.6 oz fine sea salt
- 2 organic lemons
- ½ bunch (approx. 40 g/1.4 oz) thyme

■ **EQUIPMENT**
- kitchen thermometer
- 2 baking tins, shape of your choice

method

Start by making the *poolish*, or pre-ferment. In a small bowl, dissolve the yeast in the water, then, in a new bowl, mix it with the flour. Cover, and leave overnight in the refrigerator. The volume should have doubled at least.

Cloudberries that are not inside the dough will burn. Soak the cloudberries in a bowl of warm water or a delicious (alcoholic) drink for 15 minutes, and drain. Do not pat them dry, because they should not absorb too much moisture from the dough.

Pour 600 milliliters (20.3 fluid ounces) of water into a large bowl, making sure that the temperature is around 28°C (82.4°F). Dissolve the *poolish* in this. Add the two types of flour, and make a dough. Make sure the water is fully absorbed, but do not knead. Fold the cloudberries well into the dough.

Allow to rest for 30 minutes—this is called *autolysis*. In this process, the dough creates gluten and sugars because it breaks down the starch. In a small bowl, mix the salt with 2 tablespoons (30 milliliters/1 fluid ounce) of water, so that it dissolves more easily and add to the dough.

Now we are going to fold the dough. Form 2 ears on the top of the ball, and fold them in. Do this 4 times, 1 for each side of the ball: left, right, top, and bottom. Turn the ball over. Allow to rest for 1 hour.

Meanwhile, peel the lemons, cut the peel into fine strips, and pick the thyme leaves. After the dough has rested for an hour, add the cloudberries, lemon peel strips, and thyme. Mix everything, and once more fold the dough as described above. Allow to rest for another hour. Divide the dough in two. Puff up the dough a little, and allow it to rest on the countertop for 30 minutes. Press any cloudberries that have popped out back into the dough. Any that are still sticking out after that should be removed.

Meanwhile, preheat the oven to 200°C (400°F).

Sprinkle some flour over the 2 balls of dough, and fold them a third time, as described above. Roll the dough balls into rounds using the palm of your hand. Sprinkle a little flour on top, and turn both balls over. Grease the baking tins with butter and some flour. Place the dough with the fold down in the tins, and allow the balls to rise for approx. 40 minutes.

Bake the cloudberry loaves for 25–30 minutes. Remove them from the baking tin and then bake for another 5 minutes, so they are an even golden color on both sides.

Some cloudberries may "float" to the surface or sit just below the crust and burn. That's too bad. Simply pull them out.

CLOUDBERRY PAVLOVA WITH YOGURT OR LABNEH

serves 4 people

■ FOR THE YOGURT
- 1 L/34 oz full-fat yogurt
  (also Greek yogurt or labneh)

■ FOR THE CLOUDBERRY SYRUP
  (APPROX. 300 ML/10.1 FL OZ)
- 125 g/4.4 oz cloudberries
- 75 g/2.6 oz granulated sugar
- 75 ml/2.5 fl oz water

■ FOR THE PAVLOVA
- 3 egg whites
- 150 g/5.3 oz granulated sugar
- 10 g/0.6 oz (2 tsp) cornstarch
- 5 ml/0.3 fl oz (1 tsp) lemon juice
- 5 ml/0.3 fl oz (1 tsp) cloudberry syrup
- 30 g/1 oz marigold petals

■ EQUIPMENT
- cheesecloth or tea towel

method

Start with the yogurt, as it needs to drain overnight. Place wet cheesecloth in a sieve or colander over a bowl. Scoop the yogurt into the cloth, pull the corners of the cloth toward each other, and twist tightly. Put a weight on the cloth, or hang it in the refrigerator with the bowl underneath. Leave to drain overnight in the refrigerator. You can also use Greek yogurt or labneh.

Make the cloudberry syrup. Put all the ingredients in a saucepan, bring to a boil, and simmer gently for 1 hour. Strain the syrup into a bowl and allow to cool.

Preheat the oven to 100°C (212°F).

For the pavlova, beat the egg whites in a sterilized bowl with the sugar until peaks form. Mix in the cornstarch and keep beating until you have stiff peaks.

In a small bowl, mix the lemon juice with 1 teaspoon (5 milliliters/0.3 fluid ounces) of cloudberry syrup. Gently fold this into the stiff egg whites so you can see the beautiful sight of the two distinct colors. You can keep the cloudberry syrup in the refrigerator for months, for your next pavlova.

Spoon the meringue into an attractive shape on a parchment-lined baking tray. Dry in the oven for 2 hours. Allow to cool outside the oven for another 15 minutes.

Place the pavlova on a plate, dollop a few tablespoons of yogurt or labneh onto it and sprinkle with the marigold petals. The rest of the yogurt or labneh is delicious for breakfast with fresh fruit.

Fruit and Nuts

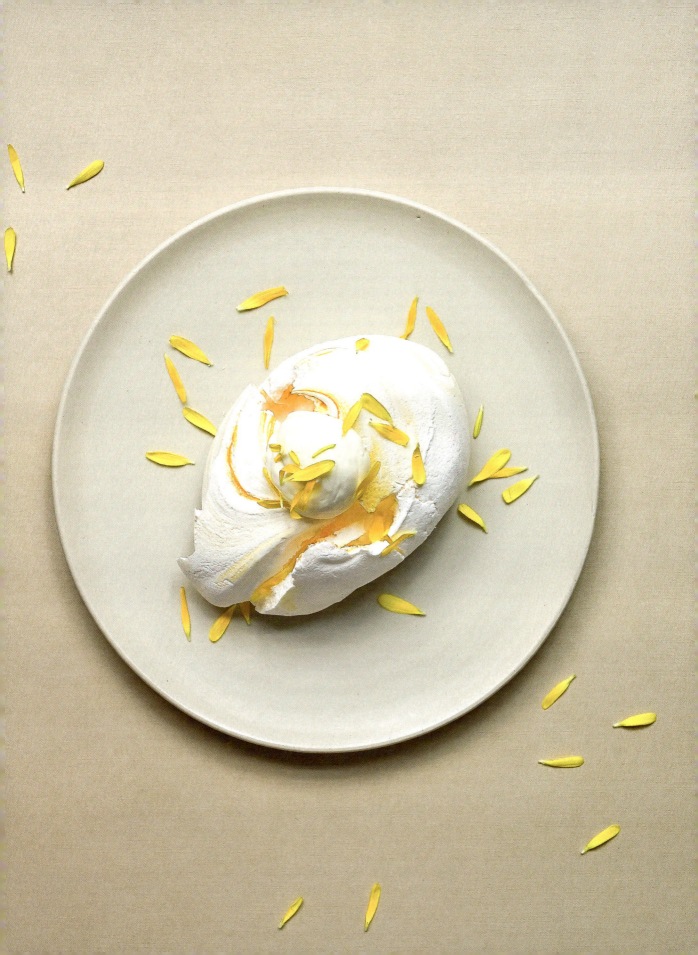

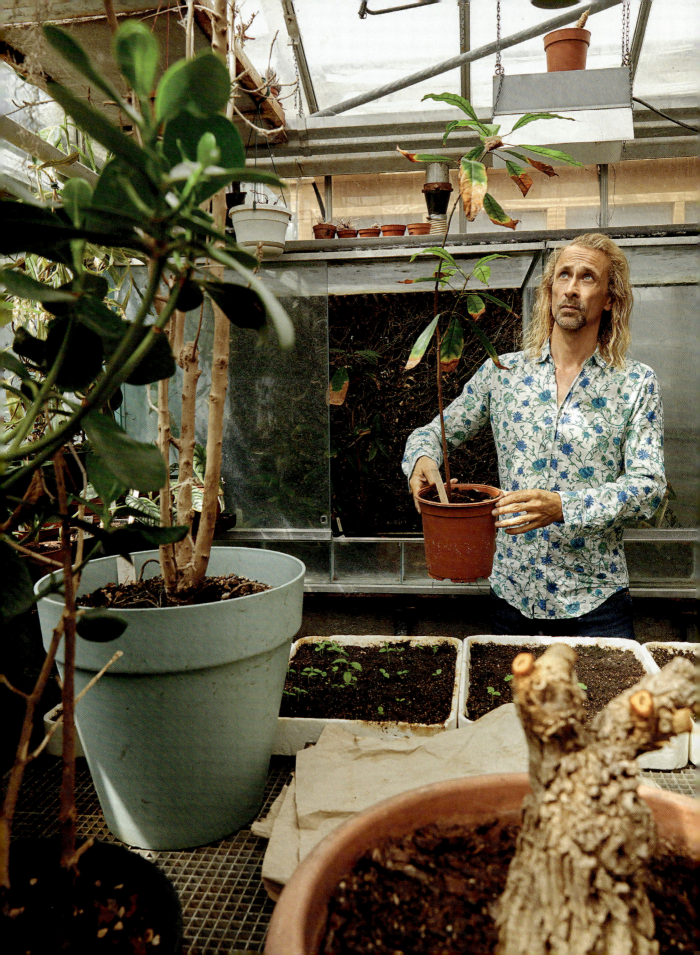

A FURTHER PLANT JOURNEYS

KOLA NUT

Cola acuminata

African Power Nut

The kola nut, with its euphoria-inducing properties, comes from West Africa. The bitter nut is chewed there mainly as a pick-me-up and has a similar, but stronger, effect to coffee, tea, and cocoa.[59] The effects can be felt for up to six hours. In many West African countries, kola nuts form an important part of the culture. Among the Nigerian Yuruba people, kola nuts are handed out at weddings and engagement ceremonies and to visitors. The Africa Museum in Berg en Dal in the Netherlands has many wooden kola nut dishes and statues on display showing kola nuts.

The kola nut gained worldwide fame with the invention of the soft drink Coca-Cola. The original recipe contained coca leaf and kola nut extract, hence the name Coca-Cola (see also Coca, page 206). Whether these extracts are still used today is not clear, because the soft drink giant guards its recipe very closely. It is more likely that the company now uses caffeine that is extracted from the decaf coffee industry. On the Internet, several recipes for Coca-Cola circulate.

Kola nuts contain caffeine, catechin, and theobromine, substances that temporarily boost concentration, cognitive functions, and alertness, comparable to the natural energy drink guayusa. Catechin is an antioxidant with a positive effect on the circulation. The antioxidants in kola nuts help prevent oxidative stress. In tests on animals, the nuts were shown to have an *analeptic* (stimulating central nervous system), *chronotropic* (affecting the heart rhythm), and lipid-reducing effect. In addition, they promote digestion.[60] They are not only used in Western Africa. During my stay in Jamaica, I learned that grated kola nut (*bisi*) is used as a remedy against food poisoning. Eating half a fresh kola nut has a powerful effect on mood and alertness.

Kola nuts can be bought in West African stores and are eaten whole or nibbled (never more than 2 nuts at a time). If you are suffering from peptic ulcers, hypertension, or heart disease, you should not eat fresh kola nuts.

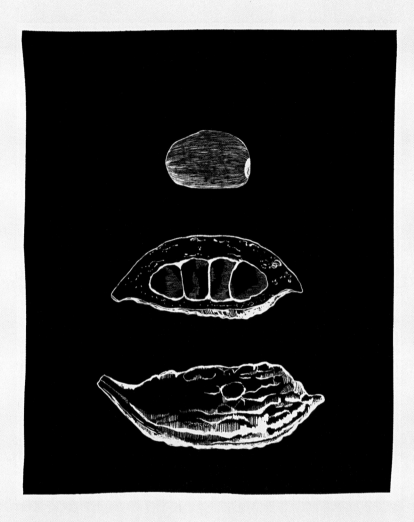

Fruit and Nuts

FURTHER PLANT JOURNEYS

CRABWOOD

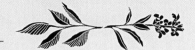

Carapa guianensis

Skin Tonic

Carapa guianensis trees can grow up to 35 meters (115 feet) tall and produce crab seeds from which medicinal oil is extracted. The name *guianensis* already tells us that the tree has its origins in the Guyanas (French Guyana, Suriname, and Guyana). The name *carapa* originates from Suriname. It comes from the Carib language and is derived from *ka*, which means "oil." Botanically, Suriname is one of the richest countries in world; at five times the size of the Netherlands, it is home to greater biodiversity than the whole of Europe.

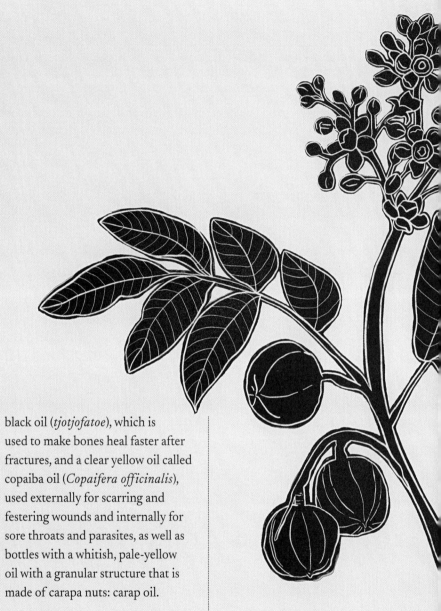

Native plant healers work alongside residents from the interior with African roots, the Maroons, and Javanese and Chinese herbalists. All these herbalists from different cultures have access to an enormous pharmacopoeia in botany, which they apply in their medicine. For every health complaint, there is a herb, tree, or fruit that can help or cure it. If you go to a Surinamese market and ask for an efficacious remedy for skin problems, the first thing herbalists will probably suggest is carap.

In among the bunches of fresh herbs and branches, market stalls always display bottles of medicinal oil. You will find plastic bottles containing black oil (*tjotjofatoe*), which is used to make bones heal faster after fractures, and a clear yellow oil called copaiba oil (*Copaifera officinalis*), used externally for scarring and festering wounds and internally for sore throats and parasites, as well as bottles with a whitish, pale-yellow oil with a granular structure that is made of carapa nuts: carap oil.

An acquaintance of mine from Amsterdam was once traveling in Suriname. To his horror, due to the tropical weather, his sweaty, clammy pants, and other unknown factors, he had sprouted cauliflower-like growths on the inside of his upper legs.

Having arrived at one of the medicinal herb markets, he asked a creole saleswoman whether she had a remedy for that. "Carap! Carap is good for everything!" she said. After two days of applying carap oil, the lumps had disappeared.

Fruit and Nuts

CRABWOOD

Carapa guianensis

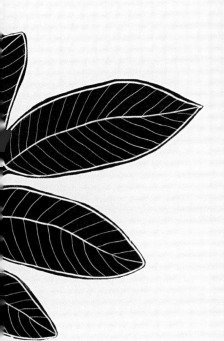

In the spring of 2022, I spent three months in Jamaica with my family, setting up The New Ark LSP Paradise, a botanical and medicinal paradise garden in the jungle on depleted farmland in memory of the record producer and composer Lee "Scratch" Perry. The undergrowth was full of ticks because of the cows, which are tick carriers. Nothing helped, until I had carap oil sent over from Suriname. Our entire team was tick-free after that. Who knows, perhaps it really is a cure-all.

To make 1 liter (34 fluid ounces) of oil, you need approximately 5 kilograms (11 pounds) of carapa seeds. In Suriname, carapa seeds are collected by Indians and Maroons and boiled in water. The seeds are then left to rest for a time, and subsequently dried in the sun. This encourages a golden-brown oil to float to the surface. This carap oil is scraped off and bottled.

Since 2004, trade in carapa seed has mushroomed as Yves Rocher acquired a patent on the seed that year. These kinds of patents are the subject of much criticism, as it is seen as biopiracy. Biopiracy is the practice of removing genetic material, such as plants, from third world countries in order to extract and process these into cultivar-worthy material, after which a patent or plant breeders' rights is requested. Farmers in developing countries, who would like to grow these varieties, are then forced to buy the expensive seeds of these varieties.

Carap oil is used to soften and care for the skin after insect bites and as an insect repellent. A little oil is massaged onto the skin several times a day until the ailment has gone. It supports the skin's ability to repair and also works to relieve eczema, acne, skin spots (red and sensitive skin), rashes, and fungal skin infections. The oil is also used for hair loss and scale (dandruff) on the scalp. Indians mix the fat of the boa constrictor with carap oil to treat joint pain. In Suriname, some people also take a drop of carap oil under the tongue to relieve stress. It is not only good for people; in Brazil, carap oil is rubbed onto furniture to protect it from termites and other wood-chewing insects.[61]

Because of its medicinal and skin benefits, carap oil is used as an ingredient in soap. In the Netherlands and Belgium, this is usually sold under the name andiroba soap. In Surinamese and herb stores, you will also find bottles of carap oil. In Surinam, people call this oil Krappa.

Fruit and Nuts

HERBS AND SPICES

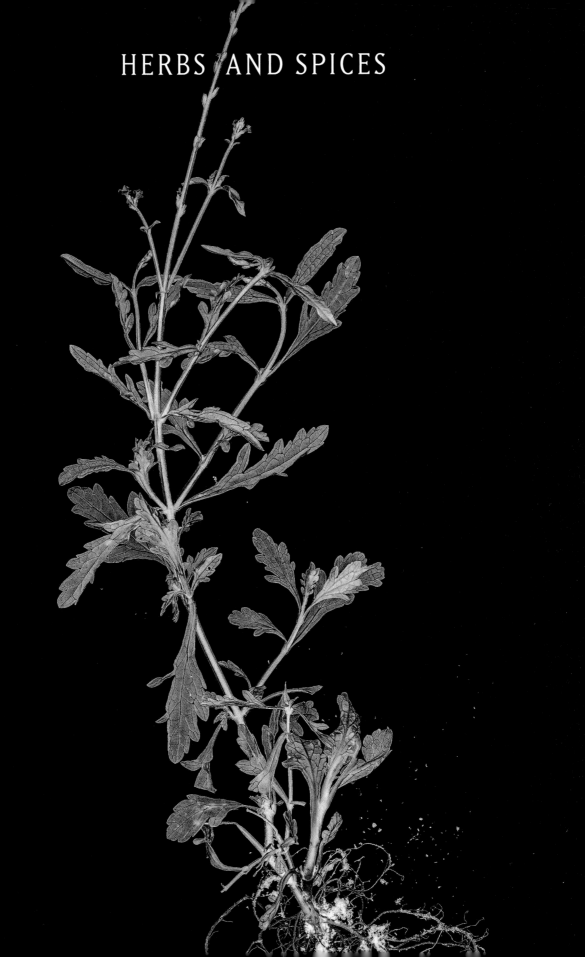

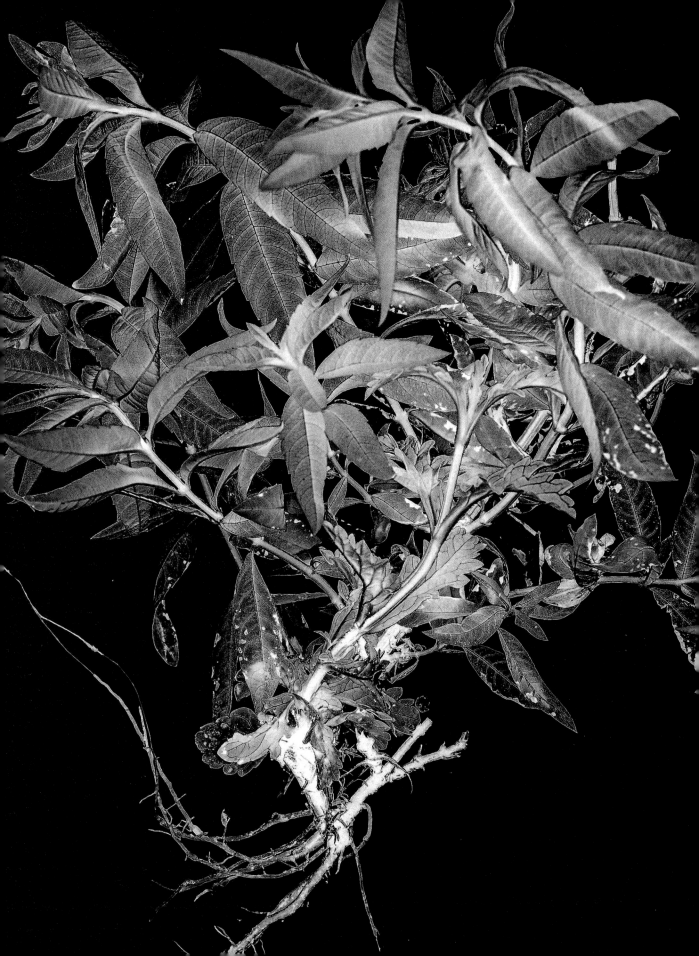

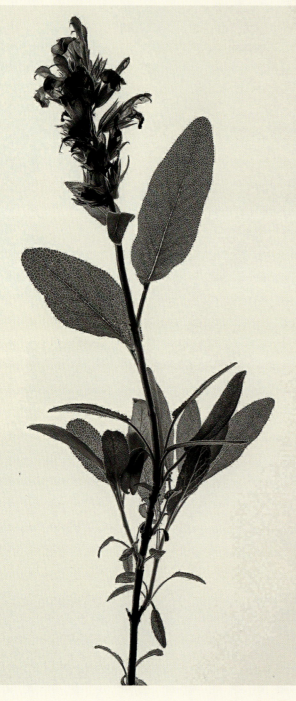

WOUTER

"In the world of plants and herbal medicine there is still much to discover. In herbal medicine, intuition and mysticism play a major role alongside science. Great scientists such as Albert Einstein readily admitted this. I see herbal medicine as a combination of art and science. When you cook, do you usually use your reason or your intuition?"

"The most fun way to cook at home is by going to the market and discovering new ingredients. The people selling them can often tell you what you can do with these ingredients. It's really great to then go home and start experimenting. Of course, some basic knowledge is welcome, but without trying things out and using your intuition you will never discover and learn new things. Is the healing effect of plants discovered in the same way?"

W "Today, using laboratory techniques such as microscopy, chromatography, and NMR, we can find what substances a plant contains. NMR, or Nuclear Magnetic Resonance spectrometry, is a spectacular advanced method of identifying substances. Initially, the plant's ingredients are all embedded in a "matrix." That means that you first have to extract them from the plant cell and then separate them them from hundreds or even thousands of other substances. Analyzing or isolating the plant substances from plant cells tends to be done with a solvent. The choice depends on the type of component you want to study. This is an enormous luxury, and as you'll understand, has not always been the case. Previously, the effect of plants was established through experiment and experience. People ate a plant, developed a stomach ache, for example, and concluded, "Ah, so it does something to your stomach." If you then start to lower the dosage and it turns out to have a beneficial effect, it becomes a drug. They also looked at the use of plants by studying (sick) animals. We are getting better and better at detecting and diagnosing diseases and finding medications that can consist of one or more (plant) substances. Do you ever use plants and herbs for their active ingredients, or do you tend to use them purely for flavor?"

J "During a beautiful trip through Peru with my wife, we were taken to a market. There were all kinds of women selling herbs. They told us nothing about their taste; only what they were good for—in the same way, we ate coca leaves for altitude sickness in Peru. So nature gives us all kinds of power ingredients that can make us feel better or stay healthy. In the professional kitchen, I'll choose an ingredient first and foremost because of its flavor. But when I make something at home, I often think about what I need. Or in other words, what my body needs. That could be a broth to pick me up or a delicious cake for some sugars and to make me happy. In fact, we use plants and herbs to revive us more than we realize. It sometimes feels to me that my body itself knows very well which plants it needs and then makes me crave them."

W "Just now, I was talking about Western methods of finding out about what substances plants contain. Living far removed from industrial societies, Indigenous people such as shamans and plant people know that plants can speak to us directly. When Kwasi, a Maroon, was looking for a medicine for malaria, the plant revealed itself to him in a dream. He saw that small cups were cut from the plant in which water or spirits absorbed the plant's bitter substances. This extract is drunk and has a strong, active effect on malaria. Meanwhile, the plant's Latin name was derived from the man who discovered it (*Quassia Amara*, see page 203), and the extract is a medicine that is officially registered with the World Health Organization (WHO).

In his 1995 book *The Cosmic Serpent: DNA and the Origins of Knowledge*, anthropologist Dr. Jeremy Narby likewise mentions medicines revealed in dreams. He spent a long time in the Peruvian Amazon and found out that Ayahuascueros acquired their knowledge about our DNA, for instance, directly through sacramental use. The shamans told him that the medicinal plants spoke to them directly. Thanks to this method, many medicinal plants have been discovered that we use in the West as well, such as curare, which is used as arrow poison but has saved many lives as a muscle relaxant because surgery under anesthetic is much easier to perform thanks to this agent. Indigenous people hardly ever receive any compensation for their discoveries. The knowledge is removed from the country of origin without thanks or recognition, copied, and used in a revenue model in the Western medical world, preferably combined with a patent. We use the knowledge but understand very little about the way in which that knowledge is obtained."

CLOVE — SYZYGIUM AROMATICUM

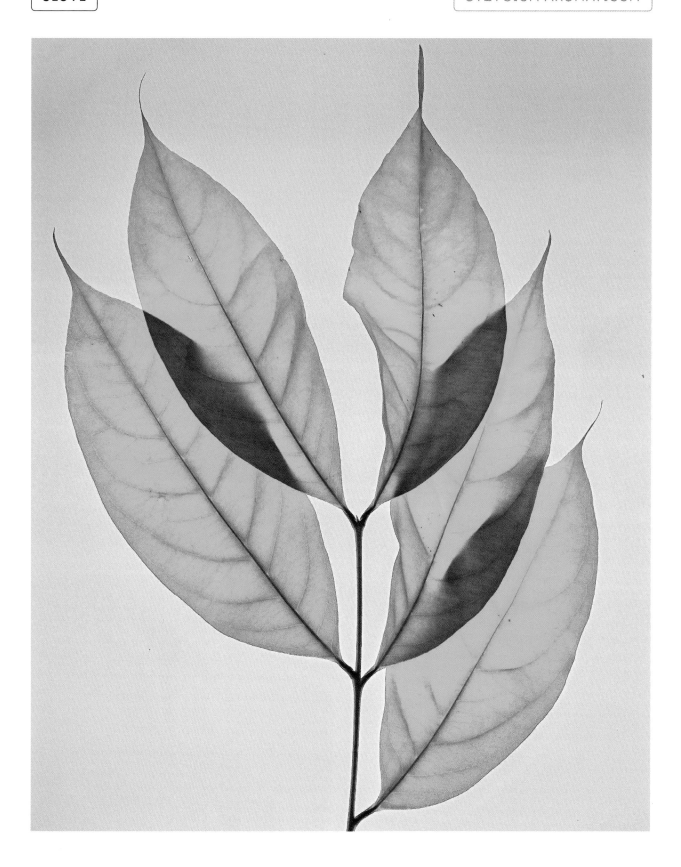

Narcotic Spice

Cloves are the unopened flower buds of the clove tree. Clove trees grow only in tropical coastal areas with an even temperature and humidity. Cloves are harvested before the flower opens, otherwise the spice is of no use. Two-thirds of the world's clove production is used for the manufacture of Indonesian kretek cigarettes. The name kretek is an onomatopoeic word for the crackling sounds these cigarettes produce when smoked.

The cloves that are also widely used in the Netherlands, albeit in food, originally come from the Moluccas in Indonesia. Around the year 1600, the Portuguese monopolized trade on the spice with much violence; later, the Dutch fought and managed to overthrow the Portuguese. During the Portuguese years, cloves were only traded in Lisbon and Antwerp. When the Dutch East Indies Company took over the trade, they also became available in Amsterdam.

Following this, the Netherlands long had the global monopoly on cloves, and in order to maintain this, cut down all clove trees outside the area of Ambon. Despite the fact that possessing or trading clove plants was punishable by death, in 1770, a Frenchman managed to smuggle a couple of cloves to Mauritius, which allowed France to start trading this spice as well. The wealth that came with the spice trade happened at the expense of the original inhabitants, who tended to earn only a few pennies or were employed as slaves on the nurseries and plantations. It was not until later that cloves were also grown in other countries, such as Madagascar and Tanzania.

Use

In the Netherlands, cloves are used as a spice in cookies, such as speculoos; in sauces; and to flavor red cabbage and beetroot, for example. Whole cloves are usually added when braising steaks, game, and stews. And then there is the hot alcoholic drink mulled wine, also known as Glühwein of course, which in the Netherlands and Germany is drunk during the days leading up to Christmas and in some regions on New Year's Eve.

In addition to their use in the kitchen, cloves have medicinal properties. Clove essential oil has a strong narcotic effect and is used for acute toothache. As a household remedy, a clove is stuck between the teeth or in the tooth's cavity to relieve the pain. When you have a toothache, you can also chew on some cloves a few times a day. The narcotic effect is due to the compound eugenol, which, by the way, is still used by dentists during root canal treatment. Eugenol is also present in basil, cinnamon, and nutmeg. In addition, clove oil has an antispasmodic, antibacterial, and carminative effect.

In China, cloves are used as a mouth freshener and aphrodisiac. Chinese eunuchs at the court of the ancient dynasties were only allowed to talk to the emperor if they had chewed on a few cloves. Cloves contain further important active compounds, including many flavonoids, and manganese, iron, magnesium, and zinc.

Some types of incense include cloves. The clove gives the incense an antiseptic effect and is said to dispel negative entities, attract wealth, and stop gossipers.

PROPERTIES
- Narcotic
- Antibacterial
- Antifungal
- Aromatic spice
- Anti-inflammatory
- Carminative
- Antispasmodic

SOURCING

Cloves can be bought at any grocery store or supermarket. Clove oil can be found in drugstores.

CAUTION

The distilled oil can provoke allergic reactions that may manifest themselves as skin rashes and itching upon contact. Clove is a good first remedy for a toothache, but then visit a dentist as soon as possible. Do not use clove longer than 48 hours for toothache.

Herbs and Spices

Appearance

Clove trees can reach a height of 20 meters (66 feet). The trees begin to bear fruit after about eight years. At the end of the branches, clusters with the unopened flowers form, which are then harvested. Cloves look like thick little nails measuring about 1 centimeter (0.4 inch). Dried cloves are black or dark brown in color, with a small brown button surrounded by four small crowns on the underside.

Extracting and Dosing

In cooking, you do not need more than two or three cloves. Cloves have a very dominant taste. When eating, you must therefore be careful that you do not end up with a whole clove in your mouth and accidentally chew on this, because cloves continue to retain their powerful flavor, even if they have been simmering in what you were cooking for several hours. In a spice jar, they keep their flavor and aroma for years .

The essential oil is present in the buds in large quantities. It is used for fungal infections, swimmer's eczema, and toothache. A tip for gum pain is to dab 1 drop of undiluted oil with a cotton swab briefly on the gums. If you have toothache, use 1 drop on the painful tooth. For fungal infections of the skin, dilute 10 drops of oil in 100 milliliters (3.4 fluid ounces) of vegetable base oil.

Use clove oil only after first consulting a doctor.

Clove oil can help with dandruff due to its antifungal, anti-inflammatory, and scalp-stimulating properties, which combat the Malassezia fungus, reduce irritation, and balance oil production.

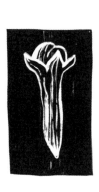

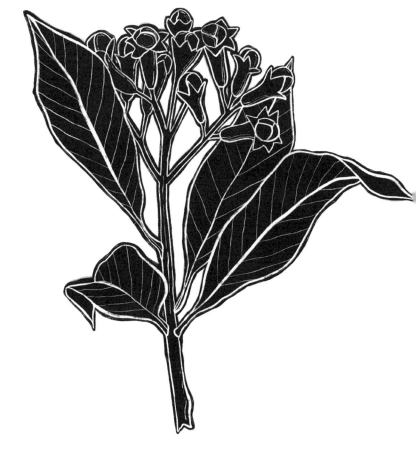

Herbs and Spices

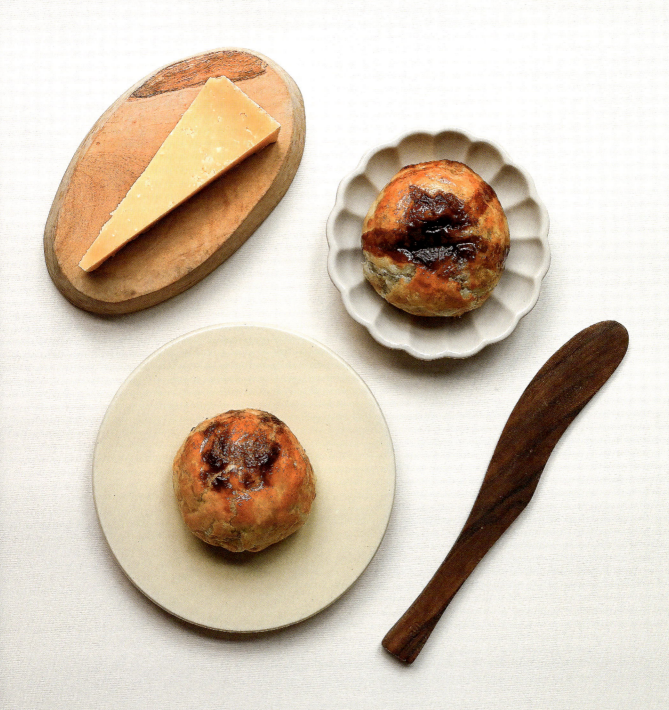

Eccles Cakes with Remeker Cheese

ECCLES CAKES WITH REMEKER CHEESE

for 8 pieces

■ INGREDIENTS
- 500 g/17.6 oz currants
- 120 g/4.2 oz butter
- 300 g/10.6 oz golden caster sugar
- 6 g/0.2 oz allspice powder
- 6 g/0.2 oz nutmeg
- 6 g/0.2 oz ground cloves
- 8 sheets of puff pastry, thawed
- 1 egg yolk, beaten
- 600 g/21.2 oz Remeker cheese, a raw Gouda-style cheese

method

Soak the currants in a bowl filled with water overnight in the refrigerator.

Put the butter in a large saucepan, add the sugar and spices, and allow the butter to melt gently on a very low heat for about 1 hour. Do not allow the butter to burn. To prevent this from happening, turn off the heat occasionally and then back on again. Remove pan from the heat as soon as the butter starts to bubble, and set aside to cool for 1 hour.

Drain any liquid from the soaked currants. Mix the soaked currants in a bowl with the cooled butter-spice mixture. If it is very dry, you can add a splash of water. Allow to cool.

Shape the mixture into 8 balls each weighing about 50 grams (1.8 ounces), and put them in the freezer for a while.

Preheat the oven to 180°C (350°F).

Remove the balls from the freezer, and wrap each ball with a sheet of puff pastry. Cut off excess puff pastry. Place folded-side down on a parchment-lined baking tray, and brush with the beaten egg yolk. Bake in the oven for 15–20 minutes until golden brown.

Serve with the Remeker cheese.

POACHED PEAR AND SABAYON WITH MULLED WINE

serves 4 people

■ FOR THE MULLED WINE
- 1 orange, sliced
- ½ lemon, peel only
- 4 cinnamon sticks
- 5 pieces of star anise
- 10 cloves
- 100 g/3.5 oz fine granulated sugar
- 250 ml/8.5 fl oz water
- 750 ml/25 fl oz red wine
- 50 ml/1.7 fl oz red port

■ FOR THE SABAYON
- 2 gelatin leaves
- 140 g/5 oz egg yolk (approx. 4 eggs)
- 120 g/4.2 oz granulated sugar
- 120 ml/4 oz mulled wine

■ AS WELL AS
- 2 conference pears
- 250 ml/8.5 fl oz water
- 100 g/3.5 oz granulated sugar
- juice of 1 lemon

■ EQUIPMENT
- kitchen thermometer

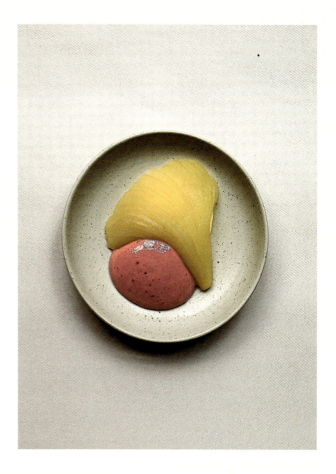

method

Start with the mulled wine. Put all the ingredients for this, except the wine and port, in a saucepan, and simmer for 20 minutes. Add the wine and port, and turn off the heat. Allow to steep for 1 hour, then strain into a bowl. Allow to cool.

Make the sabayon. Soak the gelatin leaves in a bowl with cold water. Beat the egg yolk, sugar, and mulled wine in a heatproof bowl, and place in a *bain marie* (a double boiler or hot water bath) until the kitchen thermometer reads 55°C (131°F).

Squeeze dry the gelatin leaves, and add them to the pan. Stir once more, and remove the pan from the heat. Use the sabayon as soon as possible.

Peel the pears, and place them in a saucepan with the water, sugar, and the lemon juice. Bring to a gentle boil, making sure that it does not actually boil but remains just below boiling point. The pears will be cooked and poached when they are completely glazed; this takes 30–40 minutes.

Halve the pears lengthwise, and carefully slice each half into strips without cutting them all the way through at the top. Place half a pear on each plate, and press gently down so that it fans out. Spoon the sabayon on the side.

Herbs and Spices

| PARSLEY | | PETROSELINUM CRISPUM |

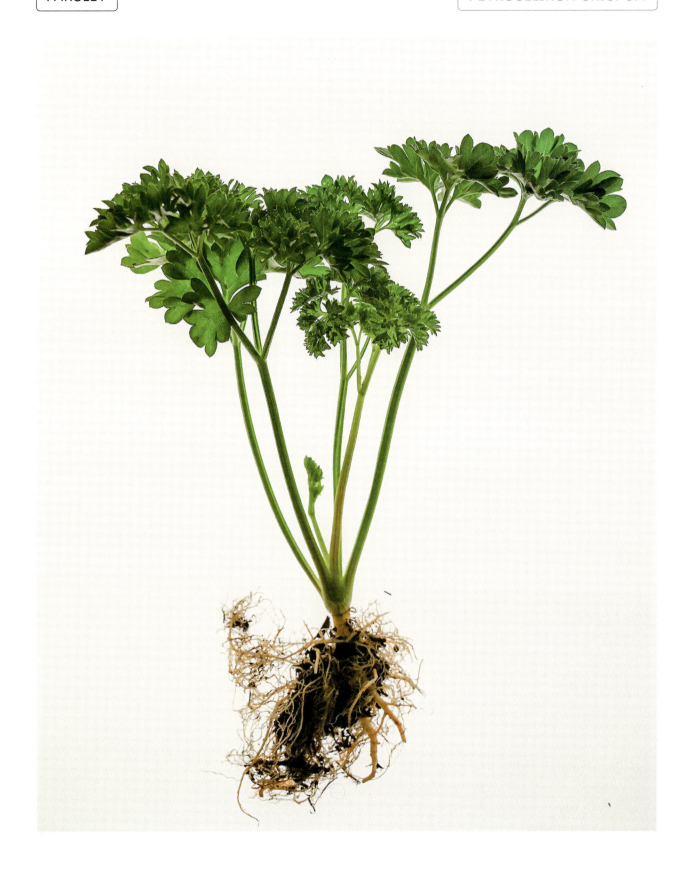

Green Iron Bomb

Parsley reached Europe from Egypt via the island of Sardinia. For the Greeks, parsley used to symbolize death and for that reason was hardly ever eaten. In antiquity, parsley played an important role in the cult of the dead and was therefore widely planted in cemeteries. Perhaps this explains why in several places in Europe, it is believed—and in some areas the belief still prevails—that you should not transplant parsley as it brings bad luck. Later, its reputation changed, and parsley was used in love rituals and at weddings, among other things, to inspire love.[62]

Three varieties of parsley exist, of which French curly parsley and Italian flat-leaf parsley are the best known. The third variety is so-called root parsley. Parsley is usually only added to a dish at the very end, so as to retain its flavor and freshness.

Use

In the Western world, parsley is the most commonly used herb for garnishing. It is widely regarded as a very healthy plant, rich in the minerals calcium, magnesium, potassium, silicon, and especially iron. Moreover, it contains many vitamins, including a large amount of vitamin C and vitamins A, E, K, and folic acid.

In addition to this wealth of vitamins and minerals, parsley's most important medicinal substances are apiol and myristicin. Myristicin is known to most people as the psychoactive and intoxicating substance derived from nutmeg. According to the *Encyclopedia of Psychoactive Plants* by Christian Rätsch, parsley is not normally associated with psychoactive substances, but it does contain powerful active ingredients. Parsley oil is used in the manufacture of psychoactive phenethylamines of the MDA and MDMA type. Taken in small quantities, myristicin helps with muscle stiffness that can arise from lack of movement. In small amounts, it is believed to also have a beneficial effect on the liver.[63] Parsley can play a role in the prevention of cardiovascular disease and has a beneficial effect on blood pressure.[64]

In herbal medicine, parsley usually is employed as a diuretic agent, useful for the removal of toxins from the body and to reduce fluid build-up and swelling in, for example, the hands.[65] It can furthermore counteract shortness of breath. Parsley's high iron content helps with increased oxygen transport in the blood.[66] In modern herbal medicine, parsley leaf is additionally used as a blood purifier, due to the large quantities of chlorophyll in the plant.[67] Herbalists also occasionally prescribe it as a menstrual stimulant and antispasmodic agent.[68]

Thanks to articles about health and nutrition in popular publications, more and more people have heard of bioflavonoids. Alongside other polyphenols, these compounds are increasingly seen as indispensable contributors to the anti-aging and health-promoting effects present in other green leafy vegetables, such as spinach. But they can also be found in berries, fruits, other vegetables, dark chocolate, and coffee.

In general, it can be said that the most colorful components of food, such as the skin of fruits, contain the highest concentrations of flavonoids. By eating industrially processed foods, many people unknowingly have a deficiency in these nutrients.

PROPERTIES
- Diuretic
- High nutritional value – a good source of vitamins and minerals
- Rich in antioxidants
- Menstrual stimulant and works as an antispasmodic on the uterus
- Absorbs the strong odor of garlic
- Blood purifier

SOURCING

Every greengrocer and supermarket sells parsley. You can also grow it easily yourself in your (vegetable) garden or in pots on your balcony or patio.

CAUTION

At a normal garnish dose, you do not need to be afraid of any side effects. Be sure to drink plenty of fluids if you eat a lot of parsley. In high doses, the myristicin in parsley has hallucinogenic properties.

Herbs and Spices

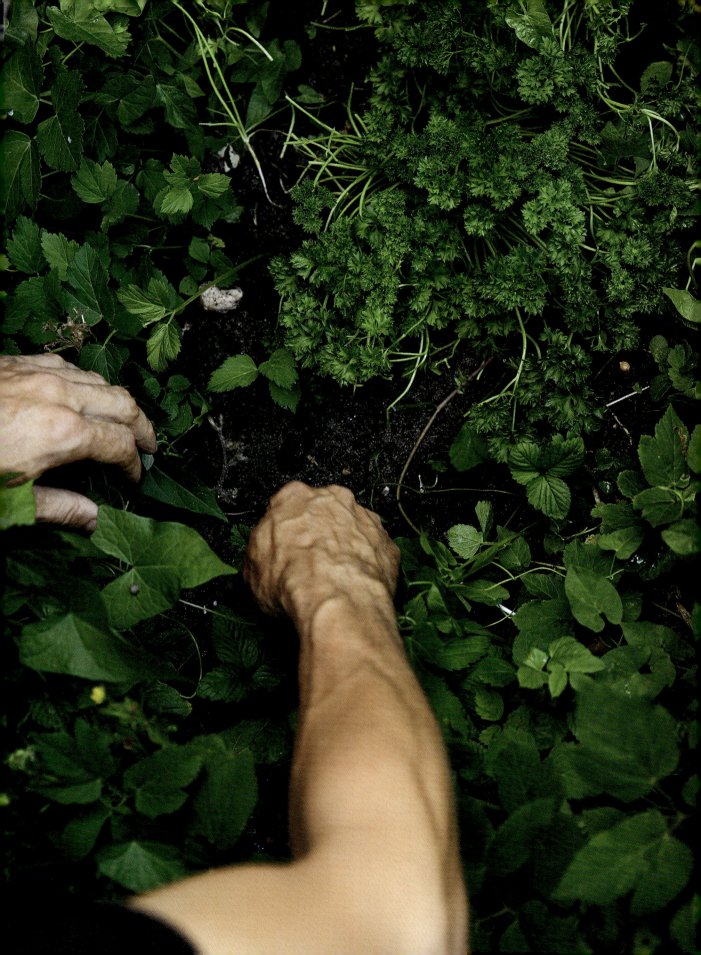

Immune weakness, which manifests as easily picking up colds or other infections, may be a sign of bioflavonoid deficiency. These bioflavonoids, by the way, are best obtained from your diet and not from a capsule bought as a dietary supplement.

Another advantage of parsley is that it is commonly known to neutralize the smell of garlic.

Appearance

Parsley is a small, bright-green, hardy, biennial plant. The seeds take a long time to germinate. Shoots of sturdy stalks develop from a taproot from which the leaves grow. They grow to about 20 centimeters/8 inches in height. The edges of the leaf tend to be irregular and curled. The Italian variety has pinnate leaves made up of several partial leaves.

Extracting and Dosing

Parsley is usually used fresh as a garnish in salad, on vegetables, or incorporated into herb butters and soups. When we were growing up, almost all vegetables were sprinkled with parsley, some salt, and flakes of butter. We always had it on hand because it grew in our vegetable garden. I now always grow it my own garden.

If you buy parsley, the bunch will keep a little longer if you put it in a glass of water as you would a bouquet of flowers.

BROCCOLI STALK WITH TOAST AND PARSLEY SALAD

serves 2 people

■ INGREDIENTS

- 1 stalk broccoli, head removed
- 60 ml/8 fl oz (4 T) olive oil
- 4 slices of sourdough loaf
- fleur de sel and freshly ground black pepper
- 1 bunch (approx. 80 g/3 oz) of leaf parsley, leaves only
- 1 shallot, cut into thin rings
- 15 g/0.5 oz (1 T) capers, finely chopped
- 30 g/1 oz (2 T) freshly squeezed lemon juice

method

Cook the broccoli stalk in a pan of simmering salted water until *al dente* (with a slight bite), about 5 minutes.

Cut the cooked broccoli stalk lengthwise into 4 equal pieces. Cut out the heart from each quarter, and roast these in a dry skillet until blackened.

Cut the blackened broccoli hearts into thick slices, and reinsert them into the stalk quarters.

Heat 30 milliliters (4 fluid ounces or 2 tablespoons) of olive oil in a skillet on a medium-high heat, and fry the slices of sourdough on both sides until they are golden brown. Sprinkle with fleur de sel.

Meanwhile, in a bowl, mix the parsley, shallot, capers, lemon juice, and the remainder of the olive oil. Season with fleur de sel and pepper.

Arrange the parsley salad on the toast, and serve with the broccoli stalks on the side.

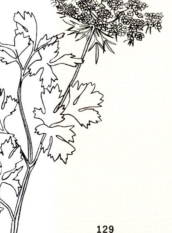

Herbs and Spices

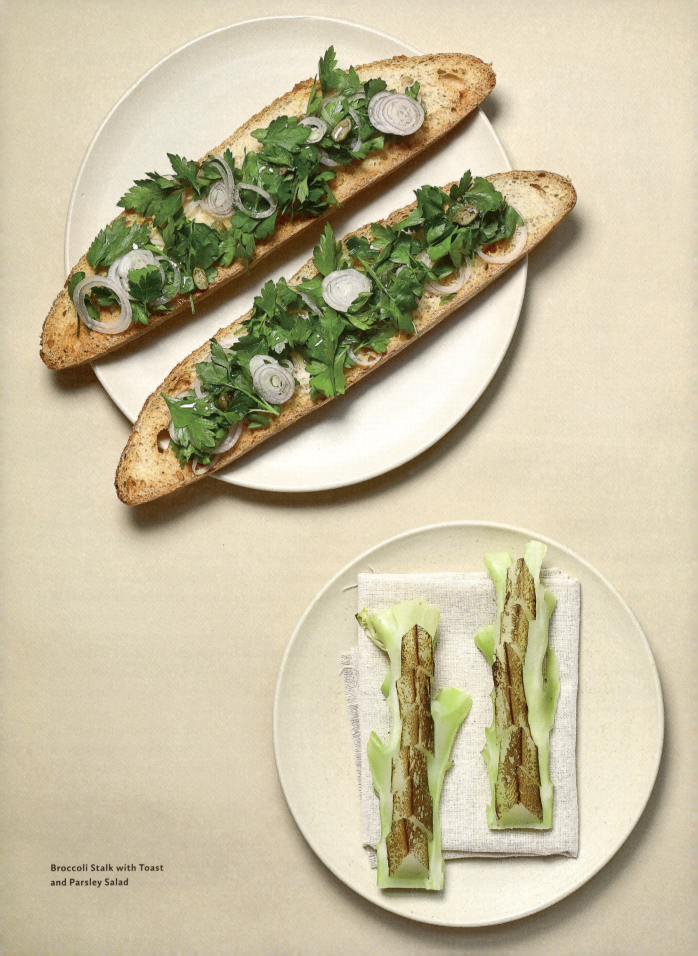

Broccoli Stalk with Toast and Parsley Salad

GREEN SALAD WITH ZUCCHINI, MINT, PISTACHIO, AND PARSLEY

serves 8 people

■ FOR THE SALAD
- ½ bunch (approx. 40 g/1.4 oz) mint
- ½ bunch (approx. 40 g/1.4 oz) flat-leaf parsley
- 1 butterhead lettuce
- 1 oak leaf lettuce
- 50 g/1.8 oz pistachios, shelled
- 30 ml/4 fl oz (2 T) olive oil
- 1 medium zucchini (courgette), sliced
- fine sea salt and freshly ground black pepper

■ FOR THE PARSLEY SAUCE
- ½ bunch (approx. 40 g/1.4 oz) curly-leaf parsley
- 250 ml/8.5 fl oz sunflower oil
- 1 egg white
- 25 ml/0.85 fl oz sushi vinegar

■ EQUIPMENT
- fine sieve

method

Wash the herbs and lettuce, and pat dry. Tear the leaves coarsely, and arrange on a large plate. Sprinkle with the pistachios.

Heat the olive oil in a skillet on medium-high heat, and sauté the zucchini slices for a few minutes. Season to taste with salt and pepper. Scatter the zucchini over the salad.

Make the parsley sauce. Wash and pick the curly parsley. Put in a blender or the beaker of a hand blender together with the sunflower oil, and whizz until you have a smooth blend. Strain the parsley oil through a fine sieve into a bowl.

Mix the egg white with the sushi vinegar in the blender, and while the blender is running, add the parsley oil until you get a firm mayonnaise.

Serve the parsley sauce alongside the salad or on top of it.

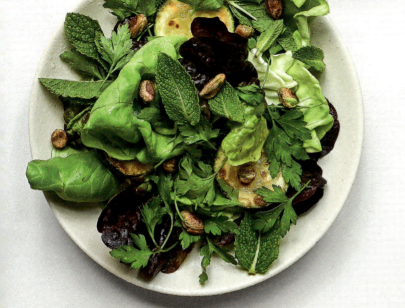

Herbs and Spices

SAGE — SALVIA OFFICINALIS

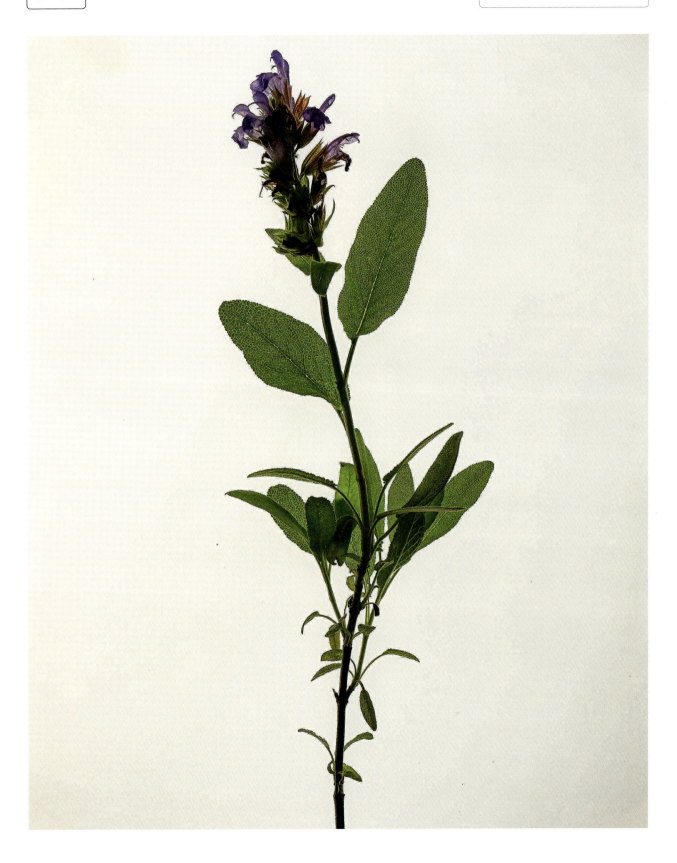

Healing Antiseptic

Sage has been praised for its medicinal properties since ancient times. *Salvia* means "healing" or "saving," and *officinalis* means that it formed part of the "official pharmaceutical inventory." In ancient herbal compendiums, sage is always associated with long life. The plant was seen as a *panacea*, a miracle remedy that helps cure all kinds of diseases, as well as a general tonic. It spread throughout Europe through monastery gardens.

The ancient Greeks believed that sage could make people immortal and that it improved memory. Egyptians saw it as a herb that bestowed life. The Romans called sage one of the *herba sacra* (holy herbs), along with verbena.

Use

Sage is native to southern Europe. In the Middle Ages, it was considered a magical plant for its wide-ranging effects on colds, sore throats, coughs, nerve weakness, digestive and fertility problems, and stimulating menstruation. No other medicinal plant has been as popular as sage.

It is still widely used for sore throat and inflammation of the mouth. The essential oils from sage are bactericidal, which is why sage is often used in toothpastes. When I feel a sore throat coming on, I usually manage to stop it in its tracks by chewing a fresh sage leaf, combined with a few drops of bee propolis and some extra vitamin C. The plant's antibacterial and anti-inflammatory properties are due to flavonoids and tannins, as well as salvin and carnosic acid compounds. These help guard against oxidative stress and strengthen immunity.

The plant is also used by mothers who want to phase out breastfeeding. Sage causes milk production to decline. This is in contrast to some other plants, such as fenugreek, and the substance thyrosinase, found in mushrooms, among others, which actually increase milk production.

During menopause, women experience a natural decrease in the hormone estrogen. Sage has traditionally been widely used to combat the unpleasant symptoms associated with the menopause.

According to Dutch herbalist Mellie Uyldert, sage's high phosphorus content helps us achieve a good night's sleep. In the Low Countries, sage milk was used as a traditional tranquilizer. In addition, sage contains vitamin K, which is important for maintaining strong bones and helps against blood clots.

Useful to know: Sage is recommended as a natural slug repellent in the garden. Also, bundles of white sage (a different species of sage) are widely used for ceremonial smudging (the ritual burning of the herb) to spiritually cleanse spaces of entities and dark energies.

PROPERTIES
- Inhibits sweat
- Anti-inflammatory
- Antibacterial
- Strengthens the stomach
- Reduces breast milk production
- Calming and promotes sleep

SOURCING

Sage can often be bought as a plant in garden centers and supermarkets. Dried and fresh sage is available from supermarkets and greengrocers.

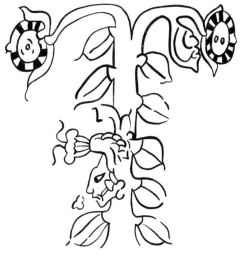

MAYA VASE – Hun Hunahpu, father of the Hero Twins from the *Popul Vuh*, obtains plant consciousness. Image from a late classic Mayan vase. The *Popul Vuh* is the sacred book and the secret guide of the Mayan Indians. The Maya were excellent astronomers, architects, farmers, and inventors of the number 0 who had a special shamanic tradition. (After a drawing from The Gods and Symbols of Ancient Mexico and the Maya: An Illustrated Dictionary of Mesoamerican Religion by Mary Miller and Karl Taube, 1993.)

Herbs and Spices

Appearance

Salvia is a hardy, evergreen, aromatic, shrubby plant. Sage bears crosswise, opposed, slightly thick leaves that can grow up to 5 centimeters (2 inches) in length. The upper side of the oblong leaf is gray-green and the underside hairy white. There are numerous cultivars of sage, with a wonderful diversity of beautiful flowers that often smell delicious.

Extracting and Dosing

You can make your own tea from both dried and fresh sage leaves. Place 5 grams (0.2 ounces) of sage leaves in 1 liter (34 fluid ounces) of water to make a pot of tea. When I have a sore throat I usually chew on 1 or 2 fresh leaves.

CAUTION

*If you drink sage tea regularly, limit your intake to 1–2 cups per day, and do not drink sage tea for more than three weeks in a row, as **Salvia officinalis** becomes addictive if consumed long term. Sage tea contains the hallucinogenic and lucid dream-inducing substance thujone, which we know as an ingredient in the drink absinthe. Artist Vincent van Gogh was fond of it and created some of his masterpieces under the influence of absinthe. In large quantities, thujone can paralyze your nervous system, so beware of the pure essential oil, which is too strong to use orally.*

Sage is hypertensive. This is helpful when you feel weak and your blood pressure is too low, but I would be careful with it if you have high blood pressure.

***Salvia officinalis** is related to **Salvia divinorum**, which is used as a vision-inducing remedy by Mexican shamans. (It can be purchased as a smokable extract in what are known as "smart shops" selling psychoactive substances in the Netherlands.) The effects can be so strong that after smoking **Salvia divinorum** you will feel thrown off balance for two weeks; see it as a spiritual beating. Smoking is actually a somewhat dishonorable way to use this sacred herb; traditionally, **Salvia divinorum**, which comes from the Mexico's Mazatec Mountains, is used fresh as a chew. In normal waking consciousness, this is followed after about 20 minutes by crystal-clear visions, which appear to be formed from white light and can be perceived if you close your eyes.*

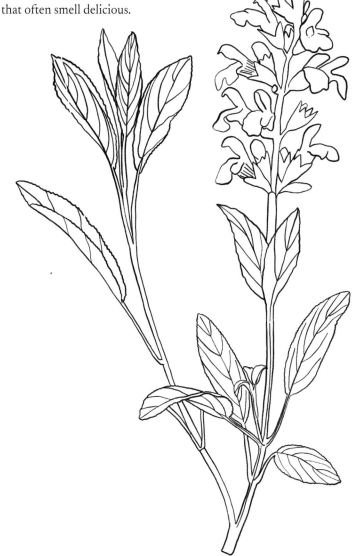

Herbs and Spices

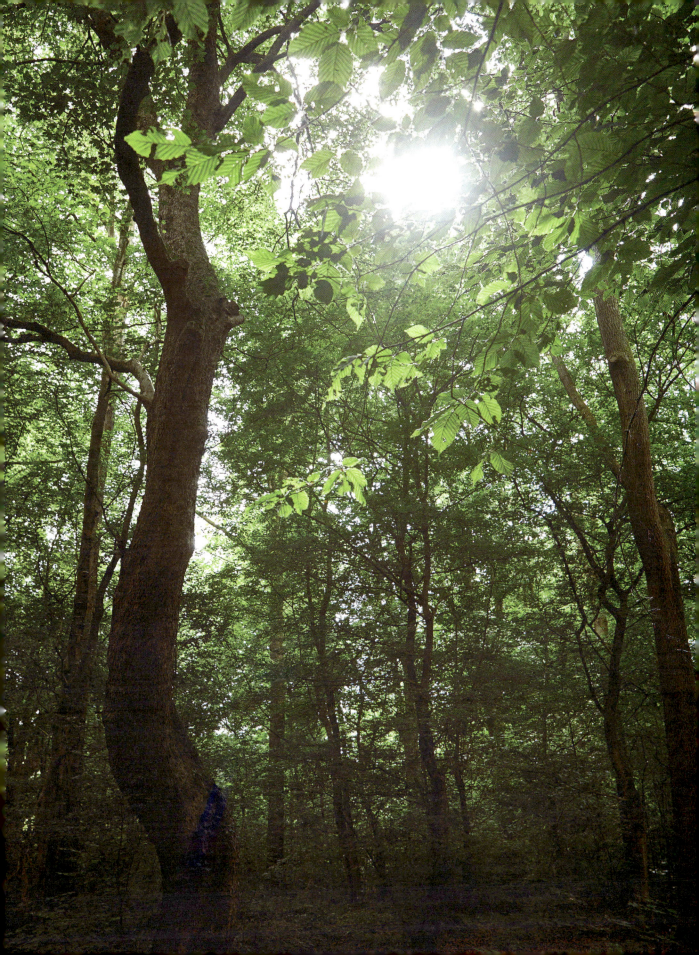

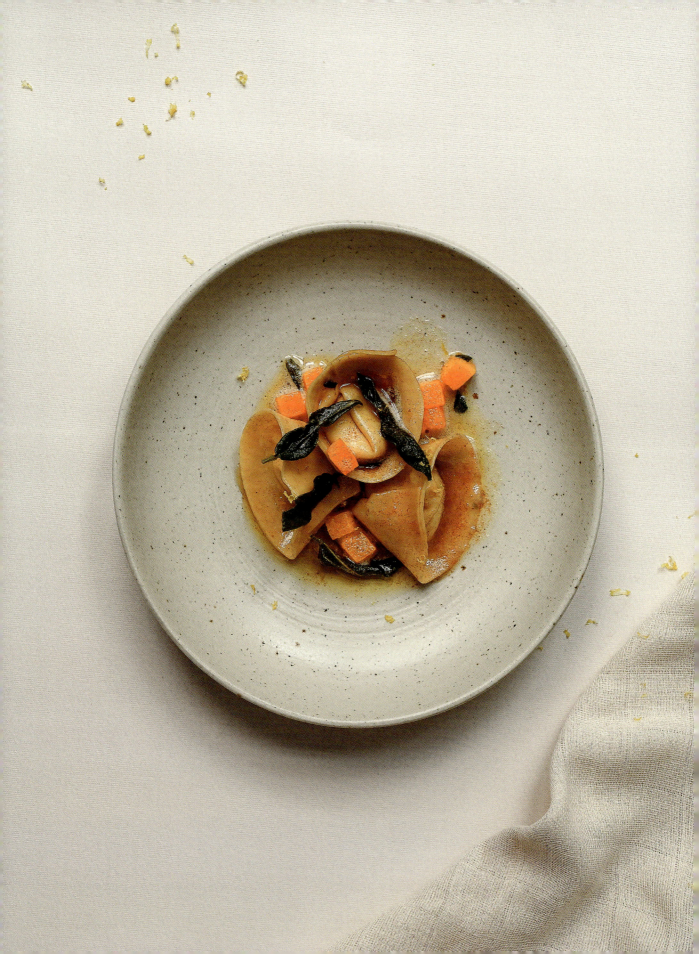

TORTELLINI WITH RICOTTA, PUMPKIN, AND SAGE BUTTER

serves 4 people (large portions)

■ FOR THE PASTA DOUGH
- 400 g/1 lb type 00 flour (finely ground Italian pasta flour)
- 4 eggs
- 15 ml/0.5 fl oz (1 T) water (optional)

■ FOR THE TORTELLINI FILLING
- 400 g/1 lb ricotta cheese
- grated zest of 1 organic lemon
- fine sea salt and freshly ground black pepper

■ FOR THE PUMPKIN AND SAGE BUTTER
- 250 g/8.8 oz butter
- ½ butternut squash (approx. 500 g/17.6 oz), peeled, seeds removed, and finely diced
- 1 bunch (approx. 80 g/2.8 oz) sage, leaves only
- grated zest and juice of 1 organic lemon
- fine sea salt and freshly ground black pepper

■ EQUIPMENT
- pasta machine or rolling pin
- skimmer

method

Start by making the pasta dough. On your countertop, pile the flour into a volcano-shaped mound. Using a spoon, scoop out a "crater," or well, in the top, and set aside the flour you have scooped out. Break the eggs into the well, and muddle the yolks with your fingertips to break them up.

Starting at the center and moving outwards, mix the flour into the eggs, drawing in a little bit more each time until all the flour has been absorbed—be careful not to break the edge of your "volcanic crater" or your entire countertop will be covered in egg. You should now have a yellowish pasta dough, slightly elastic and not too dry. If it is too dry, add a little water; if it is too wet, add the remaining flour you set aside. You must be able to stretch the dough without breaking it.

Knead the dough for another 10 minutes. Using your palm, push the dough out, and punch it back in without breaking it. Wrap the dough in plastic wrap (clingfilm), and place it in the refrigerator for 30 minutes. After it has rested for half an hour, roll out the dough with a pasta machine or rolling pin.

If you are using a pasta machine, divide the dough into 4 equal portions, and form into roughly 1-centimeter-thick (0.4-inch-thick) rectangles; this will help to create a more even shape when the pieces come out of the machine. Start with the machine's larger size (which is usually the highest number on the sprocket), and reduce the size one notch each time you the pass the dough through the machine. You should now have nice long pasta sheets. Cut them into 10-by-10-centimeter (approx. 4-by-4-inch) pieces.

In a bowl, season the ricotta with the lemon zest, salt, and pepper. Spoon the filling onto the center of the pasta sheets. Fold one corner to the diagonally opposite corner; you now have a triangle. Place the long side of the triangle facing you, with the point outwards. Now fold the point inward, toward you. Fold the outer points together, and press. You have now made a tortellino; if you make more than one you have made tortellini.

Melt the butter in a pan, and add the diced pumpkin, letting it cook for about 5 minutes. Add the sage, and let the butter brown, then deglaze the pan with the lemon juice.

Meanwhile, cook the tortellini in a saucepan with salted water for about 3 minutes, or until soft.

Using a slotted spoon, scoop the tortellini out of the pasta water, and add them to the butter sauce. Finish with the lemon zest, salt, and pepper.

SAGE "OPPERDOEZER" POTATOES WITH MUSTARD-OLIVE SAUCE

serves 4 people

■ **FOR THE OPPERDOEZER POTATOES WITH SAGE**
- 12 small Opperdoezer potatoes (baby Dutch yellow waxy boiling potatoes in the US)
- 15 g/0.5 oz (1 T) butter
- splash of sunflower oil
- 12 sage leaves

■ **FOR THE MUSTARD-OLIVE SAUCE**
- 70 g/2.5 oz butter
- 1 shallot
- 1 garlic clove
- 5.7 g/0.16 oz (1 tsp) mustard seed
- ½ bunch (approx. 20 g/0.7 oz) sage, leaves only
- 50 g/1.76 oz Taggiasca olives, pitted
- 50 ml/1.7 fl oz Ricard pastis anise liqueur
- 250 ml/8.5 fl oz vegetable stock
- 15 g/0.5 oz (1 T) coarse mustard
- 30 ml/1 fl oz cream
- fine sea salt and freshly ground black pepper

■ **EQUIPMENT**
- long match or lighter
- coarse sieve

method

Boil the whole, unpeeled potatoes in salted water for about 12 minutes until cooked and tender. Drain, and leave the potatoes to cool down a little. While they are still warm, gently rub off the skin. Allow to cool.

Heat the butter and sunflower oil in a skillet on medium-high heat, and sauté the potatoes until crispy. Slice each potato, and push a sage leaf into it for flavor.

Heat the butter in a pan on medium-high heat, and fry the shallot, garlic, mustard seed, and sage leaves for a few minutes. Add the olives, and deglaze the pan with the Ricard liqueur. Flambé briefly by carefully holding a lit match to it (make sure the extractor fan on the stove is off). Reduce the Ricard to one tenth. Add the vegetable stock, mustard, and cream, and simmer for 10 minutes. Whizz everything briefly with a hand blender or in a blender, and strain through a coarse sieve into a bowl. Season to taste with salt and pepper.

Spoon a generous ladle of sauce onto each plate, and place 3 sage Opperdoezer potatoes into this.

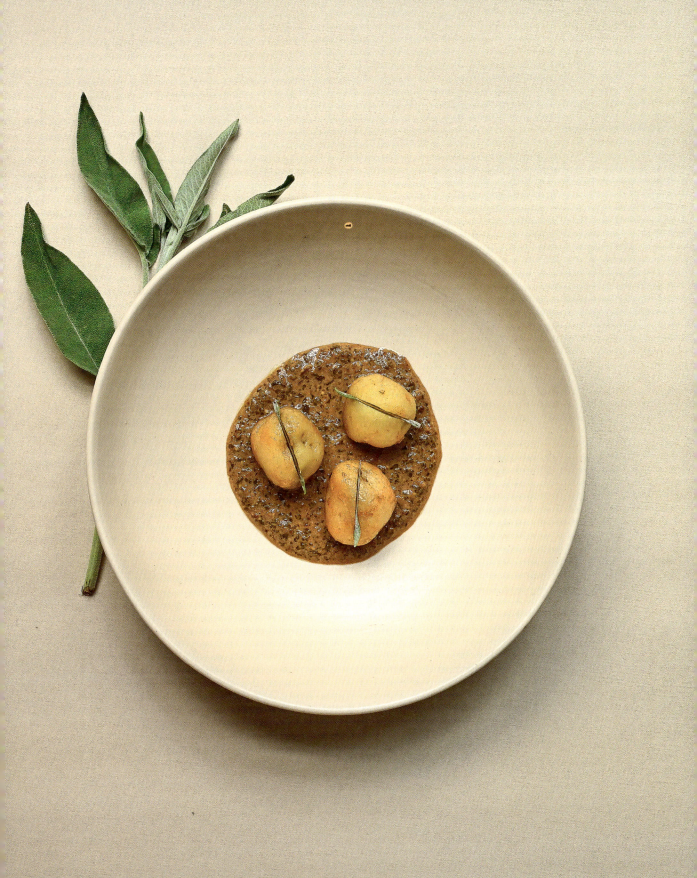

VERBENA

VERBENA OFFICINALIS / ALOYSIA CITRIDORA

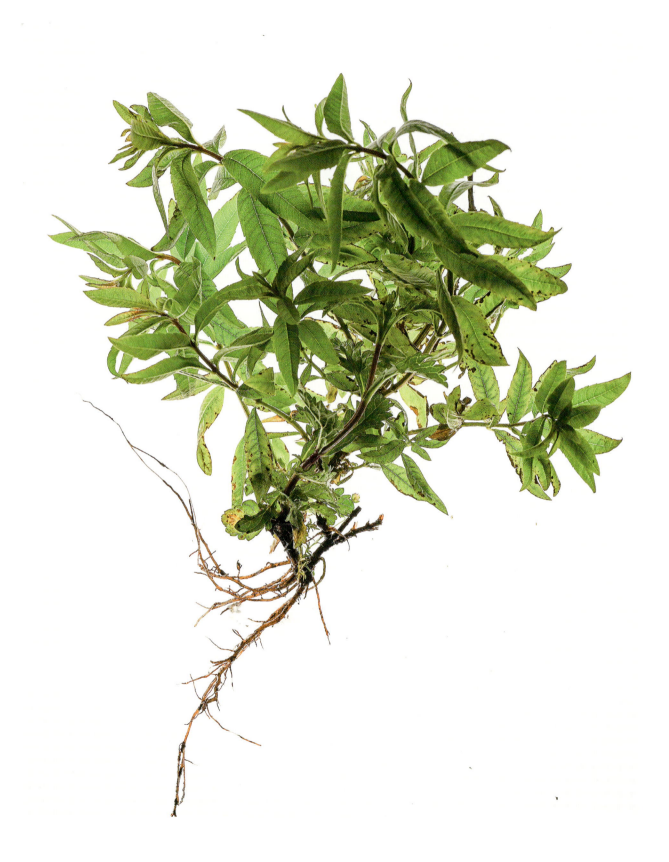

Nerve-Strengthening Herb

There is quite a bit of confusion over the name verbena. In colloquial language, it refers to many more species than botanically fall under the genus name Verbena. Vervain is equally confusing; sometimes it refers to *Verbena officinalis*, at other times a plant from a different genus. The genus name Verbena is a Latin name of unknown origin. One hypothesis is that verbena comes from the Ancient Greek *verbenaka*, which itself was derived from an ancient Indo-European word meaning "(magic) staff," a reference to the plant's appearance.[69]

The Latin variant of this is *verbeneca*, "holy twig," which referred to the twigs priests wore in their crowns during sacrificial rites: vervain, laurel, olive, and myrtle. According to Bible stories, the plant grew on Mount Golgotha and was used to staunch the blood flowing from Jesus Christ's wounds after he had been crucified. The Dutch name *ijzerhard* ("iron hard") and its German equivalent *Eisenkraut* ("iron herb") refer to use of the herb by blacksmiths, who used it to harden steel. Ironhard was also considered one of the best remedies for injuries from iron weapons.

Vervain or verbena was a sacred plant to the Egyptians, Germanic peoples, Celts, and Persians. The plant, like sage, was a sacred ritual herb for the Romans. Roman peace envoys were called *verbenarii* ("twig carriers") because they always clutched a sprig of verbena when approaching their enemies.

Before harvest time, large offerings were made to Mother Earth. Verbena was harvested in late spring, on or around June 21, the solstice. During spring festivities accompanying harvesting, there should be no sun or moon in the sky and the star Sirius had to be in ascent. Before a plant was harvested, a circle had to be drawn around it with a piece of iron, silver, or gold, for the plant then to be pulled out of the earth with the left hand. Vervain only acquired its qualities to cure almost all diseases, drive out bad spirits and to settle disagreements when it was harvested under these conditions and beeswax and honey had been offered to the earth.[70] The Teutons and Celts used ironhard in spells and also included it in love potions, because it was believed to make the drinker's member as hard as steel.[71]

The sacred plant was widely used by medieval magicians. Anyone who bathed in the undiluted juice of the plant, or rubbed themselves with the entire plant, would be rewarded. These people were said to have the gift of looking into the future; their wishes would come true; they would befriend their enemies; and they would be protected against diseases and bewitchment. In French, the plant was also called *herbe aux sorciers* ("enchanter's nightshade") or *herbe aux enchantements* ("magic herb").

Almost all the old herbal books, such as the ninth-century *La pharmacie des moines*, refer to the magical and miraculous properties of vervain. For example, if you were clutching a sprig of verbena when approaching a sick person, asked how the person was feeling, and they replied "good," then the patient would soon get better; if the answer was "bad," then the patient would soon die. This popular belief is believed to have originated from Macer Floridus' medical reference books from the 12th century.

PROPERTIES
- Neurotonic (nerve-strengthening)
- Neuroanalgesic
- Tonic (strengthening)
- Anxiety-reducing
- Sleep-inducing
- Supports digestion
- Expectorant
- Stimulates the uterus at delivery
- Compress or bandage for bruises
- Antioxidant
- Anti-inflammatory
- Antibacterial

SOURCING

Verbena is available from herbalists and as a tea in health food stores. The plant is easy to grow in the vegetable or herb garden, and can be found throughout Europe and naturalized in North America in the wild. It is hardy.

CAUTION

Pregnant women should not use verbena because it can induce contractions.

Herbs and Spices

Vervain was also one of the eight ingredients of (psychoactive) magic salves used during rites and initiations. I have been to Egypt eight times and learned there about the mystery cult of Isis. In ancient Egypt, the cult of Isis was not only a mystery cult but also a mystical healing one. Central to this was obviously Isis, the divine sorceress. She was flanked by Osiris, the shamanic god. Isis was initially human—she only became divine after initiation by the plants. One of the most important plants used in her healing cult was ironhard.[72] In Egypt, ironhard is therefore called "tears of Isis."

Use

The plant contains vitamin C, iron, essential oil, bitter substances, and various other medicinal substances, including tannins that have a preservative and astringent effect, as well as verbenalin, which is sleep-inducing. Today's Latin name shows that verbena has long been used as a medicinal plant. This applies to all plants with the term "officinalis."[73] In contemporary phytotherapy, verbena is used as a tonic, relaxant, and fever-reducing drug (as a substitute for paracetamol and aspirin). The plant (often in combination with arnica) is also still used in compresses to heal bruises.

The plant engages the parasympathetic (rest-and-digest) nervous system and has neurotonic (nerve-strengthening) and neuroanalgesic (nerve-pain-relieving) properties. The plant is prescribed for nerve exhaustion, nervousness, insomnia, and anxiety. In animals, the plant has been shown to have anti-inflammatory properties.[74]

A 2006 study and a double-blind study from 2016 showed that vervain extract could be a promising medicine for treating chronically inflamed gums.[75]

Another scientific study by Paweł Kubica, from 2020, showed that the ingredients of vervain can suppress the growth of malignant cells and that it has antioxidant and antibacterial properties.[76] Vervain is one of my favorite plants. I regularly drink a cup of vervain tea myself because of the beneficial effect it appears to have on my nervous system.

Appearance

The plant can grow to 1 meter (just over 3 feet) high and has thin, ascending, slightly hairy stems which are woody on the underside. Flowers are light pink to violet, and the unopened flower tops somewhat resemble green asparagus tops. They grow in the armpits of bracts in long thin spikes. Stem leaves are gray-green in color, and deeply incised. The plant is virtually odorless. Though a native perennial in Europe, it is rare in the Netherlands. It is widely naturalized elsewhere, including North America.

The more common lemon verbena has a fresh and sweet, lemony scent comprising a large number of components. Lemon verbena has woody round stems with small light green opposing lanceolate leaves. Flowers are pale purple. Lemon verbena is native to Chile, and in the Netherlands is called verbena, vervain, or ijzerhard ("iron hard") because, in terms of calming properties and external growth form, it resembles European *Verbena officinalis*. Page 140 has an image of lemon verbena; page 20 shows the bitter *Verbena officinalis* (with the lilac flowers).

Extracting and Dosing

The active ingredients in verbena are water-soluble. Thus the plant can therefore be drunk as a tea. To make an infusion, use approximately 3 grams (0.1 ounce) of dried leaf to 250 milliliters (8.5 fluid ounces) of boiling water.

According to physician Geert Verhelst, the dosage for a mother tincture is 40 drops taken three times daily. A mother tincture can be obtained by using 1 gram (0.03 ounces) of herb to 31 milliliters (0.001 fluid ounces) vodka, gin, or a other spirits with an alcohol percentage of 40%. For example: 30 grams of herb to 100 milliliters (3.4 fluid ounces) of vodka. Leave to steep for 2 weeks in a sterilized, airtight, sealed jar in a cool and dark place. Label the jar with the plant name and date, and every day give it a good shake. When ready, filter this macerate through a coffee filter into another sterilized jar. Due to the preservative effect of the alcohol, you can keep the tincture for at least 1 year.

Herbs and Spices

A nice suggestion from Verhelst for a refreshing bath is to add verbena extract. Add 250 grams (8.8 ounces) of dried leaves to 1 liter (34 fluid ounces) of boiling water, boil for a few minutes, take off the heat, and allow to steep for a further 10 minutes. Strain into a bowl, and add the extract to your bath water.

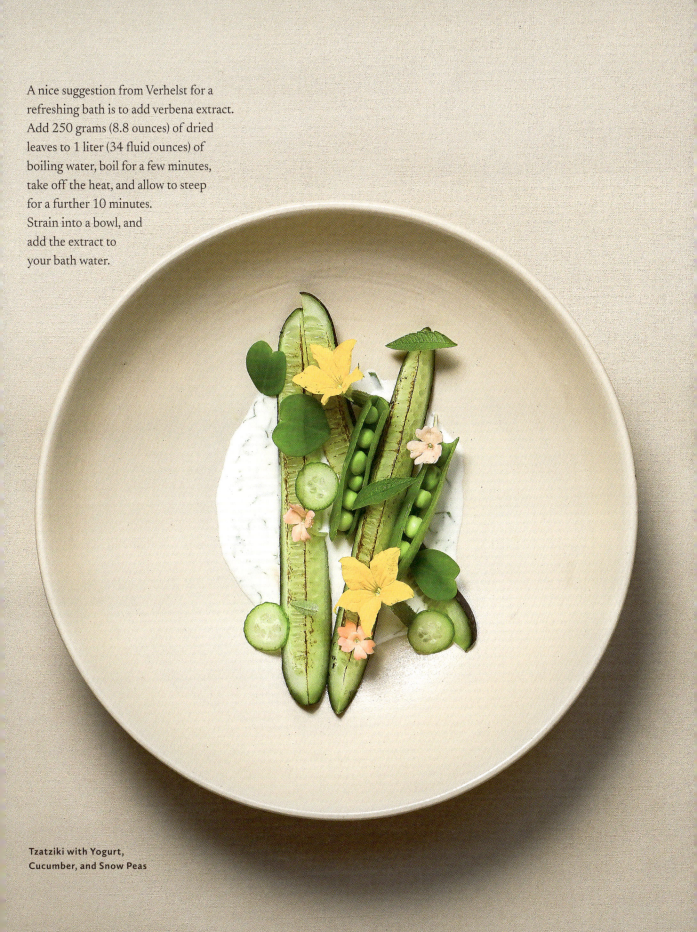

Tzatziki with Yogurt, Cucumber, and Snow Peas

TZATZIKI WITH YOGURT, CUCUMBER, AND SNOW PEAS

serves 4 people

■ **FOR THE TZATZIKI**
- 250 ml/8.5 fl oz Greek yogurt (preferably 10% fat)
- 1 garlic clove, finely chopped
- 5 g/0.17 oz (1 tsp) dried dill
- 5 g/0.17 oz (1 tsp) dried mint
- 15 g/0.5 oz (1 T) chopped fresh verbena leaves
- juice of ½ lemon
- splash of olive oil
- fine sea salt and freshly ground black pepper

■ **AS WELL AS**
- 2 snack cucumbers
- 8 snow peas
- small handful (approx. 40 g/1.4 oz) of fresh flowers and herbs, such as sorrel, vervain, and cucumber flowers

■ **EQUIPMENT**
- kitchen blow torch

method

Mix all the ingredients for tzatziki in a bowl.

Cut the cucumber lengthwise into 6 pieces, and sear with a kitchen blow torch on all sides until black spots appear—roasted cucumber is surprisingly aromatic.

Blanch the snow peas for 5 minutes in salted boiling water, then rinse under cold water. Open the pods on one side with a knife.

Place one large spoonful of tzatziki in the center of each plate. Arrange a few cucumber lengths and snow peas on top, and garnish with the flowers and herbs.

JUICE OF FERMENTED HONEY WITH PEAR, SORREL, AND VERVAIN

makes 1 liter (34 fluid ounces), or 4 large glasses

■ **FOR THE FERMENTED HONEY**
- 400 ml/13.5 fl oz water
- 100 g/3.4 oz raw honey

■ **FOR THE JUICE**
- 750 ml/25.4 fl oz pear juice
- 250 ml/8.5 fl oz fermented honey (see above)
- 1 bunch (approx. 80 g/2.8 oz) sorrel
- 1 bunch (approx. 80 g/2.8 oz) verbena, leaves only
- ice cubes

■ **EQUIPMENT**
- sterilized glass bottle or jar
- cheese or tea towel
- elastic
- sieve

method

First, make the fermented honey, because this requires a month's patience. Mix the water with the raw honey in a measuring cup or bowl, and pour into a sterilized glass bottle or jar.

Cover with a piece of clean cheesecloth, and secure with an elastic band.

Store the bottle or jar in a dark place at room temperature for at least 30 days. After that, store in the refrigerator.

Whizz all ingredients for the juice, except for the ice cubes, in a blender or in the beaker of a hand blender. Pour through a sieve into a decanter. Stir in the ice cubes, and serve immediately.

Herbs and Spices

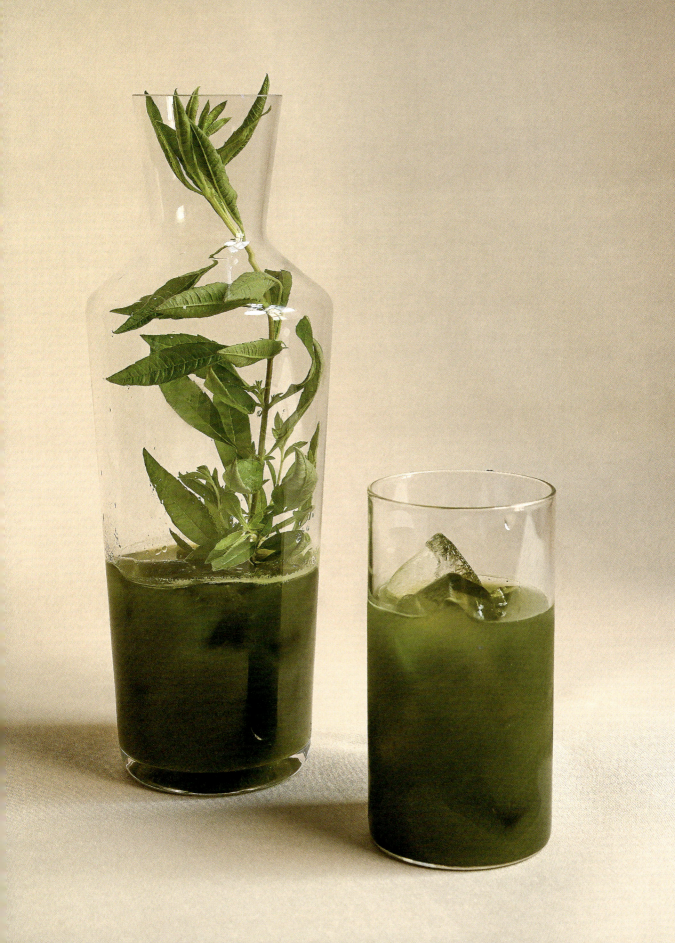

SAFFRON | CROCUS SATIVUS

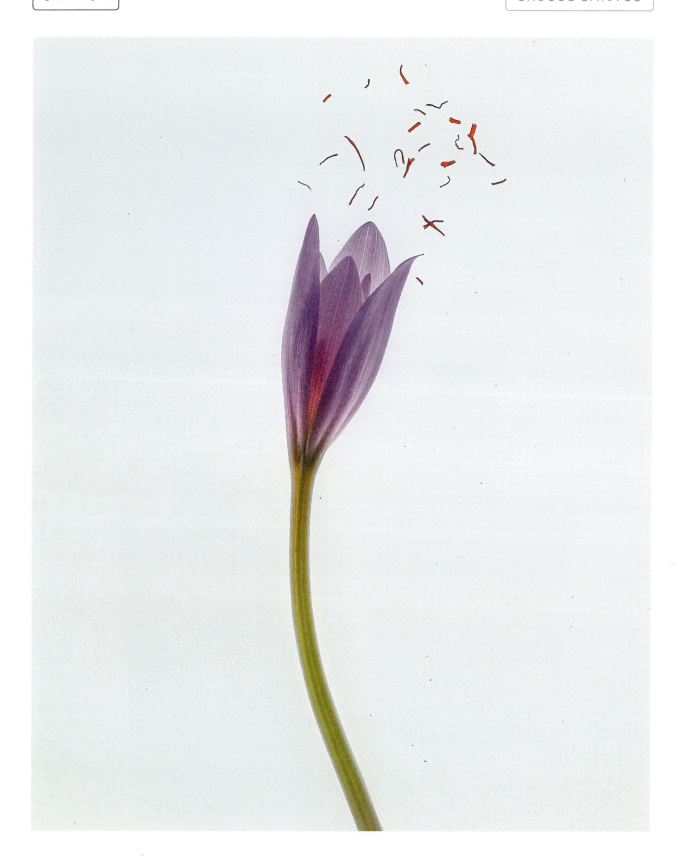

The Herb of Joy

Persia—the land of fire temples, great Sufi poets, Zarathustra, and saffron. In present-day Persia, now Iran, a veritable saffron cult exists. Iranian culture is permeated with poetry, and saffron plays an important role in this. Whereas in many other countries poetry is seen as an enthusiast's means of expression, everyone in Iran can recite some poems by Hafiz, Rumi, or Ferdowsi, and grandparents use them to teach their grandchildren as wise lessons for life.

According to Belgian professor of ethnobotany Marcel de Cleene, in the ancient herbal manuals and poetry, saffron was referred to just as often as the rose, but saffron was easier to use in the kitchen and medicinally. In ancient times, saffron was attributed magical and medicinal properties. The spice is also mentioned in the Egyptian *Ebers Papyrus* (1550 BCE).

Saffron is the most expensive spice in the world, due to its labor-intensive harvesting process. Each crocus only forms three stigmas. Saffron is related to the tulip, which also originated in Persia and Turkey. One kilo (2.2 lbs) of saffron costs 30–40,000 euros (roughly, 25,000–33,000 British pounds or 31,000–42,000 US dollars) and contains some 180,000 stigmas, which, when the saffron crocus flowers, are each picked manually with tweezers from the purple-lilac flowers.

Saffron is now grown worldwide, but Iran still controls 90 percent of global production. Other producers of the red gold include Afghanistan and Spain.[77] It is an essential ingredient of Spanish paella and the French fish soup bouillabaisse. A well-known dish has the poetic name of *morasa polow*, which means "Persian jeweled rice." It has a brilliant color palette and is a veritable explosion of all kinds of spices and special flavors that contrast and reinforce each other and make you dream about the treasures of Ali Baba and the Forty Thieves from *One Thousand and One Nights*. Jeweled rice contains small red berberis berries (barberry), flaked pistachio kernels, candied orange peel, and saffron. The bottom of the rice dish is hard and caked due to a special baking process. It is often eaten with the walnut-pomegranate-juice dish *fesenjān* (see page 104).

Use

Saffron is a medicinal plant with many therapeutic effects. Phytochemical studies have shown that saffron contains at least four active ingredients, including crocin, crocetin, picrocrocin, and safranal.[78] Two of these remarkable saffron antioxidants, crocin and crocetin, have antidepressant properties, enhance mood, and may help combat burnout, protect brain cells against progressive damage, reduce inflammation, and help with weight loss.[79]

Saffron is also known for its memory-enhancing and its anxiety-reducing properties. In Persian medicine, saffron is traditionally used for gastrointestinal problems, asthma, insomnia, depression, and memory problems.[80] Saffron was a component of the psychoactive magic salves that allowed European witches to make contact with other dimensions in the spirit realm.

Since ancient times, saffron has been thought to enhance women's libido—you could make women swoon with it.

Saffron is widely used in Asia as a fabric dye. Robes worn by Buddhist monks and Hindu ascetics, for example, are died yellow-orange with saffron.

PROPERTIES
- Antidepressant
- Aphrodisiac
- Sharpens the memory
- Anxiety-reducing
- Anti-inflammatory
- Flavoring
- Dye

SOURCING

Available in supermarkets but often cheaper in Middle Eastern and Asian supermarkets or online.

CAUTION

Do not use saffron in large amounts—just 10 grams (0.35 ounces) is a lethal dose. Saffron is used to induce laughter, sometimes with fatal consequences; according to many testimonies in old herb manuals, you can laugh yourself to death with it.

Herbs and Spices

In India, saffron water is often used to write down *mantras* (a specific word or sound repeated to aid in concentration during meditation). Just one thread of saffron is enough to turn a liter (34 ounces) of boiling water deep yellow in an hour.

Appearance

The saffron crocus blooms in autumn for eight days. It is a bulbous plant with a green smooth stem alongside which thin, elongated, green leaves grow to approximately the same height as the flower. The stem bears a purple flower, which houses the three red-orange stigmas that are harvested. The stamens, also located in the center of the flower, are not used and have no culinary value.

Extracting and Dosing

Saffron threads are traditionally ground into powder in an Iranian-style mortar. A splash of hot water is poured over this precious powder to dissolve it and make saffron water. This liquid is sprinkled over rice, among other things. I myself find it easier to rub a few saffron threads between my thumb and index finger, and dissolve these in a glass of water.

I find the taste of saffron a bit like honey or pollen: earthy and somewhat dull but full of flavor ending in a bitter twist. In short, the taste is unique. I love it and, therefore, always have saffron in the house. One of my favorite breakfasts is oatmeal with saffron.

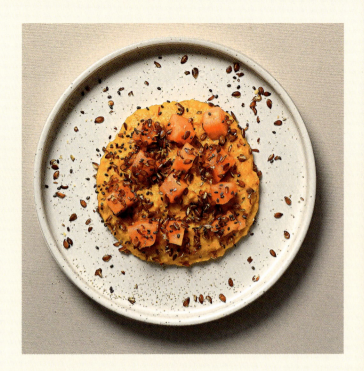

WOUTER'S OATMEAL WITH SAFFRON

serves 4 people

■ INGREDIENTS

- about 400 ml/13.5 fl oz whole milk
- 10 strands saffron
- 100 g/3.5 oz rolled oats
- 100 g/3.5 oz papaya
- 15 g/0.5 oz (1 T) chia seeds
- 15 g/0.5 oz (1 T) ground flaxseed

method

In a saucepan, bring the milk to a boil. Add the saffron, followed by the rolled oats. Simmer until the porridge has reached the desired thickness; keep an eye on it, because this does not take long. If you want it creamier, add a little extra milk.

Meanwhile, dice the papaya.

Ladle the oatmeal into bowls or deep dishes. Spread the papaya on top, and sprinkle with the chia seeds and ground flaxseed.

Herbs and Spices

JEWELED RICE WITH CANDIED ORANGE, PISTACHIO, AND SAFFRON

serves 4 people

INGREDIENTS

- 200 g/7 oz basmati rice
- 250 ml/8.5 fl oz water
- 100 g/3.5 oz Afghani green raisins (check Turkish or Moroccan supermarkets or online)
- 1 cinnamon stick
- 5.7 g/0.17 oz (1 tsp) saffron threads
- 50 g/1.75 oz green peeled pistachios (check Turkish or Moroccan supermarkets or online)
- 25 g/0.9 oz candied orange peel (check Turkish or Moroccan supermarkets or online)
- 50 g/1.75 oz flaked almonds, toasted
- 50 ml/1.8 fl oz rosewater (check Middle Eastern supermarkets or online)
- fine sea salt

method

Wash the rice several times under cold running water, and place in a rice cooker or saucepan. Add the water, raisins, cinnamon, saffron, pistachios, and candied orange peel. Give all the ingredients a good stir, and turn on the rice cooker or put the saucepan on the stovetop. If you are using a saucepan, bring the rice to a boil and simmer gently.

Once the rice is cooked (in the saucepan, this will take about 20 minutes), add the toasted flaked almonds and rosewater. Season with salt and more rosewater to taste.

Serve immediately.

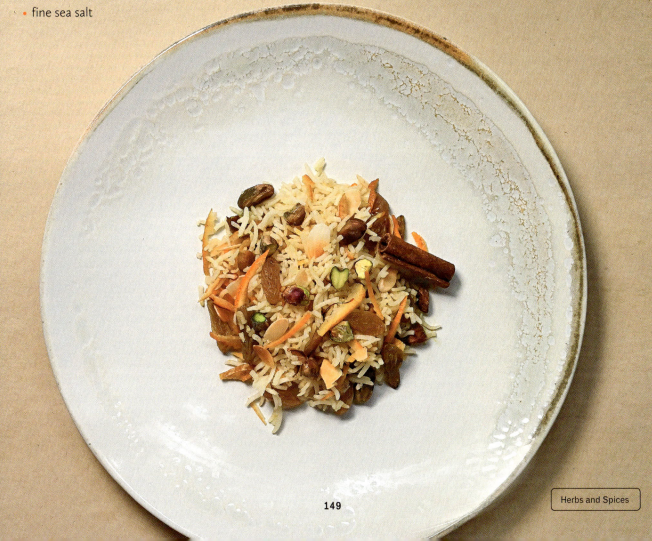

Herbs and Spices

VALERIAN

VALERIANA OFFICINALIS

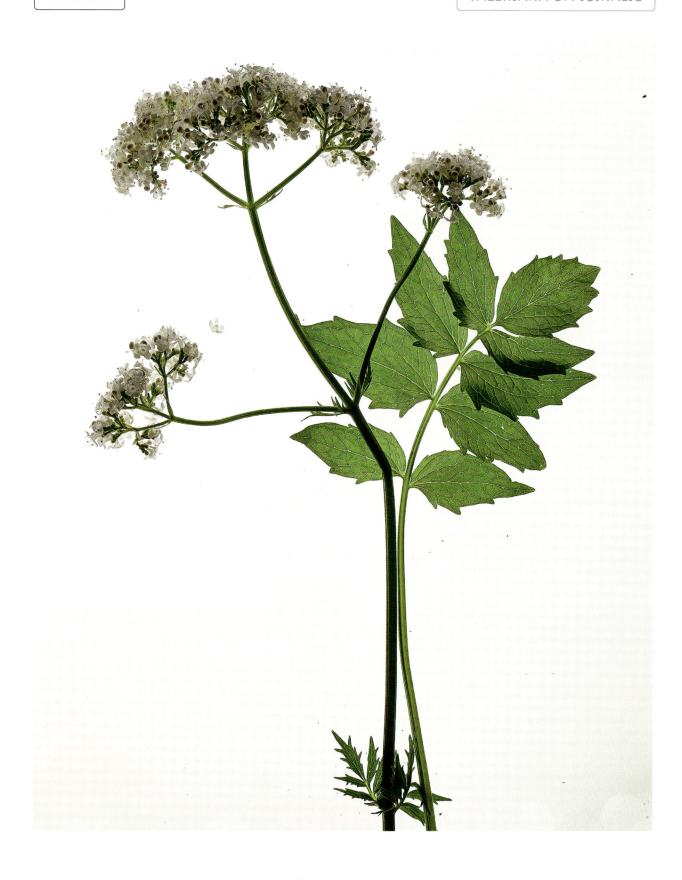

Calming Herb

The name valerian is derived from the Latin *valere*, meaning "to be healthy." Valerian has been used as a sedative herb for centuries and as the second part *officinalis* in the name already indicates, it would be found in the herbal or medical pharmacy. Valerian was recommended by Hippocrates (460–377 BCE) as a tranquilizer, and it is still being used for this in modern herbal medicine. According to legend, the Pied Piper of Hamelin had valerian in his pockets. The scent of the plant was traditionally used as a lure for rodents and feral cats. Beehives were protected from predatory bees by placing valerian near them.

Among the ancient Germanic peoples, Hertha, the goddess of the flowering earth, seated on her red deer wreathed with hop vines, held a valerian stem in her hand. She was honored on Heart's Day at her shrine at Kraantje Lek in the dunes near Haarlem in the Netherlands with festive dancing and fires. This feast is still always celebrated on the second Monday in August; it is essentially the culmination and the conclusion of summer.[81]

A relative of the European valerian is the *Nardostachys jatamansi*; an oil extracted from its roots is known to us as "nardus." The plant grows in the Himalayan Mountains and has been used for centuries for its medicinal properties. It takes 50–100 pounds of roots to distil one kilogram (2.2 pounds) of essential oil. In ancient times, the plant and the oil enjoyed great prestige among the wealthy. In Roman arenas, its scent was sprinkled around to calm people down. Nardus is also mentioned in the Bible, in the Song of Solomon, and as part of Jesus's foot-anointing by Mary Magdalene. That last story shows how precious nardus was, as the alabaster bottle represented a value of 300 pennies (Mark 14:5)—over 15,000 euros (around 12,500 British pounds or 15,700 US dollars) today. Nardus is still used in magical and religious rites. The oil is used in Ayurvedic medicine to treat hysteria, epilepsy, and as an antispasmodic. I sometimes use nardus oil in my magic shows for its special fragrance and effect.

Use

Preparations from valerian roots have a long-standing reputation as sedatives, mind-altering (medicinal) agents.[82] Valerian is a herb that, in addition to calming—it makes falling asleep easier and in a somewhat higher dose to sleep longer—also has anxiety-reducing properties. Valerian extracts appear to influence the chemical messengers in the brain, reducing the number of stimulating nerve signals. Valerian is being investigated as a potential aid in withdrawing from addictive drugs like benzodiazepines.[83]

Appearance

Valerian flowers fragrantly from June until the end of August with white or pink flowers. The plant reaches about 1.5 meters (34 feet) in height.

PROPERTIES
- Calming
- Sleep-inducing
- Anxiety-reducing
- May help with withdrawal from addictive substances

SOURCING

You can grow valerian yourself or buy it as tinctures or capsules at drugstores. You can also go out into nature and look for the plant itself. Make sure to bring a shovel so that you can dig out the root.

CAUTION

Because valerian is calming and can therefore cause drowsiness, you should not take it when driving or operating machinery. Pregnant or nursing women and children under the age of 3 should not use it either. Also, do not use it if you are a liver or kidney patient, as it can overload these organs.

Valerian is not particularly habit-forming or addictive, but in phytotherapy, interrupting use every now and then is recommended. According to herbalists Mellie Uyldert and Geert Verhelst, it is better not to take valerian for longer than three weeks at a time.[84]

In the Netherlands and Belgium, it grows on moist, nutrient-rich, and calcareous soils, such as those found in meadows, damp forests, and along rivers and streams.

Herbs and Spices

The inside of the root is whitish-yellow; when dried, it releases its special fragrance. Its leaf consists of 11–19 lanceolate partial leaves.

Extracting and Dosing

If you want to grow valerian yourself, doing this in a pot will make harvesting easier. In the fall of the second year, lift the plant from its pot, harvest some of the roots, then put the plant back in the pot. Thoroughly clean the harvested roots in water. Pat them dry with a cloth, and dry on a rack or in a dehydrator (below 40°C/104°F!), and use to make a tea, powder, or tincture.

It is best to use a cold-water infusion of the root. Leave the dried root to macerate for 6–8 hours (see page 26). If you want make a tincture, use an alcohol solution of 60–70 percent alcohol.[85] The recommended dose is the equivalent of 2–3 grams (0.07–0.10 ounces) of dried root and is taken 1–5 times a day.

FLOWER BUTTER

makes about 200 g/7 oz

■ **INGREDIENTS**
- 200 g/7 oz butter
- 10 g/0.35 oz nasturtium flowers
- 10 g/0.35 oz nasturtium leaves
- 5 g/0.18 oz cornflowers (bachelor buttons)
- 10 g/0.35 oz valerian flowers

method

Allow the butter to come to room temperature. Loosen it using a whisk or a food processor. Carefully fold all the leaves and flowers into the butter, except the valerian, so that they do not bruise and brown.

Use a spoon to form the butter into a quenelle (smooth, oval shape) on a plate, or put it inside a dish and smooth it out. Sprinkle with the valerian flowers.

The butter tastes best when eaten within 3 days.

Herbs and Spices

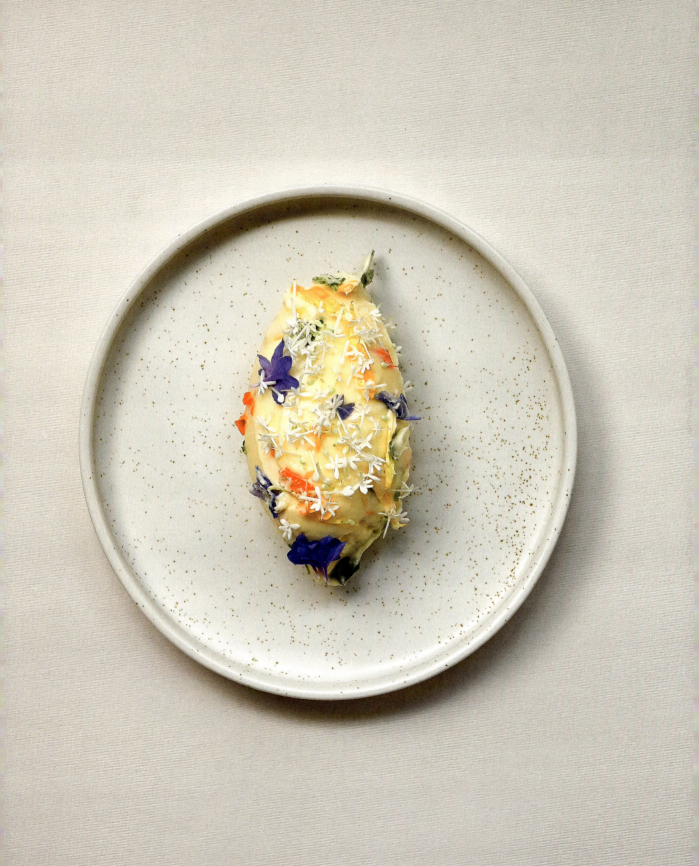

HOT CHOCOLATE WITH VALERIAN

serves 4 people

■ FOR THE LOLLIPOPS
- 400 g/14 oz dark chocolate

■ FOR THE CHOCOLATE MILK
- 30 g/1 oz (2 T) valerian root
- 1 vanilla pod, halved
- 2 pieces of star anise
- 15 g/0.5 oz (1 T) fennel seeds
- 1 cinnamon stick
- ½ organic orange, peel only in strips
- 1 L/34 fl oz whole milk

■ EQUIPMENT
- 4 sticks

method

Start by making chocolate lollipops. Chop the chocolate into coarse pieces, and place in a heatproof bowl. Place in the microwave, and heat at full power for 20 seconds. Give the chocolate a good stir. Place the bowl back in the microwave, and reheat for 20 seconds, then give it another good stir. After repeating this 3–4 times, you will see that the first chocolate is beginning to melt.

Once the chocolate really starts to melt, shorten the time in the microwave from 20 to 10 seconds. Keep stirring in between heating it.

When most of the chocolate has melted but you can still see some pieces of chocolate, there is no further need to microwave the chocolate. Keep stirring until the last pieces have melted and blended into the rest of chocolate so that it is ready to use.

Pour the melted chocolate into a piping bag, and pipe 4 discs of approximately 10 centimeters (4 inches) in diameter on a flat surface lined with parchment paper. Insert the sticks in these discs.

Put all the ingredients for the chocolate milk in a saucepan, and bring to a boil. Turn off the heat, put the lid on the pan, and leave to steep for about 15 minutes. Strain the milk into a bowl. Insert a chocolate lollipop into each glass, and pour the warm milk over the lollipops. Stir until you have a smooth chocolate milk.

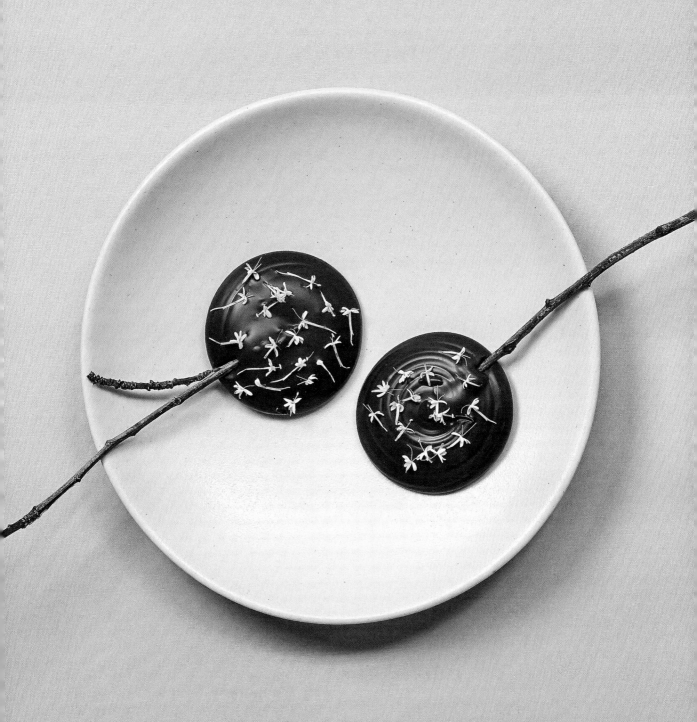

FURTHER PLANT JOURNEYS

CANNABIS

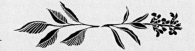

Cannabis sativa

Marijuana as a Folk Remedy

Entire libraries have been written about cannabis. It has been used by humans as a food source, medicine, stimulant, and for making rope and clothing from the plant's fibers. The seeds offer excellent nutrition as they contain important essential fatty acids. Cannabis, or hemp, is a useful plant with many applications. Perhaps the greatest gift bestowed by this ally of humanity is paper and textiles.

Cannabis' medicinal powers were first documented by Shen Nung (Shennong), a great master on our path, around 2800 BCE. He also cautioned against its excessive use.[86] Some of the plant's medicinal aspects had already been described in ancient times. Cannabis extract lowers eye pressure associated with glaucoma and appears to have helped various people I know who needed eye surgery. It is interesting to note that as early as the time of Pharaoh Ramses III (1194–1163 BCE), a cannabis recipe for treating eyes was known.

The 1960s saw the emergence of a new youth culture in the Netherlands, and hashish and marijuana (weed), as well as other psychedelics, became popular. As in old shamanic times, the public began to consume the same power plants as entertainers.

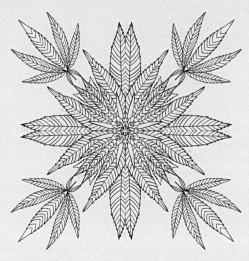

"The essence of Sixties pop music was drug oriented. The audience became psychedelically 'active.' As John Lennon once remarked: 'We don't seem to play for them, they play us.'"[87] Young people initiated themselves (and this is happening once again now in the house music scene). Young people underwent a rite of passage that elders were not aware of. Whereas, in the past, young people were initiated by tribal elders, they now began to self-initiate with mind-expanding substances such as cannabis. In 1972, the first Dutch coffee shop opened, and marijuana and hashish have since become a regular feature of Dutch culture. In September 2003, it became possible to obtain cannabis on prescription from pharmacies for certain conditions.

The Netherlands is the first country in which this was possible. In the meantime, cannabis became legal in a number of countries, including many US states. In the Netherlands, this is oddly enough still not the case, but legalization is getting closer and closer.

Cannabis grows all over the world. From the Altai and Himalayan Mountains, the plant was spread by nomads across the world. Cannabis plants are among the first crops that mankind began to cultivate. It is a holy sacrament for Hindu holy men in India known as *sadhus*, and for followers of the Rastafari religion in Jamaica who are known as Rastafarians.

For many people, cannabis is a means to expand their consciousness and become aware of themselves and their thought patterns. Many call cannabis a "plant teacher." According to the Amsterdam psychiatrist Bart Hughes, you can think of cannabis as a "psycho vitamin," because it aids brain metabolism and boosts cerebral blood supply, sharpening perception.[88] Some people believe that cannabis makes you apathetic, but it can also make you curious—about yourself, the universe, and life's mysteries. Other people become more creative.

Herbs and Spices

FURTHER PLANT JOURNEYS

CANNABIS

Cannabis sativa

You do not always have to get stoned to experience the benefits of cannabis. The use of cannabidiol (CBD) oil, for example, allows you to experience certain medicinal properties of marijuana without the high. CBD oil is legal and now widely available at drugstores and online in the Netherlands as long as it contains less than 0.05 percent psychoactive tetrahydrocannabinol (THC). In the United Kingdom, CBD oil is legal as long as it contains less than 1 milligram (3.5 ounce) of THC per pack. In the United States, both cannabis and CBD oil are currently legal in 18 states (2023), but each state varies as to usage (medical or recreational) and quantity of THC permitted.

Many studies have shown that CBD has antioxidant properties, which means that there might be a role for CBD in the prevention of both neurodegenerative and cardiovascular disease. In low doses, cannabis has a calming effect. In addition, it also produces a sense of euphoria and in some cases could therefore be used for depression. Cannabis can have side effects, however. Your eyes may become red due to enhanced blood flow, you can develop a dry mouth, and you might feel more hungry. Some people get the giggles when they first use cannabis. Long-term cannabis use may lead to memory loss.

THC and CBD are phyto (plant) cannabinoids. Our bodies themselves make cannabinoids, and our cells have numerous cannabinoid receptors. Cannabis contains more than a hundred different cannabinoids. It is not known what the effect a large part of these cannabinoids is, except that many of them have antibiotic properties. THC is the plant version of the substance anandamide, the body's own happiness molecule. The word anandamine comes from the Sanskrit word *ananda*, which means "bliss." Anandamine was the first of the body's cannabinoids to be discovered.

In large amounts of THC, cannabis can lead to psychedelic experiences involving hallucinations that may be experienced as visions. Be particularly careful when eating cannabis, such as in "space cake," a popular cannabis sponge in the Netherlands, or "hash brownies" found in the UK and US. When eating cannabis in food, it is easy to make the mistake of not waiting long enough for the high to kick in, leading you to unintentionally ingest high doses of THC and get very stoned. THC only begins to work an hour or two after consumption, so pace yourself.

THC has numerous other properties; it is known to be an antiemetic, for instance.[89] It therefore can help with nausea when undergoing chemotherapy, for example. When using THC, some people experience anxiety, because their perception of the world changes. In that case, it is best to stay calm and realize that what you are going through is caused by the cannabis and that the feelings will disappear when the THC wears off. Interestingly, CBD oil can reduce the anxiety that some people feel after consuming THC, as it mitigates the effects of THC, though in a complex way. Also note that CBD and THC may amplify each other.

In the Netherlands, because it is still illegal, only pharmacists, phytotherapists, and doctors may prescribe cannabis for numerous conditions.[90] (It is hoped that the Dutch government will decide to legalize cannabis soon.) In the UK and US, in general, doctors and therapists write prescriptions for drugs (including for cannabis if medically and legally required), and pharmacists typically just dispense what is prescribed; however, pharmacists with appropriate qualifications and training may prescribe drugs in certain situations in both countries.

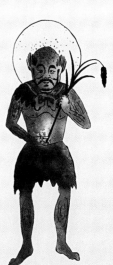

SHÊN-NUNG – This Chinese emperor is said to have discovered the properties of many plants. In his pharmacopoeia (2,737 BCE) he already points out that *Cannabis sativa* plants have male and female genders. (After a drawing by Thomas Christensen.)

Herbs and Spices

FURTHER PLANT JOURNEYS

SWEETGALE

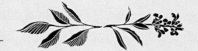

including *Myrica gale*

Ancient Healing Herbal Beers

During the time the sacred poems and prose of Iceland and Norway, the *Edda*, was recorded, Europe was still as verdant as the Amazon in Suriname and covered in one enormous continuous primary forest. At that time, a squirrel would be able travel from treetop to treetop all the way from northern Europe to southern Spain without once having to hit the ground.

Before humans started farming, they were primarily nomadic hunter-gatherers for thousands of years, obtaining their food as needed on a daily basis by moving great distances around the landscape, following game and other prey and collecting wild plant foods seasonally. This lifestyle changed with the advent of agriculture and the domestication of grains.

According to the most common theory, this also involved people allowing grains to ferment and beginning to brew beer. It is possible that drinking beer was invented much earlier and that people began to settle down and grow cereals because they wanted to have a constant supply of beer, bread, and porridge. Natufians, who lived in the area that is now called Palestine, Jordan, Israel, and Syria 13,000 years ago were the first people known to have brewed beer.[91]

The old beers that were made 10,000–30,000 years ago were quite different from the ones we have today. Many were sacred beers and contained medicinal and psycho-tropic herbs. To make beer, which is more difficult than wine, you must first ferment your grain to release the sugars from the starch.[92]

In order to be able to ferment grain and convert the starch into sugars, it is usually first malted with natural enzymes that are already present in the grain. In many cultures, people chewed on grains and starchy roots to get this process going. Later, people discovered that you can also malt grains by letting them germinate. After a few days, the fermentation process of grain was sufficiently underway and the grains were then dried.[93]

The first written texts about the fermentation process of grain are probably those in the Finnish Kalevala, *Rune XX* (1000 BCE), which describes how a semi-divine woman started the fermentation process for beer with the help of the saliva from a bear. So the word "beer" might just derive from "bear." Also, Sumerian clay tablets have been found with inscriptions showing grain fermenting for beer making.

In the Amazon rainforest, a primal beer is made from cassava tubers, and the fermentation process is started using human saliva. Cassava beer is called *casiri* in Suriname. After I had helped Trio Indians in Suriname whom I had befriended on their allotment, where they cultivated cassava, they invited me to their home to drink casiri.

Herbs and Spices

FURTHER PLANT JOURNEYS

SWEETGALE

including Myrica gale

BREWERY – The first brewery known to us dates back to 3500 BCE and was located at a Sumerian trading post on the Silk Route in the Zagros Mountains (the mountain range between Iran and Iraq). This illustration shows Sumerian beer tasters. (After the seal of Hammurabi, 1913 BCE).

Together with Kupyas and his family, deep in the eastern Amazon of Suriname in Kwamalasamutu, I drank my first three bowls of casiri and experienced a pleasant intoxication.

Casiri is made by women by chewing on pieces of cassava, which they then spit into a bowl of water mixed with grated cassava. This is done in the morning. As a result of the heat, time, and enzymes from the saliva, the casava ferments and its sugars are converted into alcohol in just a few hours. The casiri is handed out at around two in the afternoon after work as payment for activities such as tending the soil. Drinking is accompanied by extensive music-making and dancing.

Likewise in other countries, such as Burma, beer is still made by women,[94] as was the case in ancient Europe. Alongside bread baking, beer brewing was one of women's regular household tasks. If they successfully completed the brewing process, women commonly placed a broom outside the door to indicate that the beer was ready for consumption. They brewed their beer in kettles and often wore a tall black pointed hat so that they could be easily identified at markets where some of them sold their beer. The broomstick, top hat, and kettle are three features that we have come to associate with witches, partly through the work of the 16th-century Dutch painter Pieter Bruegel the Elder. The church eventually banned women from brewing beer, because they believed women were acquiring too much power and earning too much money through these endeavors. It started to spread misinformation, claiming that the women-brewers engaged in witchcraft.

Female brewers became fearful and stopped brewing beer, afraid of being accused of witchcraft and facing execution, such as burning at the stake or hanging; consequently, beer brewing increasingly became a male profession. Because of these developments, much knowledge has been lost. Later, the Protestant Church only allowed brewing to be carried out by men. The first brewing guilds also sprung up in these times.

Female herbalists who were using various medicinal and psychoactive plants (in "flying ointments"), inexorably ended up at the stake, usually together with their daughters. These women took along with them into the fire a huge wealth of knowledge about healing and vision-inducing plants. Knowledge about precise dosages and plant ratios are now scarcely available, if at all. Through the Inquisition and later the strict Protestant Church, their ancient plant and mushroom knowledge almost completely disappeared. Composer Ludwig van Beethoven's great-great grandmother Josyne was thus also burned at the stake in Brussels.

Herbs and Spices

SWEETGALE

including Myrica gale

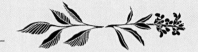

FURTHER PLANT JOURNEYS

Previously in Europe, we had a tree cult in which women who were called *tooveresse* (sorceresses) and *sabias* (sages) played a central role. They had a very high status, evidenced by the many figurines of goddesses that have been found. In ancient Egypt, and even earlier, it was priestesses who tended to be the most knowledgeable about the sacraments and medicine plants. Only later, during the Middle Ages, were these wise women demonized and called "witches," when people in Europe began to fear their knowledge and power. Even before these women and their knowledge had largely disappeared, sacred trees had often been cut down first.

In the Netherlands, this process has remained in people's memory through an event that occurred in the eighth century in the Frisian town of Dokkum. At the time, a tree cult existed in Europe in which a number of tree species were sacred. The Christian missionary Boniface used his axe to cut down the first sacred old oak tree (Donareik) to build a church in its place. He made his first attempt to convert the Frisians in AD 716, but was chased away. Forty-eight years later, an elderly man by then, he tried again, along with a delegation of associates. He paid for his plan with his life, when he was thrashed to death with branches from the oak tree he had just felled. Writer Atte Jongstra refreshingly described his death as "ecological resistance." The Frisians' symbolic choice of oak branches instead of swords or other weapons says it all as far as I'm concerned.

Back to beer . . .

In the Belgian Ardennes, many beers are still brewed according to old recipes. Around the first Sunday of spring between Easter and Pentecost, many villages around the town of Vielsalm traditionally light large night-time bonfires, the so-called "*grand feux*." Around these fires, there is dancing, partying, and beer drinking. In the middle of the pyramid of pine trees and pruned fruit wood, a stick is erected with a replica of a *macralle* (witch). The fire is lit by the last man to marry in the village. At some point during the festivities, the stick with the macralle drops to one side, pointing at the next person in the village to marry. This tradition shows that ancient European rituals from the pre-Christian era live on, along with a few ancient beer recipes.

In Europe, several types of sacred and mind-expanding beers were made with all kinds of psychoactive and medicinal plants that, as a result, had different psychotropic effects from the common Pilsner beer or lager. In the latter, the only psychoactive plant usually added is hops. The original early Pilsner contained very different mind-expanding plants.

Not many laws continue to be in force after half a millennium, but still in the Netherlands today, by law your beer must contain hops. A brewer at Jopen brewery in Haarlem told me it cannot be sold as beer otherwise. In 1516, the German Duke Wilhelm of Bavaria banned the use of any ingredients other than barley, hops, and water for making beer, so that beer brewers were not able to include special (sometimes toxic but also medicinal and hallucinogenic plant-based) herbal mixtures in their beer.

One of these was the bitter herb sweetgale (*Myrica gale*) which was included in so-called *gruit* beer for its hallucinatory and vision-inducing effect. There were also various other primal beers incorporating all kinds of different plants that, for instance, would increase your stamina and make you run faster, be strongly intoxicating or aphrodisiac, or psychotropic and vision-inducing. These drinks probably played a crucial role in the development of humankind.

Viewed thus, the so-called *Reinheitsgebot* (German Beer Purity Law) of 1516 was one of the first consumer protection and information laws. It was also Germany's first drug law. Some academics suggest that the Bavarian law was intended to suppress the use of pagan ritual plants. Be that as it may, it was the case that German brewers could only buy their hops from Duke Wilhelm. In addition,

Herbs and Spices

FURTHER PLANT JOURNEYS

SWEETGALE

including Myrica gale

he himself was the only brewer allowed to continue making wheat-based beer. As a result, it became extremely difficult for German beer brewers to experiment with different types of beer.

Sweetgale is still used by some Native cultures in Eastern Canada as a traditional remedy against abdominal pain, fever, bronchial complaints, and liver problems. Essential oil from sweetgale is used as a remedy for acne and sensitive skin.[95] *The Dutch Herbarius* by Stephaan Blankaart from 1756 stated that sweetgale ale will make you drunk quickly.[96]

Just like the recipe for Coca-Cola, gruit recipes were well guarded and therefore highly cherished secrets. Gruit, also sometimes called *grut*, usually contained a grain (for conservation purposes and to create a high alcohol content), as well as a combination of various narcotic herbs, such as bog myrtle (also known as wild sweetgale), wild rosemary, heather, laserwort, laurel berries, or refined resin. The resin was usually taken from the resin glands of the psychoactive wild sweetgale.

Each gruit beer was different and had its own secret formula. But there were also gruit beers and true original German Pilsners that contained hallucinogenic nightshade species, such as the painkilling and hallucinogenic henbane.[97] The German word *pilz*

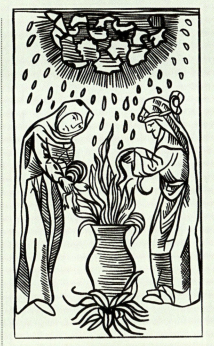

PSYCHOACTIVE BEERS – The witches of medieval Europe induced drunkenness with a wide variety of brews, most of which had a psychoactive component from a type of nightshade and often gale. Here, two witches ask for rain and thunder and prepare a potion to help them with that. (After a 1459 block print.)

means "mushroom." The very earliest Pilsner, in fact, also contained magic mushrooms, probably Psilocybin (see page 67). In addition, there were brewers who used magic plants to create healing and psychotropic primordial beers and gruit, but almost all knowledge has been lost and the recipes have either been destroyed, perished, or lost.

As far as I know, there are currently only two or three brewers in the Netherlands who make gruit beer. A brewery from Gouda uses a recipe

from the 14th century, and Jopen brewery from Haarlem one from 1407. Both are still obliged by Dutch law to include a trace of hops. In the Ardennes, you can order sweetgale beer from Mr. Roland in the village of Comanster; he serves Cervoise. Gageler Brewery in Belgium also continues to brew sweetgale beer. You can get recipes through beer clubs and from small brewers to make your own.

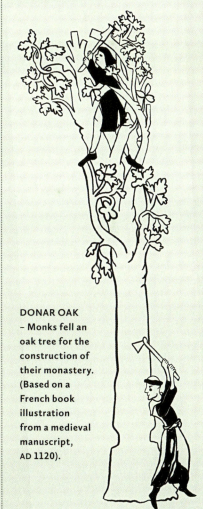

DONAR OAK – Monks fell an oak tree for the construction of their monastery. (Based on a French book illustration from a medieval manuscript, AD 1120).

Herbs and Spices

LEAVES AND FLOWERS

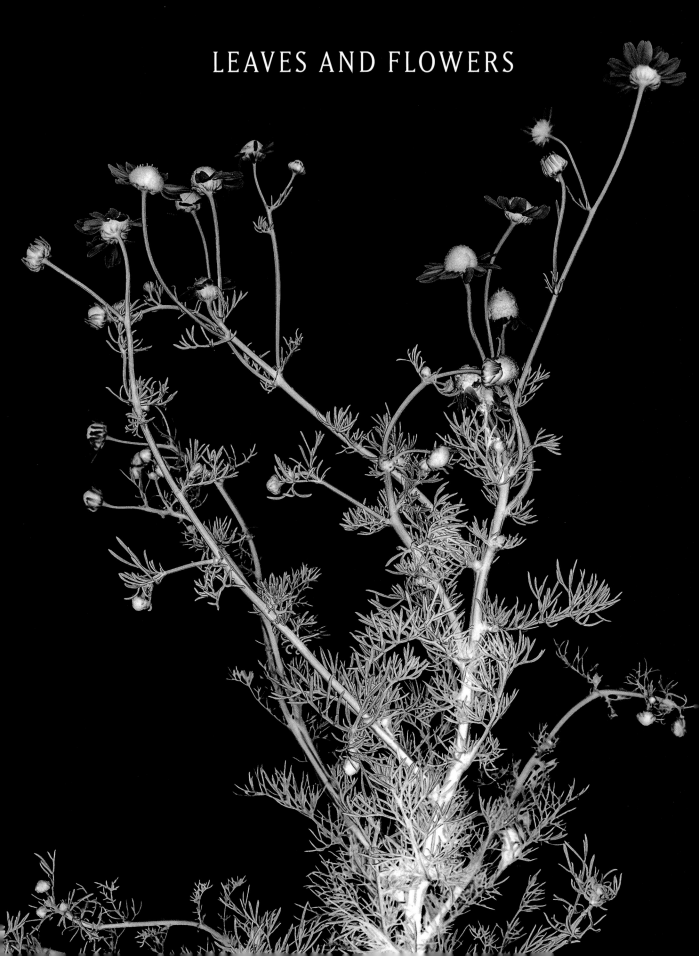

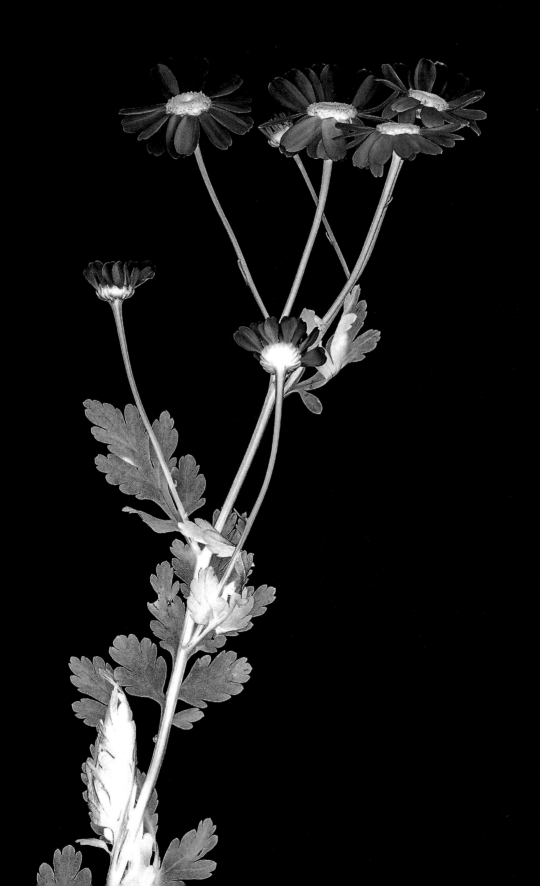

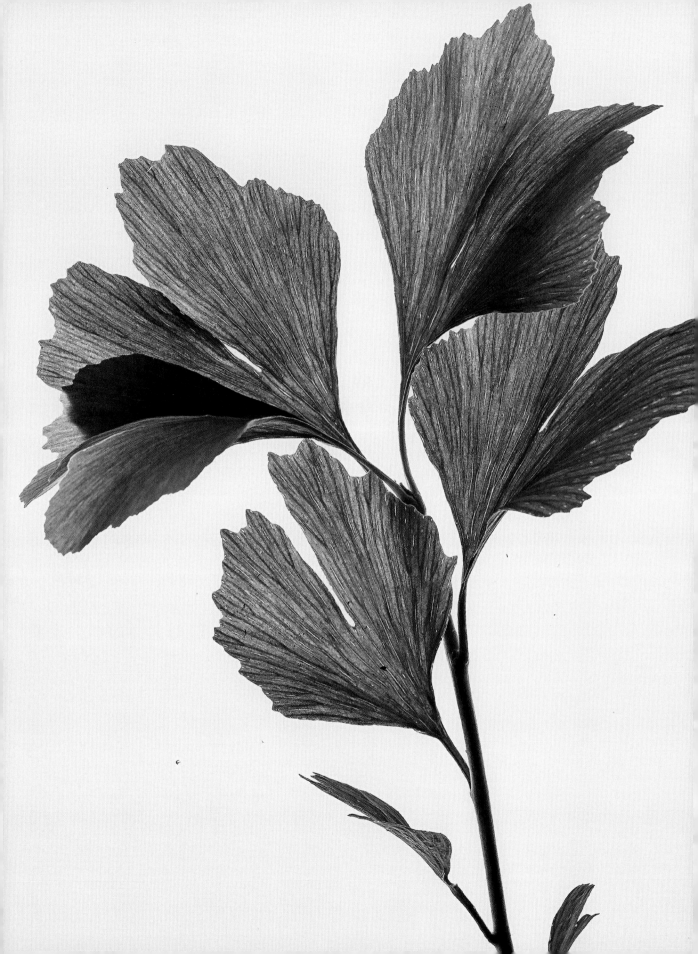

WOUTER "The plant kingdom is capable of producing an enormous diversity of substances. We can only guess at the quantity. We estimate that the plant kingdom comprises some 400,000 different plant species. At present, we know of some 14,000 species of mushrooms, and I'm sure that many more have yet to be discovered. Plants that have been extensively analyzed are known to be capable of producing hundreds of thousands of different substances, most of which are unique to that particular species of plant. This implies that an infinite source of substances is stored in nature, which could be of great importance to human beings.

At the moment, we only know about a very small part of this. That's why it is so important that biodiversity on Earth remains intact, so that we will continue to have access to the sources of power from nature. What's more, nature has been much better at creating more diverse substances than we could recreate in a laboratory. We can obviously come up with numerous other reasons for why keeping up biodiversity is so important, although I want to mention one specifically: the active ingredients in plants can differ quite substantially. The same plant or mushroom in a different climate or environment can have a different compound composition. With the products you use in your kitchen, do you ever notice a difference in their taste, even though they come from the same supplier?"

JORIS "The same plant tasting differently when it has been grown in another environment is something we call *terroir* in the kitchen. This French word is perhaps best known in relation to wine. You can taste it when the grape has enjoyed a lot of sun. The same goes for coffee. Beans that grow in high, cold areas are slightly fruitier and more acidic than the beans from warm, low-lying regions, which are more full-bodied and bitter. All peaches are different. Similarly, every region, every piece of land even, has a unique climate. The way the wind blows and the sun shines—it all plays into how the final product tastes. Does *terroir* also affect the plant's healing power?"

W "The plant's composition is determined among other things by where it is found, the soil in which the plant has grown, the altitude at which the plant spent its life, the temperature, and the amount of sunshine it received there. In Europe, sunlight contains about 10,000 lux, but around the equator it is 140,000 lux. That can have quite an impact on the presence of medicinal substances. The plant's age and when it is harvested during the season; what part of the plant (root, bark, flower, leaves, et cetera) is being picked also affects the presence of substances. What's more, different substances may be found on different parts of a plant. And it doesn't end there, because ways of drying or preserving also affect the substances and how they work. Interesting, isn't it?"

STINGING NETTLE | URTICA DIODICA

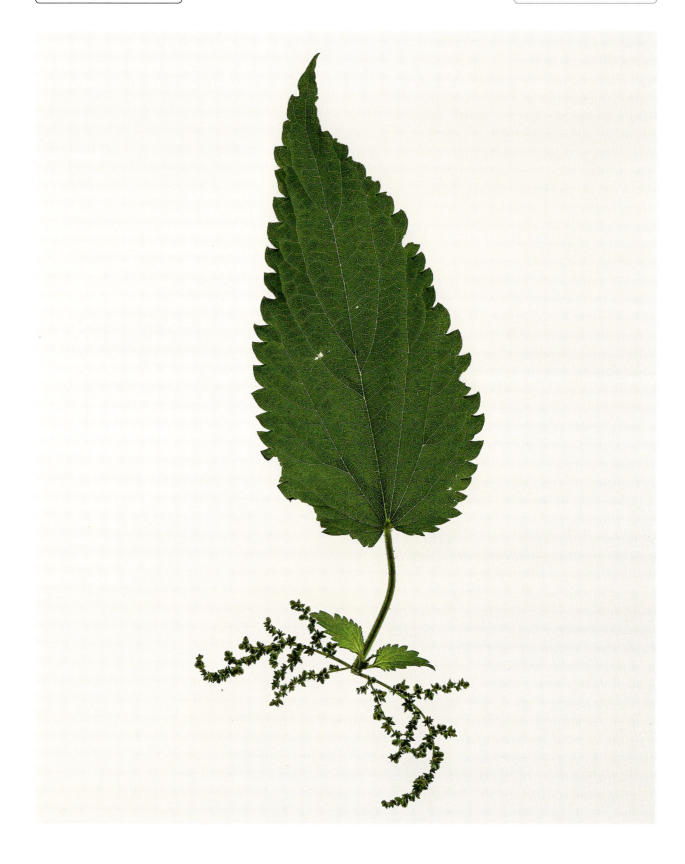

Cunning Healer

The stinging nettle is native to Africa and West Asia and has now spread across the globe. I imagine that everyone's childhood memories are colored by nettle stings. My mother would helpfully rub some plantain or purple dead-nettle leaves on my burning skin. Rather conveniently, these plants tend to grow near nettles and function as a natural antidote. By rubbing, you remove the nettle's barbs from your skin; they will however already have released their poison by then.

The itching is brought on by a combination of histamine, serotonin, acetylcholine, formic acid, and oxalic acid. You can squeeze out the juice of the dead-nettle or plantain with a trick I was taught by a Rastafarian elder in Jamaica. Take some leaves, crumble them together into a wad, put this in a piece of cloth or an old T-shirt, twist the fabric into a tight ball, and squeeze or wring this into a bowl. You can also use this extraction method for other plants, such as "leaf of life" (*Bryophyllum Pinatum*, also known as *Kalanchoe Bidentata*) which is used for colds, flu, and throat ailments. In Suriname, leaf of life is called "miracle leaf." You can easily grow this plant on your windowsill at home.

In the Netherlands and Belgium, mystical forces have been attributed to its most common plants since time immemorial. Stinging nettle is cunning, but also beneficial, a typical witch's herb. The plant was used to ward off curses, so it was thrown into the fire for protection and placed underneath children's pillows on their first birthday. It was believed that you could tell if a sick person would get better or succumb to their illness by putting fresh nettle leaf in their urine: If the leaf turned black, it meant doom; if it remained green, they would soon recover. The first Germanic people linked nettle to Thor, the god of thunder and fertility. In AD 77, Pliny the Elder wrote that many people regarded nettle as a sacred plant and ate it to stay healthy.

In antiquity, prickly plants were often seen as a remedy against the unwanted presence of demons. A common name for this stinging plant in the Low Countries was therefore "devil's weed." The presence of nettle at a crossroads was believed to have been evidence of witch gatherings. It was long thought that if nettles grew tall in summer, the coming winter would be severe. All in all, a special plant, therefore, surrounded by many stories.

Use

This "weed" is both nutritious and beneficial. Most of us prefer to pull it straight from the ground and throw it on the compost heap or in the trash for fear of the stinging urticating hairs. A great shame, because nettle contains plentiful minerals, trace elements, calcium, zinc, selenium, silicon, sulfur, and vitamins, including vitamins B2, B5, and B9, which have a hair- and nail-strengthening effect, among other things. So, instead of discarding nettle in your garden, consider using it in a soup or as a base for a homemade herbal tea.

PROPERTIES
- Depurative (blood and lymph purifying, detoxifying, deacidifying)
- Helps prevent kidney stones
- Anti-inflammatory
- Anti-rheumatic
- Immunomodulating
- Stimulates blood formation
- Source of minerals
- Supportive in osteoarthritis
- Strengthens hair and nails

SOURCING

Stinging nettles grow throughout America, England, Belgium, and the Netherlands on nitrogen-rich soil, so basically always near buildings. Wear gloves when you pick them. Nettle tea can also be purchased ready made at drugstores and health food stores.

CAUTION

For normal doses of nettle (1 cup of tea a day) there are no known side effects. Do keep its mild diuretic properties in mind. For pregnant women, it's better not to drink nettle preparations, because too little research has been done on possible effects on the pregnancy.

Leaves and Flowers

Early on, the stinging nettle was already seen as a beneficial edible spring green. Ancient Romans processed the plant in their spring cures to boost their health and vitality. According to alternative healer Mellie Uyldert, drinking nettle tea, along with a number of other herbs, helps drive away typical spring ailments and drain mucus. The plant is also said to have a cleansing effect on blood vessels.

Fresh nettle leaves were slapped onto rheumatic knees in order to expel the acids. Nettle roots were seen as a stimulus for people who wanted to have children; an extract was made with it.[98]

In the past, the plant's fibers were used like hemp and made into textile. In large parts of Europe, before the advent of cotton, this was the most important fiber material for making clothing, rope, and substances.

You can obviously also just leave it in the ground, because birds benefit greatly from eating nettle seeds. Many butterfly species lay their eggs on the leaves. The stinging nettle is a precious food source and host plant for animals and insects (a "host plant" is a plant on which an animal finds the substances essential for their growth and wellbeing).

Appearance

The greater stinging nettle is dioecious; that is, there are separate male and female plants. They belong to the *Urticaceae* family. The stinging nettle has green, serrated leaves with downy undersides covered in hairs. It is the hairs on the leaves and stems that, on contact, secrete substances that give a burning sensation and rash. The hairs have a barb at the end that causes them to hook into the skin. The plant grows to between 30 centimeters (a foot) and 1.5 meters (5 feet) in height. In the Netherlands and Belgium, they shoot up early in the spring and flower from May until July. The nutritious plant likes to grow on nitrogen-rich soil and therefore seems to tread on the heels of humankind.

Extracting and Dosing

Always wash nettle before you work with it. You can make tea from it, which you can basically drink every day. Use 3 grams (0.1 ounces) of dried leaves to 250 milliliters (8 fluid ounces) of hot water. Or use it like spinach in hot dishes, or add it to soups. Once you have heated nettle by blanching, cooking, or stir-frying, it loses its stinging effect. The leaf is also easy to dry; this is another way to get rid of the sting.

Leaves and Flowers

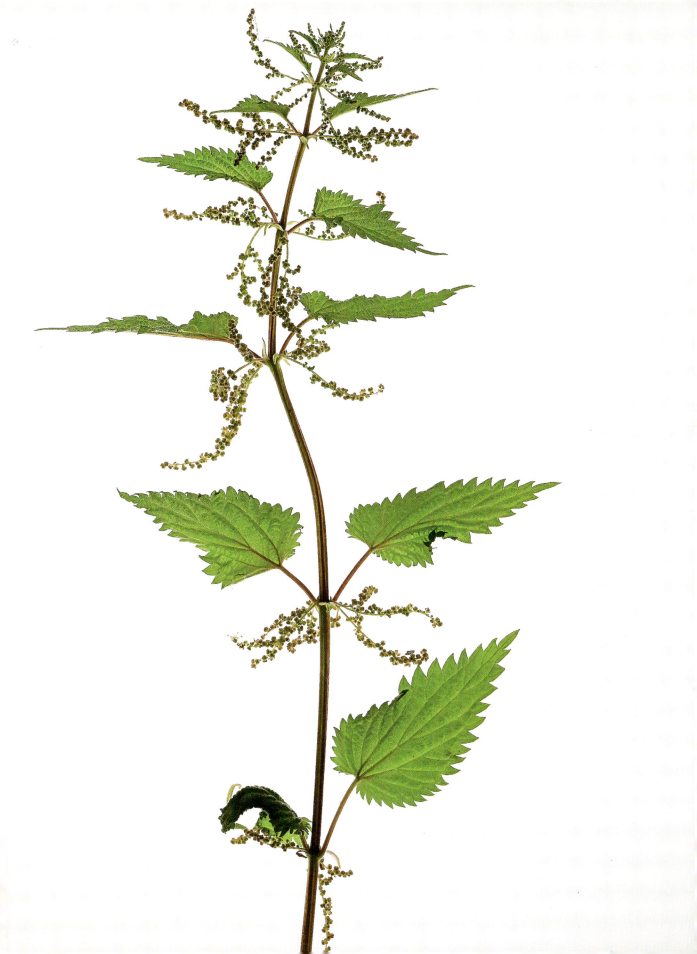

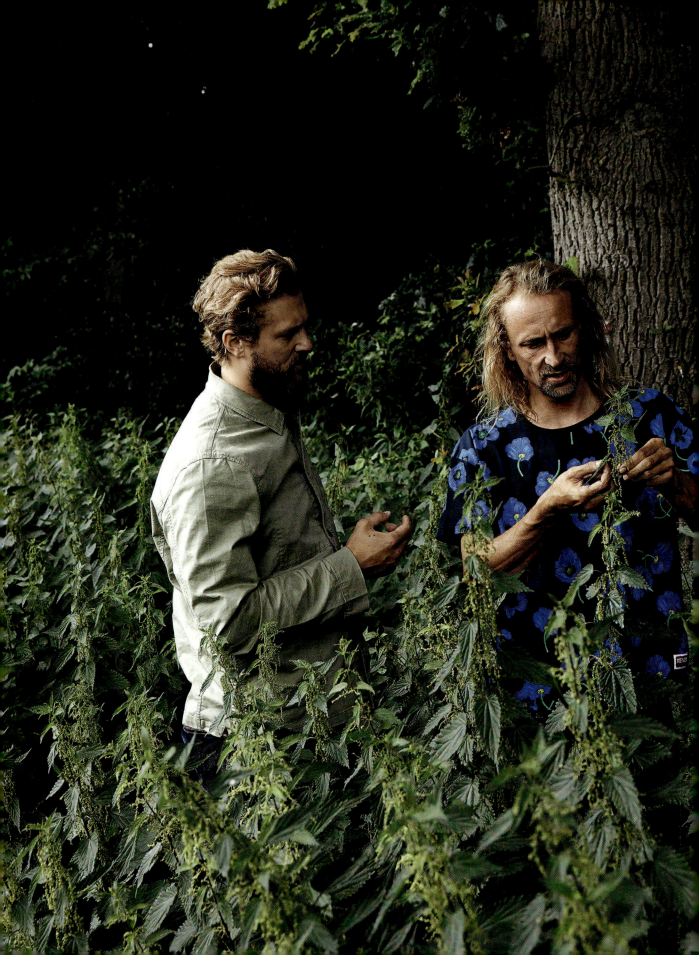

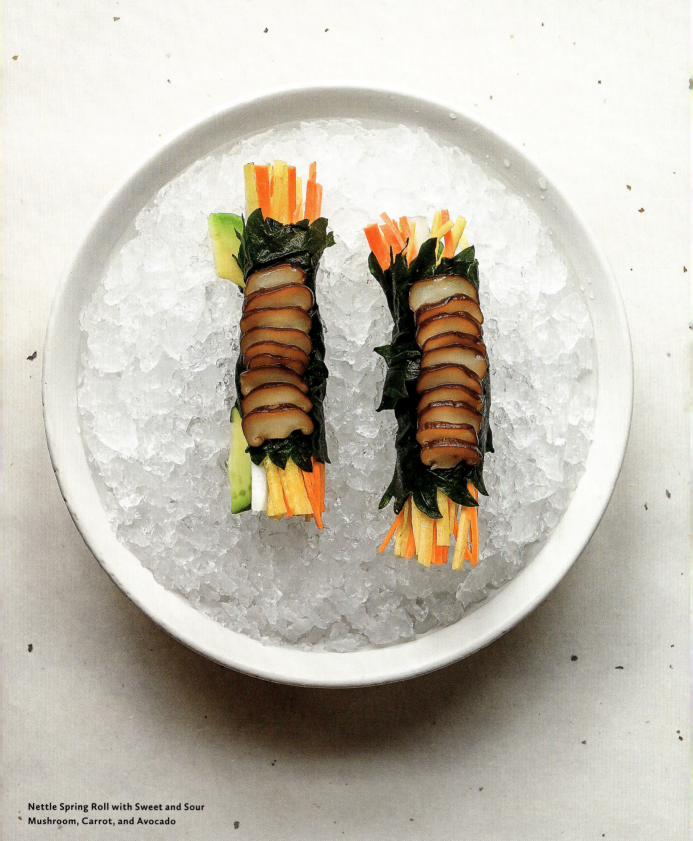

Nettle Spring Roll with Sweet and Sour Mushroom, Carrot, and Avocado

NETTLE SPRING ROLL WITH SWEET AND SOUR MUSHROOM, CARROT, AND AVOCADO

for as many as you like

■ FOR THE SWEET AND SOUR MUSHROOM
- 10 small shiitake mushrooms
- 50 g/2 oz granulated sugar
- 50 ml/2 fl oz white wine vinegar
- 50 ml/2 fl oz white wine

■ FOR THE SPRING ROLLS
- nettle leaves
- sesame oil
- yellow root
- orange root
- avocado

method

In this recipe, I do not give weights and quantities for the spring rolls, because you can make them as big, small, fat, thin, and as many as you like. The important thing is that you use raw crunchy vegetables, so that could also be (giant white) radish. This will be juxtaposed with the creaminess of the avocado and, of course, the nettle leaf.

For the sweet and sour mushrooms, remove the stalks from the mushrooms and place the caps in a heatproof bowl. In a saucepan, bring the sugar, white wine vinegar, and white wine to the boil. Pour the hot mixture over the mushrooms, and allow to cool completely.

Blanch the nettle leaves for 15 seconds in a pan with plenty of salted boiling water, and rinse immediately in ice water. Pat them dry, and lay them flat on the countertop; drizzle with a few drops of sesame oil.

Finely julienne the crisp and creamy vegetables, arrange on the nettle leaves, and wrap the nettles leaves around the filling to form spring rolls. Thinly slice the shiitake, and arrange on top of the spring rolls.

For a dip, you can use the delicious parsley aioli on page 62.

Leaves and Flowers

STIR-FRIED NETTLE LEAVES WITH AVOCADO AND SESAME SEEDS

serves 4 people

■ INGREDIENTS

- 500 g/1 lb of nettles, washed
- 45 ml/1.5 fl oz (3 T) olive oil
- 30 g/1 oz (2 T) sesame seeds
- 2 avocados, peeled, pitted, and cut into 8 equal segments
- 1 garlic clove, finely chopped
- fine sea salt and freshly ground black pepper

method

Wash and dry the nettles. Be careful, as they will still sting—this only disappears when they are heated.

Heat the olive oil in a skillet on low heat, and fry the sesame seeds until golden-brown. Do not leave unattended, as they brown very quickly. Add the avocado segments, and sauté for a moment until they have colored a little. Add the garlic, and sauté briefly without it coloring. Now add the nettles, and simmer. The leaves will shrink a little like spinach, but should be cooked for 3 minutes, otherwise they will stay too tough. Season with salt and pepper.

Divide among plates, and serve immediately. Eat as a hot salad or as a vegetable side dish at dinner.

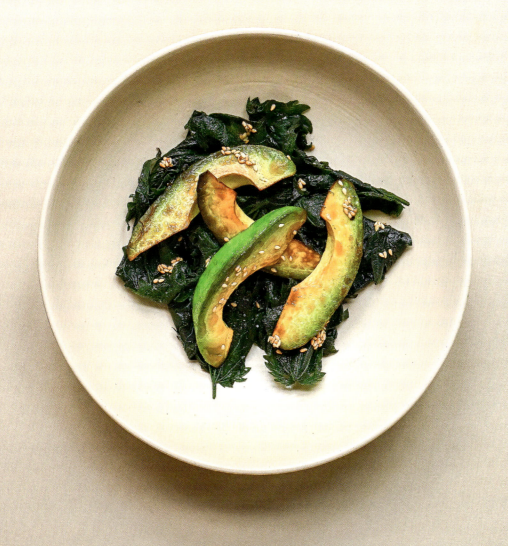

| GINKGO | | GINKGO BILOBA |

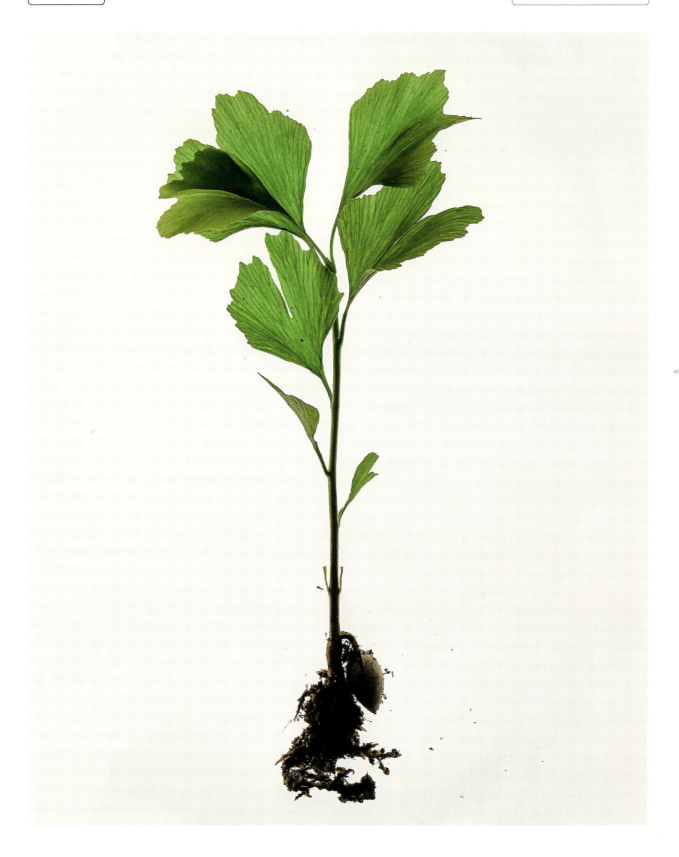

Anti-Aging Tree

Ginkgo biloba can be thought of as a living fossil. It is the last surviving member of its family and has lived on Earth for 250 million years. Ginkgo biloba is the only type of gingko to survive the Pleistocene Ice Age (between 2.6 million and 11,700 years BP, and then only in China. The plant survived the dinosaurs and does not mutate when subjected to nuclear radiation. In Hiroshima, ginkgo was one of the first plants to start growing again following the nuclear catastrophe. Partly because of this, ginkgo is seen as a symbol of strength and life.

In Japan, ancient ginkgo trees were worshipped as gods. They are very long-lived, after all—China boasts a specimen that is 3,000 years old. Trees were often planted at Buddhist temples. One of the largest trees in Korea, in the Yongmun-san temple, stands 60 meters (197 feet) tall and has a diameter of 5 meters (16.4 feet). This tree is said to have been planted in the ninth century in order to preserve the species from extinction. People still make pilgrimages to this tree.

Use

The first traces of medicinal usage can be found around 2800 BCE in the Chinese materia medica *Pen Tsao Ching*. Legend has it that the emperor was prompted to prepare an infusion of ginkgo leaves for the cognitively declining members of the imperial court in order to make their minds lucid again.[99]

Herbalist Geert Verhelst believes that the plant's strong resistance against all kinds of extreme external influences is indirect proof of its strength and the presence of antioxidants. It is the flavonol glycosides in ginkgo that give it its antioxidant, anti-inflammatory, and neuroprotective properties. As far as I know, the plant has only been in use in Western herbalism since the 20th century.

The leaves of the plant contain ginkgonosides. These are water-soluble and help improve the blood flow in the small capillaries. The plant is often prescribed to stimulate the memory, because the ingredients affect blood flow to the brain. Leaf extract of ginkgo has been used for many years to treat age-related memory problems, including Alzheimer's disease and dementia. Experimental and clinical studies have demonstrated its favorable effects on a wide range of pathological disorders.[100] Because ginkgo protects blood vessel walls against aging and improves memory, the plant is often touted as an anti-aging remedy.

There is some scientific evidence and further indications that ginseng (see page 224) and ginkgo can improve cognitive performance. A recent double-blind study proved that the memory capacity of Alzheimer's patients improved significantly when they regularly used ginkgo extract.[101]

PROPERTIES
- Promotes blood flow of the small capillaries
- Blood-thinning
- Antioxidant activity
- Enhances brain function through improved blood flow
- Improves memory
- Helps against asthma
- Protects blood vessel walls

SOURCING

Ginkgo extracts can be purchased at drugstores. In summer, you can also pick fresh ginkgo leaves from a tree (in the Netherlands and Belgium or other places where gingko commonly grows). Some herbalists believe that the most active ingredients in the leaf are present in autumn when the leaves turn yellow. The seeds of these trees do not easily germinate when they stem from trees grown at a latitude north of Geneva, Switzerland. So buy them at a Chinese supermarket or grocery store.

CAUTION

In people with poor cerebral blood flow, a light headache may develop when they first begin to use gingko biloba. Do not use ginkgo before or just after surgery because of its blood-thinning action. Also, don't use ginkgo when you have bleeding stomach ulcers

Leaves and Flowers

But these are not ginkgo's only powers. In Japan, people are trying to cure infertility by taking pulverized ginkgo blossom under specific conditions,[102] while in Chinese medicine one of ginkgo's most important applications is for asthma.[103] Many people believe that because the plant has survived so many tribulations, it contains knowledge that is ingested when it is consumed.

Appearance

The ginkgo tree has a gray-brown, corky bark. Its leaves are fan-shaped and leathery and resemble butterflies. They are green in spring and summer and fall in autumn. There are male and female trees. Only the female trees form fruit. Of these, the flesh is not edible, but the ivory-white nuts inside are. These are considered a delicacy in Asia.

If you would like to grow your own ginkgo tree, so that you always have fresh leaves to pick, buy fresh seeds from a Chinese supermarket or grocery store. In China, the seeds are used to make soup. Place a handful of seeds in the freezer (or refrigerator) for 6 weeks so that the seeds think it is winter and then sow them 2–3 centimeters (about 1 inch) deep. After that, it is a matter of patience. I had no trouble growing two small trees from a handful of seeds; I can now pick from these. The ginkgo tree will only bear fruit after 30 years.

Extracting and Dosing

For a clear effect, ginkgo preparations should be taken for some time, at least 6–8 weeks.

You can make your own tea from ginkgo and drink it as a maintenance dose. A stronger effect can be obtained by buying standardized extracts. Discuss the right dosage for you with your doctor.

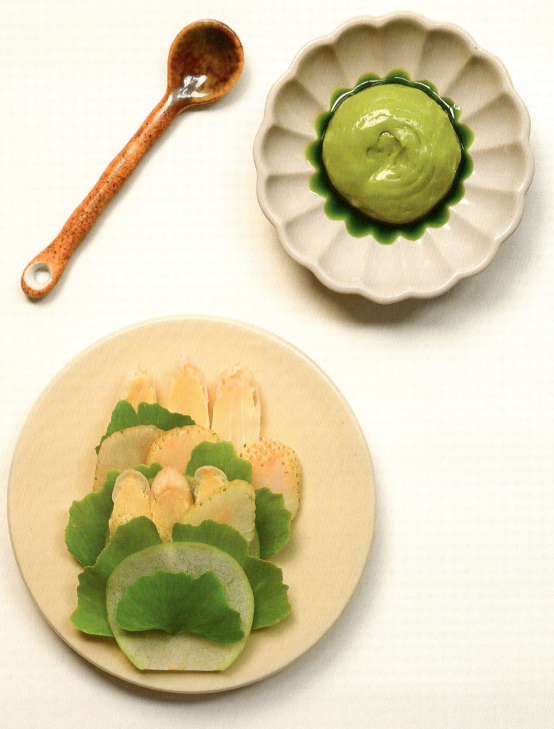

Salad of Ginkgo with White Asparagus and Granny Smith Apples

SALAD OF GINKGO WITH WHITE ASPARAGUS AND GRANNY SMITH APPLES

serves 4 people

■ **FOR THE PARSLEY CREAM**
- 1 bunch (approx. 80 g/2.8 oz) leaf parsley
- 200 ml/6.8 fl oz sunflower oil
- 1 egg white
- 25 ml/0.8 fl oz sushi vinegar

■ **FOR THE SALAD**
- 4 spears white asparagus
- 2 Granny Smith apples
- 5 green strawberries
- 25 ginkgo leaves

■ **EQUIPMENT**
- cheesecloth
- peeler
- mandolin

method

First make the parsley cream. Pick the green leaves from the parsley; without stalks this will leave you with about 40 grams (1.4 ounces). If you have less, add some more parsley leaves. In a blender, whizz the leaves with the sunflower oil for 30 minutes until as smooth as possible. This process causes the oil to heat up, which is what we want. Strain the parsley oil through a piece of cheesecloth into a bowl, squeeze well. In a tall beaker, mix the egg whites and the sushi vinegar with a hand blender and while mixing, slowly pour in 200 milliliters (6.7 fluid ounces) of parsley oil until you have a nice firm cream.

Peel the white asparagus spears using a vegetable peeler. Cut the spears into three pieces, then thinly slice each piece lengthways using the mandolin. Thinly slice the unpeeled Granny Smith apples using the mandolin. De-stem the green strawberries and cut into thin slices with a sharp knife.

Place the asparagus pieces side by side on a plate so that they are touching. Arrange the gingko leaves on top. Place the green apple slices and then the green strawberry slices on top of these. Repeat with one more layer, and prepare the other plates in the same way.

Serve the parsley cream in a bowl on the side with some drizzled parsley oil around it.

Leaves and Flowers

RICE PUDDING WITH GINKGO NUT, RED DATE, AND CRANBERRY POWDER

serves 4–6 people

■ INGREDIENTS
- about 700 ml/24 fl oz whole milk
- 150 ml/5 fl oz whipped cream
- 1 vanilla pod, halved
- 200 g/7 oz pudding rice
- 40 g/1.4 oz ginkgo nuts
- 8 red dates (Asian supermarket or health food store)
- 70 g/2.5 oz granulated sugar
- fine sea salt
- pinch of cranberry powder (health food store)

method
In a saucepan, bring the milk, whipping cream, and halved vanilla pod to a boil. Add the rice, ginkgo nuts, and red dates, and put the lid on the pan.

Gently cook the rice for about 15 minutes until soft. Stir frequently, and add additional milk if necessary. Do not add the sugar until the rice is cooked, along with a pinch of salt.

Spoon the rice pudding into deep plates, and sprinkle with some cranberry powder.

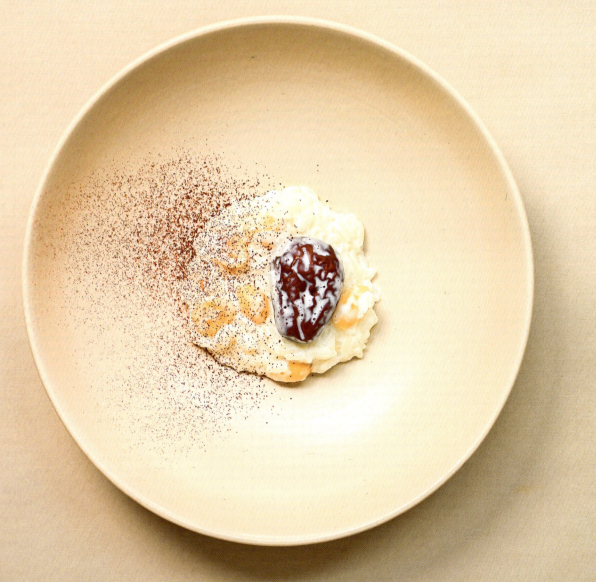

| GERMAN CHAMOMILE | | MATRICARIA CHAMOMILLA |

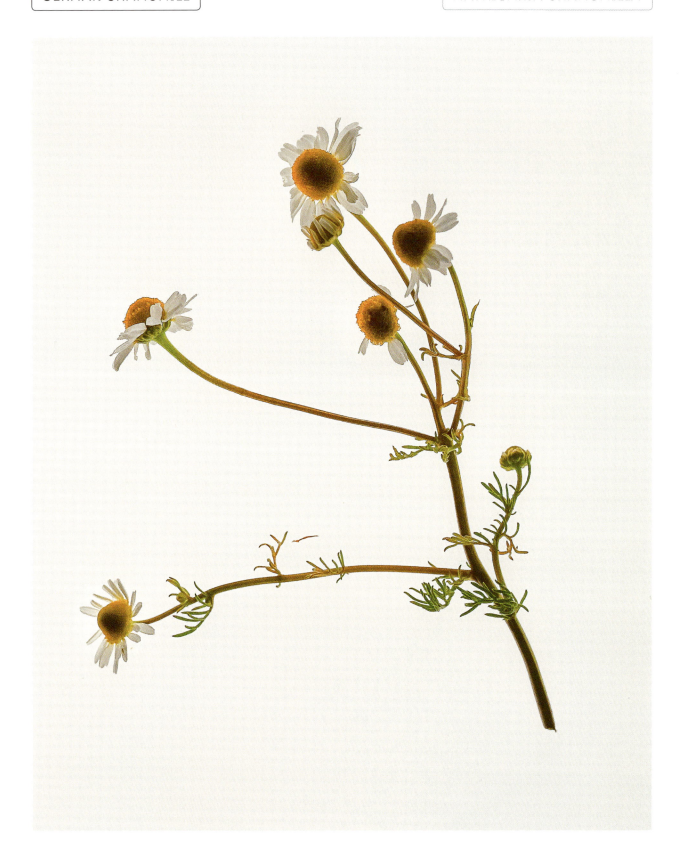

Sun Messenger

German chamomile's scientific name is composed of several words. *Matricaria* stems from the Latin word *matrix*, which means "womb," and *caria* means "care." This plant was consequently used for women's diseases, especially childbirth and uterine problems. The species name *chamomilla* is derived from the Greek *chamai*, which means "on the ground," and from *melon*, which refers to "apple," so literally "ground apple," as its flower heads resemble apples and its crushed leaves smell like apple.[104] German chamomile grows in the United Kingdom and Europe as far north as the Caucasus in western Siberia, as well as in North Africa and North America.

The ancient Egyptians considered true German chamomile a flower of the sun god Ra due to its fever-reducing and anti-inflammatory properties. This comparison is partly because the appearance of the flowers is associated with the bright sun. Alternative healer Mellie Uyldert says about German chamomile: "The little plant with the golden heart leaping to the sun is a sun messenger. German chamomile dissolves cramp and allows heartening solar strength to flow through you again."[105] Many of German chamomile's traditional applications have been supported by scientific laboratory research. This is especially true of its antibacterial, antifungal, antiviral, sedative, and anti-inflammatory properties.[106]

Use

With its various applications, true chamomile is one of the most-used medicinal herbs. German chamomile works mainly for inflammation, to relieve pain, to calm, and is used as a component in cosmetics.[107] It is added to shampoo to make hair blonder, for instance.

In general, only German chamomile's flower heads are used. Chamomile tea is often taken as an inhalant for colds; you hold your head over a pan with flower heads steeped in hot water with a cloth draped over your head in order to breath in the steam. This has a soothing effect on the throat, dissolves trapped mucus, and expedites the healing of colds. German chamomile also has a beneficial effect on the stomach and may assist with abdominal pain and stimulate digestion. Due to its anti-inflammatory and disinfecting properties, it protects against stomach ulcers. The tea soothes the gastrointestinal system.

In addition, German chamomile tea is often drunk in the evening for a good night's sleep. It has a favorable effect on the nervous system and is mildly hypnotic and relaxing. I myself often drink it in the evening. German chamomile strengthens the nervous system and is used as a remedy for agitation, restlessness, stress, and irritability.

Chamomile is also used as a mouth rinse in cases of gum inflammation and tooth nerve pain and is believed work for mild gastrointestinal mucosal inflammation.[108] But it is not only good for human beings; if you sow it in your garden, it improves the health of the soil and other plants in its vicinity.

PROPERTIES

- Antibacterial
- Antifungal
- Antiviral
- Calming
- Anti-inflammatory
- Antispasmodic (also menstrual cramps)
- Digestive stimulant
- Stomach-strengthener
- Nerve-strengthening
- Relieves itching (external)
- Bleaching (externally on the hair)

SOURCING

German chamomile is easy to grow in your garden or on your balcony or patio. The tea is available from drugstores, tea stores, supermarkets, or markets.

CAUTION

Excessive use of German chamomile can lead to insomnia—curious, when you consider that it promotes sleep in smaller doses. If you are finding that you cannot sleep when using chamomile, then stop using it for a while. Use chamomile only in moderation when pregnant, and never use essential oil of chamomile during pregnancy.

Leaves and Flowers

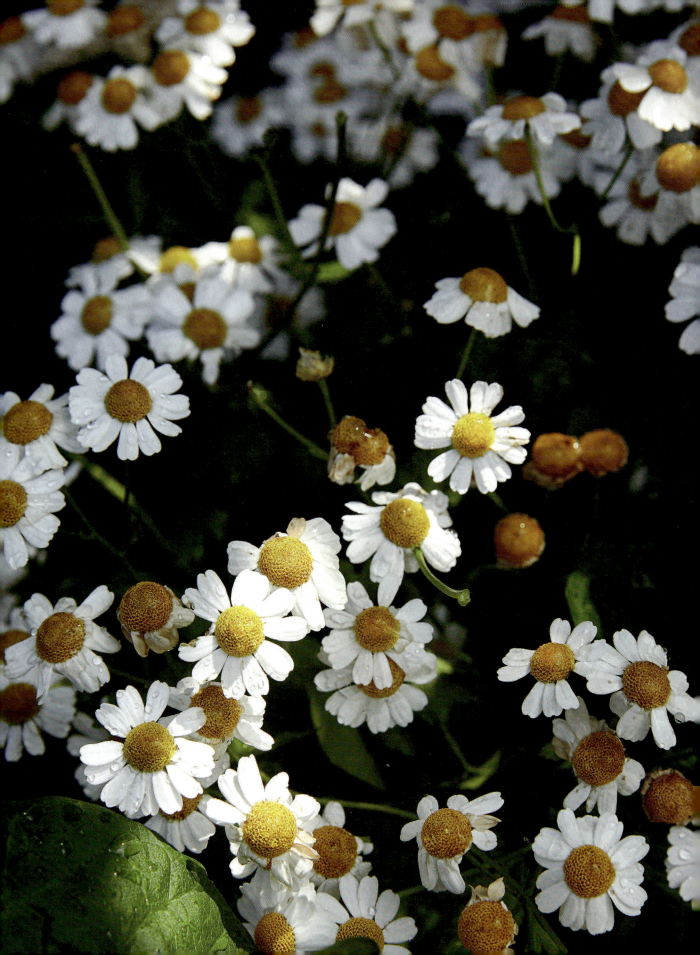

Appearance

To make sure that you are dealing with genuine German chamomile, it is best to grow it yourself in your garden or on your balcony. Genuine German chamomile has daisy-like flowers. The flowers have a heart of yellow florets which are surrounded by white petals. The plant flowers from May to September. The composite leaves are bipinnate or tripinnate.

Its stems grow 15–50 centimeters (6–19.5 inches) tall. Other varieties are Roman chamomile, scentless chamomile, corn chamomile, and wild chamomile or pineapple weed. On the face of it, they are not very easy to distinguish from each other, but true German chamomile can be identified by its sweet apple-like fragrance. In the Netherlands, United Kingdom, and North America, the plant also grows in the wild and likes neutral to slightly acidic sandy, loamy soil in the sun.

Extracting and Dosing

Remove the stems from the German chamomile flowers, or just pick the flower heads. Dry the flower heads on an untreated wooden board.

Make German chamomile tea by gently steeping 2–8 grams (0.071–0.28 ounces) of flower heads in 500 milliliters (16.9 fluid ounces) of hot water for 10 minutes. Put a lid on the teapot, bowl, or saucepan while the tea is steeping; this stops the oils from dissipating too quickly.

Drink a maximum of 2–3 cups of German chamomile tea a day; it is said to be an effective relief for (menstrual) cramps.

Use 200 milliliters (about 7 ounces) German chamomile tea mixed with 1 drop of clove oil externally against candida, which relieves the itching and can kill the fungus.

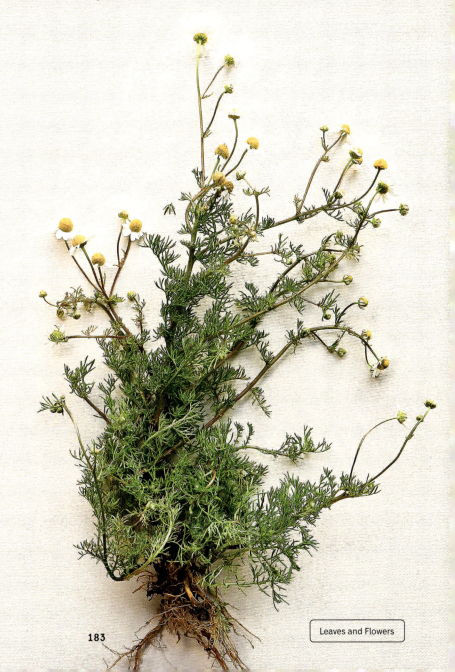

Leaves and Flowers

TURNIP IN CHAMOMILE SALT CRUST WITH RAVIGOTE

serves 4 people

■ **FOR THE TURNIP IN CHAMOMILE SALT CRUST**
- 500 g/approx. 17 oz flour
- 150 g /approx. 5 oz fine sea salt
- 50 g/1.8 oz coarse sea salt
- 2 handfuls (approx. 40 g/1.4 oz) chamomile, flowers and leaves finely chopped
- 2 eggs
- 4 turnips

■ **FOR THE RAVIGOTE SAUCE**
- 1 boiled egg, passed through a sieve
- 40 ml/1.3 fl oz mayonnaise
- 30 ml/1 fl oz creme fraîche
- ½ shallot, chopped
- 7.5 g/0.25 oz (½ T) finely chopped capers
- 7.5 g/0.25 oz (½ T) finely chopped gherkins
- 7.5 g/0.25 oz (½ T) chopped curly parsley
- 7.5 g/0.25 oz (½ T) chopped chervil
- fine sea salt and freshly ground black pepper

■ **EQUIPMENT**
- small brush
- fine sieve

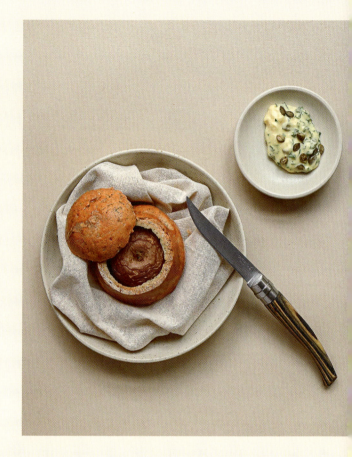

method

Preheat the oven to 170°C (325°F)

In a bowl, make a pastry with the flour, two kinds of salt, chamomile, and eggs. Roll out one-third of the dough into 4 discs for the turnips. Brush with a little water, and place 1 turnip on each disc. Roll out the rest of the pastry, cut into 4 pieces, and cover each turnip with a piece of the pastry.

Press the pastry firmly down at the edges, and trim any excess. Bake the turnip in the salt crust for 1 hour in the oven.

Remove the turnip pastries from the oven, and allow to cool completely.

Meanwhile, for the ravigote, mix all the ingredients in a bowl, and season with salt and pepper.

Cut off the tops of chamomile salt crust covering the turnips. Remove the turnips, and cut each one into wedges. Serve with the ravigote sauce.

Leaves and Flowers

CHERRIES WITH CHAMOMILE GRANITA AND OUDWIJKER LAZULI CHEESE

serves 4–6 people

■ **FOR THE CHAMOMILE GRANITA**
- 250 ml/8.5 fl oz chamomile tea (you can make the tea as strong as you like; it tastes best made with fresh chamomile)
- 75 g/2.6 oz granulated sugar
- 20 g/0.7 oz honey

■ **FOR THE CHERRY JAM**
- 500 g/about 17 oz cherries
- 100 ml/3.4 fl oz cherry lambic (kriek) beer

■ **AS WELL AS**
- 100 g/3.5 oz cherries
- 200 g/7 oz Oudwijker Lazuli cheese (soft Dutch blue cheese like Gorgonzola), room temperature
- 10 chamomile leaves

■ **EQUIPMENT**
- kitchen thermometer

method

Start with the chamomile granita. Put the chamomile tea in a saucepan, and bring to a boil. Add the sugar and honey, and stir. Making sure everything is well dissolved, remove the pan from the heat, and place in a container in the freezer. After 1 hour of freezing, stir with a fork. Repeat every 30 minutes. At some point you will have granita, usually after about 3 hours.

Wash the cherries for the cherry jam, stone and cut them up as finely as you like. Put them in a pan together with the beer, and bring to a boil. Remove the pan from the heat when the kitchen thermometer reads 105°C (220°F). You can also test the jam by spooning a little onto a cold plate. If it is still runny, cook it a little longer. Allow to cool.

Halve and stone the rest of the cherries. Spoon a small circle of cherry jam onto each plate, crumble some cheese on top, and arrange the halved cherries around it. Sprinkle with chamomile leaves. Remove the granita from the freezer, loosen with a fork one last time, and scoop some chamomile granita onto each plate.

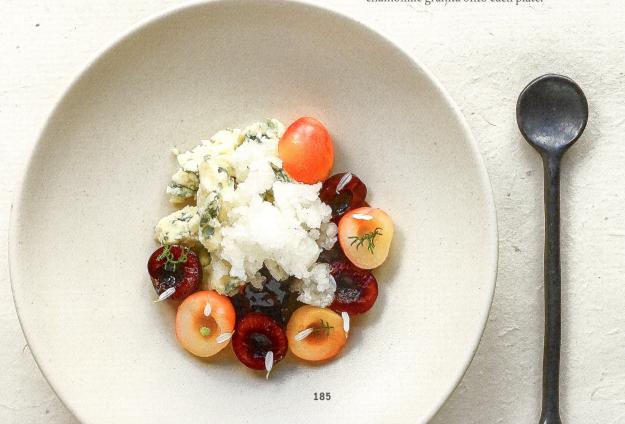

MATCHA TEA

CAMELLIA SINENSIS

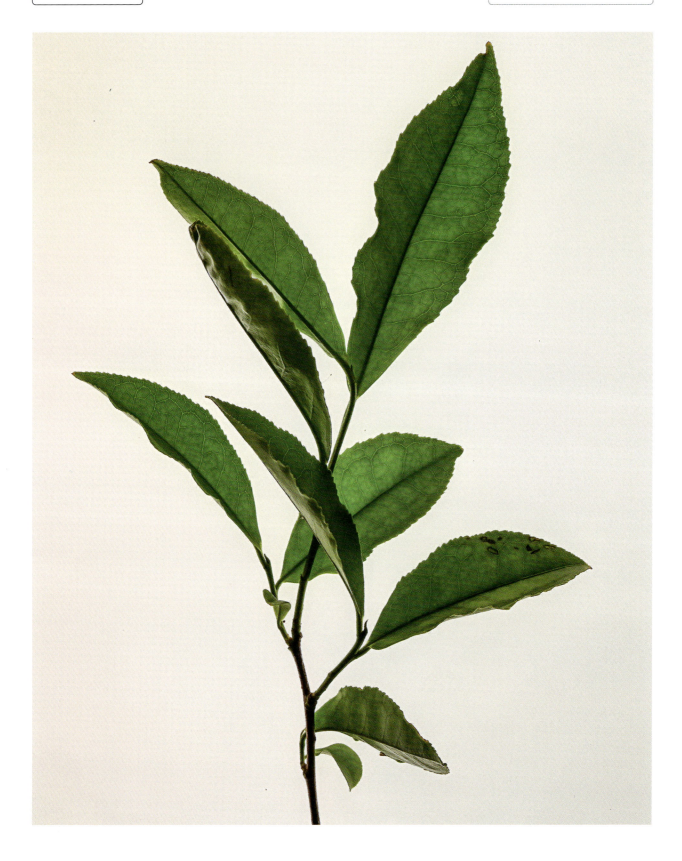

Queen of Tea

Matcha tea as we know it comes from Japan, but the history of matcha begins in China. During the Song dynasty (AD 960–1279), making powder from dried and steamed green tea leaves and whipping this up with hot water became popular. Japanese Zen monks then took this method of making tea back with them from China to Japan. They drank the tea to stay alert and awake during their meditations. In Japan, matcha took on a life of its own and specific rituals and ceremonies sprang up around it. The preparation and drinking of matcha during a tea ceremony in Japan can easily take an hour.

All types of tea, including matcha, come from the same plant: *Camellia sinensis*. It is the processing of the tea that gives it its unique taste and color. For the best matcha, only the small upper leaves of the tea bush that have grown in the shade for a few weeks are used. The tea is picked by hand, and the leaves' veins and stems are likewise removed by hand. The leaves are steamed to arrest the fermentation process and then dried. Just grinding the leaves to make 30 grams (1 ounce) of matcha powder takes an hour. This is usually done on the tea plantations themselves using millstones that rotate very slowly so that all the flavor is retained. Now you understand why matcha is so incredibly expensive and why it is called the "queen of tea."

Use

Matcha is extremely rich in antioxidants that help remove free radicals and slow down our bodies' aging process. Matcha thus helps to counteract cardiovascular disease and keep our skin and blood vessels supple. Matcha contains a great deal of calcium, potassium, vitamins A and C, iron, and proteins that strengthen your immune system.

Most green teas are prepared by extracting the dried tea leaves in water. Matcha is a tea you drink whole, which means that the pulverized tea can release the theine, theobromine, and caffeine in your body. These substances therefore remain active in your body for much longer. The clarifying effect of a bowl of tea can be felt for up to six hours. The real effect of the caffeine in a cup of coffee essentially only lasts for 10 minutes.

Green tea and matcha contain cathecin, an antioxidant substance that has a beneficial effect on the blood circulation system. The substances caffeine, L-theanine, and epigallocatechin gallate (a particular type of catechin) improve cognitive function and alertness. L-theanine improves sleep in the long term and also has a relaxing effect. Green tea and matcha boost our immune system, as has been demonstrated in several studies including one by Keiji Matsumoto and colleagues in 2011.

PROPERTIES

- Rich source of antioxidants
- Clarifying
- Promotes concentration
- Stimulates the nervous system
- Good for the prevention of cardiovascular disease
- Reduces damage to DNA
- Source of calcium, potassium, vitamins A and C, and iron

SOURCING

For sale in good tea stores and Japanese stores. You can only really buy the best matcha (of ceremonial quality) in Japan. Compared to ordinary green tea, matcha is often seen as expensive. The real potency of matcha is only present for the first two weeks; after that, the tea is perfectly okay to drink, but its fragrance and potency will have degraded.

CAUTION

Due to the caffeine and theine, green tea may lead to insomnia if you drink the tea late in the day. Green tea in excessively high doses can also lead to reduced uptake of minerals.

Appearance

Matcha tea is made from the *Camellia sinensis plant*. The tea plant has dark green, lightly serrated, leathery, oval leaves with fine hairs on the underside. The plants are highly bifurcated. The plant is pruned to a height of 80–120 centimeters (31–47 inches). In order to produce matcha tea,

Leaves and Flowers

the bush grows under shade nets for at least three weeks; this intensifies the leaves' taste and increases the number of substances compared to ordinary green tea. The ideal elevation for growing tea plants is at 1000 meters (3,280 feet) above sea level. The plant likes to grow on slopes in sun and partial shade and requires a great deal of precipitation. It grows best in the tropics and subtropics. Once ground, matcha powder is bright green in color.

Extracting and Dosing

For the preparation of matcha, a splash of warm water is mixed in a bowl (chawan) with a small amount of powder into a homogeneous substance by beating and stirring it with a special bamboo whisk (chasen). You can make thick or thin tea from matcha powder. For thin tea (usucha), whisk 1.75 grams (0.06 ounces) matcha powder with a splash of water with a bamboo whisk. Add 75 milliliters (2.5 fluid ounces) of water heated to 60–75°C (140–167°F), and whisk until you see a light-green frothy layer.

For thick tea (kotcha), pour 40 milliliters (1.35 fluid ounces) of water heated to 60–70 °C (140–158°F) over 3.75 grams (0.1 ounces) matcha powder. Mix gently with the whisk. Always drink matcha immediately, but quietly and attentively.

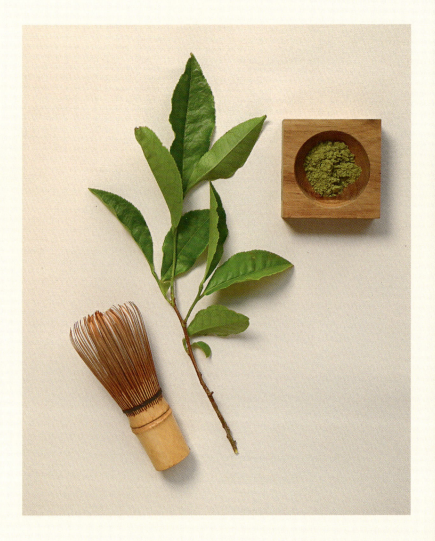

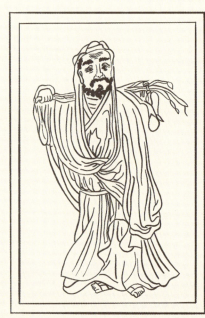

BODHIDHARMA – Old Chinese drawing of Bodhidharma, a Buddhist teacher, carrying a tea plant. (After a drawing from Folklore and Odysseys of Food and Medicinal Plants by Ernst and Johanna Lehner, 1962.)

Leaves and Flowers

ENERGY BALLS WITH SEEDS, NUTS, DRIED FRUITS, AND MATCHA

for the whole team

INGREDIENTS
- 20 g/0.7 oz dried figs
- 80 g/2.8 oz pitted dates
- 20 g/0.7 oz pistachio kernels, shelled
- 20 g/0.7 oz sunflower seeds
- 20 g/0.7 oz white almonds
- 25 g/0.8 oz honey
- 25 g/0.8 oz coconut oil
- 10 g/0.35 oz bee pollen
- 15 g/0.5 oz (1 T) matcha powder

EQUIPMENT
- fine sieve

method

Finely dice the figs and dates and finely chop the pistachios, sunflower seeds, and almonds. Heat the honey with the coconut oil, and mix all the ingredients, except the matcha powder, in a bowl. Knead into a "dough."

You can form this mixture into any shape you like, but I like to roll them into balls about 3 centimeters (just over an inch) in diameter. Using the sieve, dust the energy balls with the matcha powder. If you store them in the refrigerator in an airtight container, they will keep for at least 2 weeks.

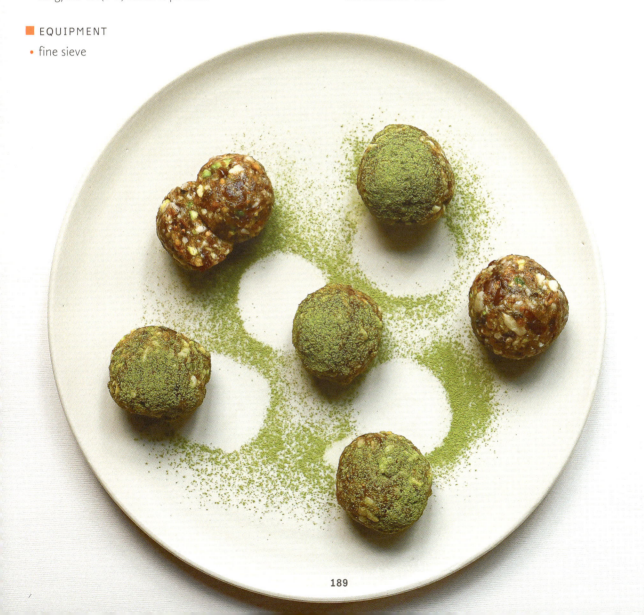

TEMPURA OF SHISO AND SHIITAKE WITH MATCHA SALT

snack or appetizer for 10 people

■ FOR THE TEMPURA
- 3 egg yolks
- 250 ml/8.5 fl oz ice-cold sparkling water
- 80 g/2.8 oz flour, plus extra
- 1.5 L/51 fl oz of sunflower oil
- 10 shiso leaves (Asian supermarket)
- pinch of fine sea salt
- 100 g/3.5 oz shiitake mushrooms, stalks removed

■ FOR THE MATCHA SALT
- 14 g/0.5 oz (1 T) matcha powder
- 42.5 g/1.5 oz (3 T) Maldon salt flakes

■ EQUIPMENT
- pan for deep-frying
- kitchen thermometer
- skimmer

method

Make the tempura batter by whisking the egg yolks, the ice-cold sparkling water, and flour together in a bowl. A few lumps of flour is not a disaster, but it is better if you do not have too many.

Meanwhile, heat the sunflower oil to 180°C (350°F) in a deep saucepan with a thick bottom.

Dip the shiso leaves into the tempura, making sure they do not have too much tempura batter on them, although they do need to be covered. Place them in the hot oil for about 30–40 seconds, until they are nicely browned. Scoop them out, and sprinkle with salt. Drain on kitchen paper. Do the same with the shiitake mushrooms. Meanwhile, mix the matcha powder and Maldon salt flakes in a bowl.

Arrange the shiitake mushrooms on the plates with the shiso leaves on top. Sprinkle with the matcha salt.

Leaves and Flowers

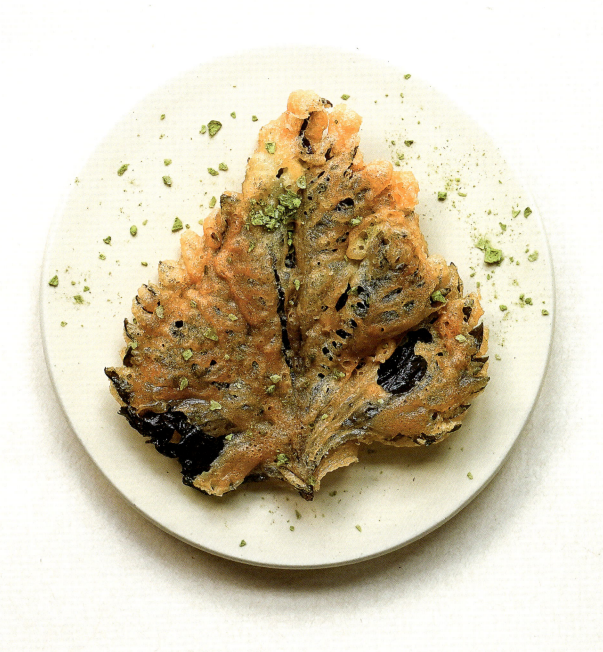

MEADOWSWEET · FILIPENDULA ULMARIA

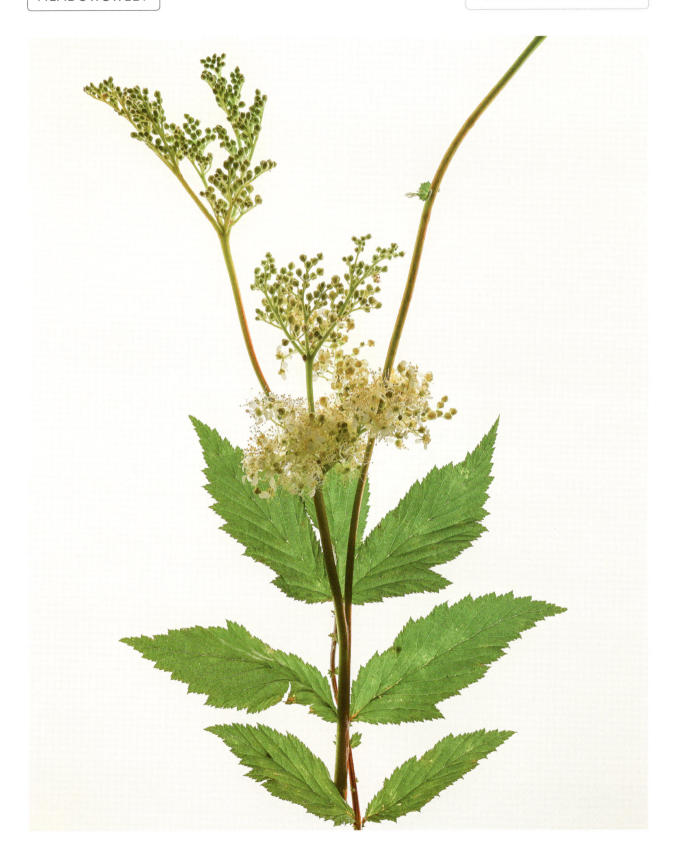

Queen of the Meadows

Together with water mint (*Mentha aquatica*) and verbena (*Verbena officinalis*), meadowsweet was one of the three sacred herbs of the Druids. In French, it is called *la reine des-prés*, "the Queen of the Meadows." Meadowsweet was the favorite plant of England's Queen Elizabeth I—she had it strewn on the floors of her chambers as a vermin repellent and for its pleasant fragrance. Not surprisingly, the plant's flower buds are nowadays used in the perfume industry.

Traditionally, the flowers' most common use was medicinal. Meadowsweet's fruits are spiroid, hence the name spirea. The other plant parts contain active compounds.

Use

Meadowsweet was the first plant in which aspirin-like substances were discovered. The name of the synthetically made medicine aspirin was derived from the plant's original Latin name *Spirea ulmaria*. Meadowsweet does not affect the stomach the way synthetic aspirin does. Thousands of people die every year as a result of internal bleeding caused by synthetic aspirin. The plant does not have these side effects, because it does not contain any blood thinning substances.[109]

In pharmacognosy and in practice, the plant has been proven to be anti-inflammatory and to have muscle-relaxing and analgesic properties. When the plant is taken for a somewhat longer time, it also has a lasting effect on joint pain. Meadowsweet is therefore known for its anti-rheumatic properties. In addition, the plant is used to treat flu.[110]

Appearance

Meadowsweet tends to grow in damp soils along streams and ditches and can be found throughout Western Europe, the United Kingdom, and the eastern United States. The flowers can be harvested between the months of June and August. The plant grows to a height of 1–1.5 meters and has small creamy-white flowers. The flowers grow in funnel-shaped clusters at the top of the plant's stems and give off a soft almond-like scent that is also redolent of honey. The small fruits are spiral-shaped. The bright green leaves are interruptedly pinnate and consist of 5–15 loose independent leaflets.

Extracting and Dosing

Every summer, I like to harvest a few meadowsweet flowers in order to have my own natural aspirin at home. It is one of my favorite medicinal plants. When picking, I always leave 75 percent of the plants where they grow.

Once I've harvested the flowers, I dry them in a dark room for 2 weeks by hanging them from horizontally stretched strings. I keep the dried flowers in a plastic Ziplock bag in a dark closet so that no light and oxygen can get to it. This way they will keep for longer.

Herbalist Geert Verhelst recommends taking the plant for an extended period of time for joint complaints. The recommended daily amount is approximately 3 grams (0.1 ounces) of dried flowers. If you drink the plant as a tea or use it as a substitute for aspirin, then do not exceed this dose.

PROPERTIES
- Anti-inflammatory
- Muscle-relaxing
- Analgesic
- Helps with flu
- Anti-rheumatic

SOURCING

It's best to go out into nature yourself and pick the flowers along the banks of rivers and ditches during the months of June to August. Dried flowers are also occasionally available on the market or in health food stores.

CAUTION

Do not exceed the recommended dose. You may develop a headache when you drink several cups of tea in a day. Do not use meadowsweet if you are hypersensitive to aspirin or are pregnant.

Leaves and Flowers

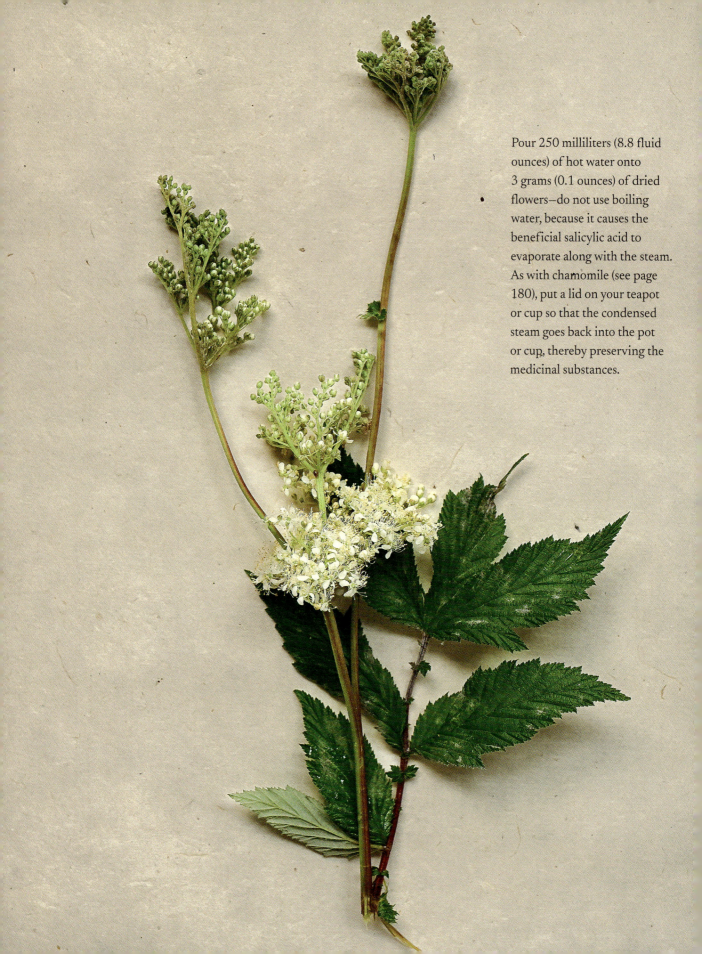

Pour 250 milliliters (8.8 fluid ounces) of hot water onto 3 grams (0.1 ounces) of dried flowers—do not use boiling water, because it causes the beneficial salicylic acid to evaporate along with the steam. As with chamomile (see page 180), put a lid on your teapot or cup so that the condensed steam goes back into the pot or cup, thereby preserving the medicinal substances.

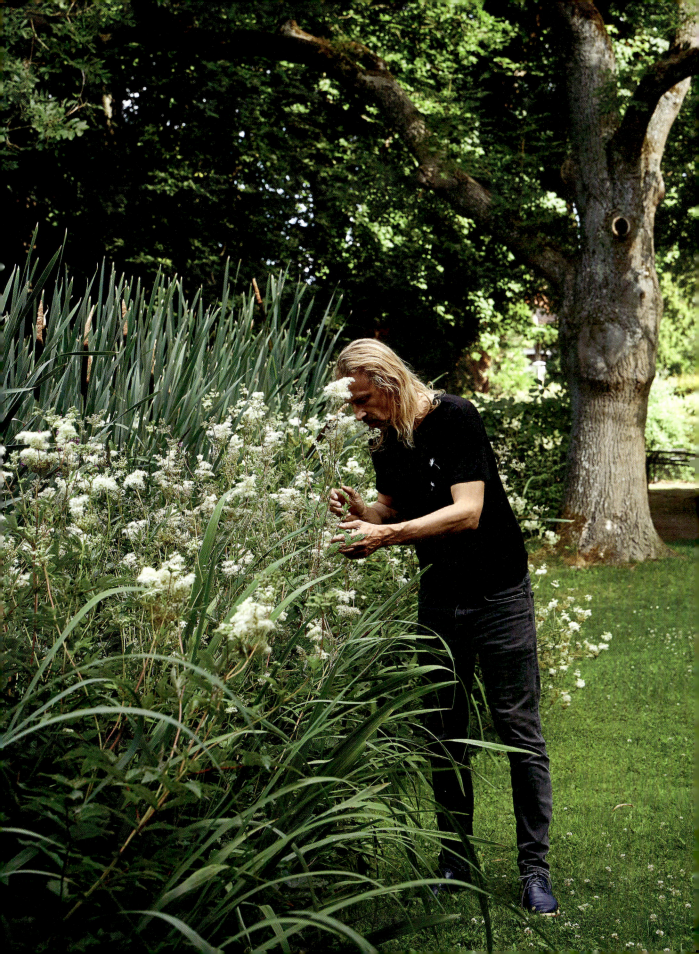

FETA WITH PEAS AND MEADOWSWEET

serves 4 people

■ **FOR THE MEADOWSWEET DRESSING**
- 25 ml/0.8 fl oz apple cider vinegar
- 25 ml/0.8 fl oz natural vinegar
- 100 g/3.5 oz meadowsweet

■ **FOR THE PARSLEY OIL**
- about 1 bunch (approx. 80 g/2.8 oz) leaf parsley
- 200 ml/7 fl oz sunflower oil

■ **AS WELL AS**
- pinch of fine sea salt
- 500 g/17.6 oz peas in the pod (optional: including shoots)
- 250 g/8.8 oz feta cheese

■ **EQUIPMENT**
- cheesecloth

method

Start by making the meadowsweet dressing. Put both types of vinegar together with the meadowsweet in a pan, and bring to a boil. As soon as it has reached boiling point, turn off the heat, and cover with a lid. Set aside for 1 hour, then strain the contents of the pan into a bowl.

Pick the green leaves from the parsley; without stalks this will leave you with about 40 grams (1.4 ounces). If you have less, add some more parsley leaves. Whizz the leaves in a blender with the sunflower oil for 30 minutes until it is as smooth as possible. This will heat up the oil, which is what we want. Sieve the parsley oil through a piece of cheesecloth over a bowl, squeeze well.

Fill a saucepan with plenty of water, and bring to the boil. Stir in the salt. Add the pea pods, and blanch for 2 minutes. Rinse immediately in ice water. Halve the pods—not at the seam but on the other side so that the peas are cut exactly in half.

In a bowl, mix the meadowsweet dressing with the parsley oil, and pour onto a deep plate. Arrange the halved pods over this mixture, and crumble the feta cheese on top. You can use the shoots from the pods as additional garnish.

Leaves and Flowers

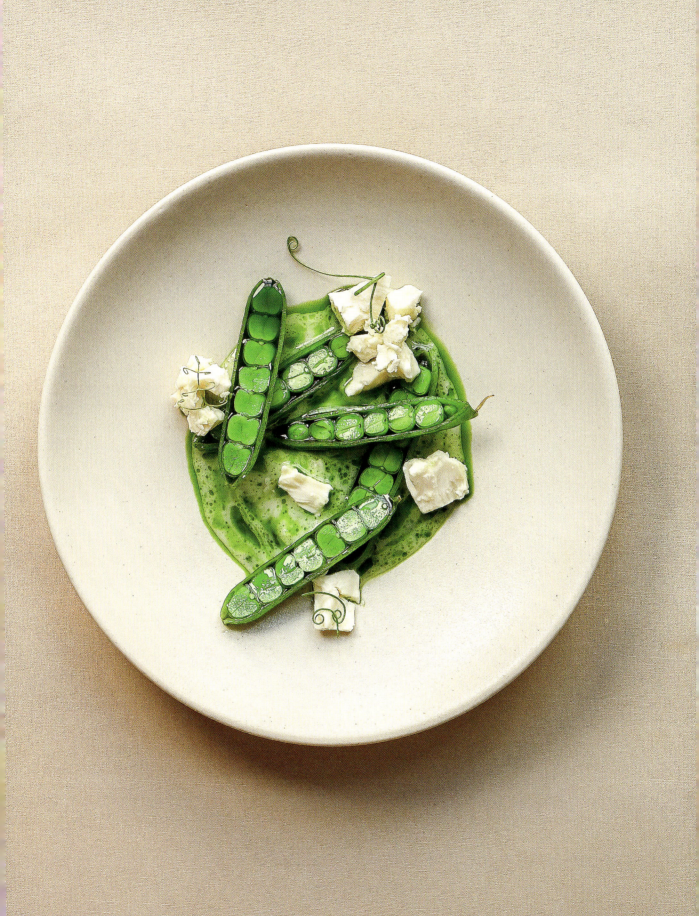

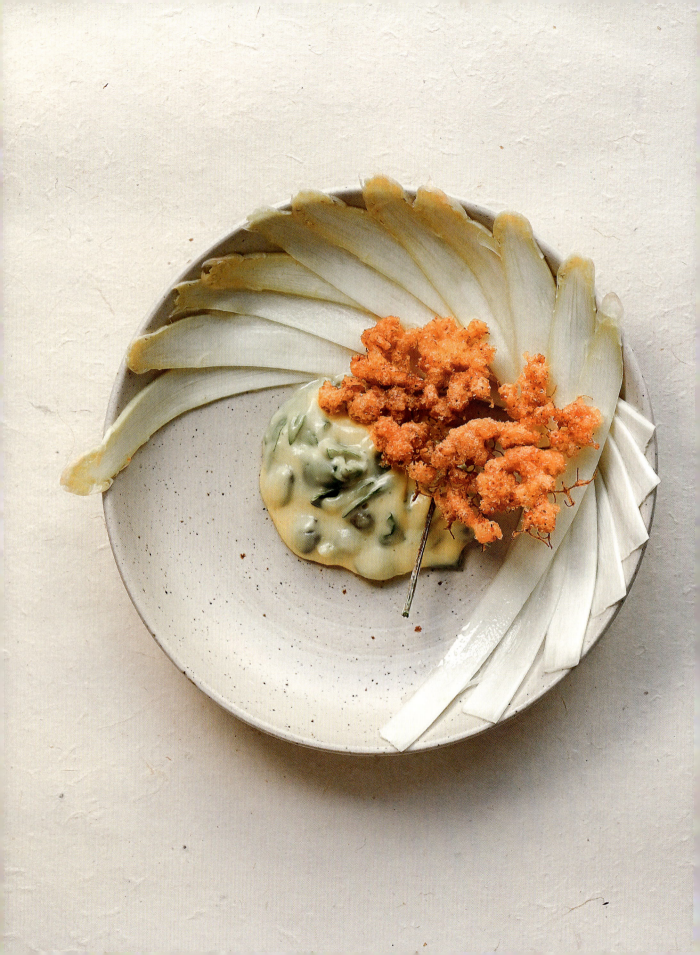

TEMPURA OF MEADOWSWEET WITH WHITE ASPARAGUS AND GRIBICHE SAUCE

serves 4 people

■ FOR THE GRIBICHE SAUCE
- 1 egg
- 15 g/0.5 oz (1 T) Dijon mustard
- 15 ml/0.5 fl oz (1 T) red wine vinegar
- 5 ml/0.16 fl oz (1 tsp) balsamic vinegar
- fine sea salt and freshly ground black pepper
- 250 ml/8.5 fl oz grapeseed oil
- 15 g/0.5 oz (1 T) finely chopped capers
- 15 g/0.5 oz (1 T) finely chopped leaf parsley
- 15 g/0.5 oz (1 T) finely chopped chervil
- 15 g/0.5 oz (1 T) finely chopped tarragon

■ FOR THE ASPARAGUS
- 8 spears white asparagus
- 1 lemon

■ FOR THE TEMPURA
- 2 egg yolks
- 90 ml/3 fl oz ice-cold sparkling water
- 40 g/1.4 oz flour
- 1 L/34 fl oz sunflower oil
- 4 tops with meadowsweet blossoms
- pinch of fine sea salt

■ EQUIPMENT
- peeler
- mandolin (optional)
- pan for deep-frying
- kitchen thermometer
- skimmer

method

Gribiche sauce is a cold egg sauce made by emulsifying hard-boiled eggs with mustard and oil. Boil the egg for 8 minutes, then plunge it in cold water to stop cooking—the egg white will be firm and the yolk semi-soft. Peel the egg, and mash with a whisk in a bowl. Add the mustard, the two kinds of vinegar, and a pinch of salt and pepper. Beat until as smooth as possible and, while whisking, add the grapeseed oil drop by drop. This will create a mayonnaise. Stir in the capers and fresh herbs.

Peel the asparagus stalks with a peeler, and thinly slice lengthways. This works very well with a mandolin or a vegetable peeler. Squeeze the juice of the lemon over the asparagus slices, and leave to marinate for 3 minutes.

Make the tempura batter by whisking the egg yolks, the ice-cold sparkling water, and flour in a bowl. A few lumps of flour is not a disaster, but it is better if you do not have too many. Meanwhile, heat the sunflower oil to 180°C (350°F) in a deep saucepan with a thick bottom.

Dip the meadowsweet blossoms into the tempura. Place them carefully in the hot oil. Remove the crispy meadowsweet after about 2 minutes, and drain on kitchen towels. Season with a little salt. Note: For best results, it is important that the meadowsweet blossom is dry and that the oil remains hot and the tempura batter cold. To keep it that way, do not fry everything at once, which causes the oil to cool down too much.

Arrange the asparagus slices on deep plates, and serve with the gribiche sauce and the tempura of meadowsweet.

Leaves and Flowers

DANDELION | TARAXACUM OFFICINALE

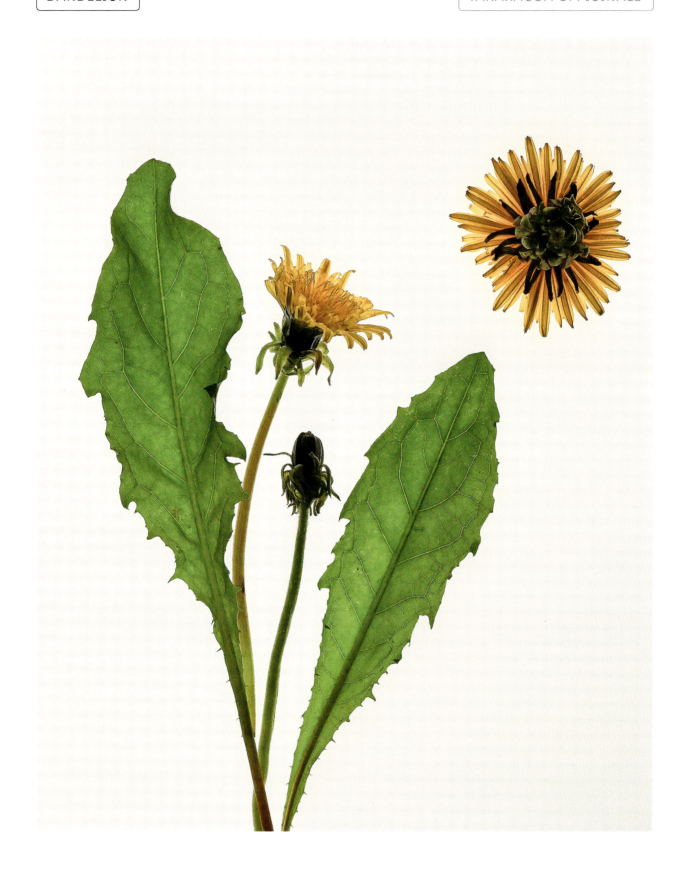

Blood Cleanser and Liver Tonic

I still enjoy blowing away the spent seedhead of a dandelion. As children, we looked for them in the meadow. Blowing away the fluff was a magical experience to me. They are carried on the wind like mini parachutes to create new life somewhere else. At home, we sometimes used the young leaves in a salad, and I occasionally eat a fresh bitter yellow dandelion to help me stay healthy. In spring, I transform the root into a powerful and cleansing elixir.

Dandelions were well known among the ancient Egyptians, Greeks, and Romans and have been used in traditional Chinese medicine for more than a 1,000 years. Although the dandelion is nowadays regarded a weed, it is also a symbol of happiness. How many times have you not wished for something you would like to come true while blowing on a dandelion head? Alongside daisies, they also add cheerful uplifting color to monotonous lawns. Dandelions and chamomile are known as "soil doctors," because they help plants growing near them.

The *officinale* part of the Latin name shows us that this plant was also included in the ancient healers' apothecary. The word *Taraxacum* comes from the Greek *taraxis*, which means "disorder," while *akas* means "remedy"—a remedy for disorder in the body. The English name "dandelion" is derived from the French *dent-de-lion* (lion's tooth), referring to its serrated leaves.[111]

The yellow flowers are a good source of nectar for bees, the basis for delicious dandelion honey. As a beekeeper, I know that when you see the first dandelion come into flower in spring, the bees may start to swarm. The roasted root of the dandelion used to be a popular coffee substitute (and alcohol tincture) and is available in many health food stores. The plant was also used to dye fabrics a yellowish-brown.

Use

Dandelion is one of the most useful medicinal plants, because all of its parts are effective and safe to use. The plant is rich in potassium and calcium and vitamins A and C. The leaves are a powerful diuretic. Its sap is a very strong remedy for warts and corns.[112] For this, you can rub the sap on the area to be treated daily; it also works for eczema and ulcers. The sap additionally supports the treatment of cardiovascular disease. The flowers contain constituents that are good for your lungs. They can be boiled with honey as a cough remedy but are also delicious for quenching thirst.

Traditional application methods are based on centuries of experimental research. Because of their various pharmacological properties, the identification, isolation, and characterization of the phytochemicals in dandelions are the subject of great interest and importance to the medical profession.

PROPERTIES
- Spring cleanser
- Blood cleanser
- Helps against osteoarthritis and rheumatism
- Bile-forming
- Diuretic
- Bitter agent
- Liver and kidney tonic
- Antioxidant
- Anti-nausea

SOURCING

You can pick dandelions yourself in nature. You can also dig out the roots. Be mindful of the plant's next generation when you take it; the rule of thumb is that you leave in place 75 percent of the plants you pick. Some drugstores and health food stores sell dried dandelion roots, flowers, and tea.

CAUTION

Overdosing can cause diarrhea. Do not drink more than 2–3 cups per day. Watch carefully how you respond to it. It has a detoxifying effect, which brings with it certain phenomena, such as a light headache when you have just begun to use it. According to Verhelst, very large doses can cause electrolyte imbalance that can lead to cardiac arrhythmias and intestinal and stomach disorders. Do not use dandelion preparations any longer than 4–6 weeks, as they can be extremely powerful.

Leaves and Flowers

The inulin mainly present in its roots helps stabilize blood sugar fluctuations. In addition, the plant contains flavones. Flavones have anti-aging, anti-inflammatory, and cardioprotective properties.[113]

Young spring leaves have a pleasantly bitter flavor and are sometimes used in salads. Eating and tasting the bitter leaves activates overall digestion and thereby helps improve food uptake. The plant stimulates the appetite, promotes the secretion of gastric juices, and has a detoxifying effect.[114] It helps prevent gas, nausea, and constipation. The plant is also used to cleanse the liver and as a blood cleanser to treat arthritis and relieve rheumatoid symptoms.

In short, dandelion contains substances that stimulate many glands and organs and have a particularly strong effect on the kidneys and liver. It is known as a liver and gallbladder tonic (a tonic is the name for an invigorating agent that stimulates and strengthens the whole body or specific parts). An extract of the root can be used as a hair tonic, thus vitalizing it.

As a bittering agent, dandelion stimulates the secretion of all digestive juices. This helps revitalize the entire body with better nutrition uptake, helping you to regain your strength after winter or an illness. The bitter substances in dandelion ensure that digestive substances are excreted more effectively. These substances act on the tongue's receptors, which in turn sends a signal to the brain. In order to enjoy their effect, you need to taste bitter substances properly and not swallow too quickly.

Dandelion is rich in many bioactive compounds with medicinal effects, including flavonoids. Because too high an intake of flavonoids in the form of dietary supplements and products with added flavonoids is potentially harmful, some doctors discourage taking them indiscriminately. Certain flavonoids in isolated form are known to potentially affect the action of some medications, for instance. If you use dandelion extracts with isolated components, it is important to discuss this with a doctor and experienced phytotherapist. Be careful of just taking flavonoid extracts; it is much better to get nutrients directly from eating as many diverse, healthy, fresh organic foods as possible. You can pick dandelions yourself almost anywhere, and add these to a salad or other dish. They contain the flavonoid luteolin, which is a strong antioxidant. This substance is also present in parsley and nettle.

Another medicinal action of the dandelion is its effect on stimulating the passage of urine. Dandelion extract causes the body to heat up, causing sweating. The blood is purified in the process, and water is discharged through sweat and urine. Uric acid—in part the cause of rheumatism and what supports it—is drained away along with the

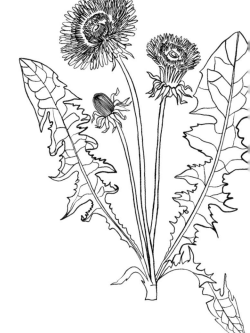

water, and this is effective in reducing the effects of rheumatoid arthritis. In phytotherapy, dandelion is often used to improve excessively low blood sugar levels and for its cholesterol-lowering and detoxifying effects.

The Swiss physician and natural healer Dr. Alfred Vogel thought extremely highly of dandelion, saying: "Dandelion has a wonderful effect on the liver, and helps to strengthen the liver, one of our most important organs."[115] He recommended using it in spring cures but in low doses, like the winter radish. Our kidneys and liver are the organs that help purify our body and blood. The active phytochemicals from dandelions activate both the kidneys and liver; because of this, blood flow to and through our connective tissue is also much greater. Connective tissue is not only located around muscles but also inside muscles, muscle fibers, around organs, bones, and nerves, and underneath our skin. Connective tissue is like a kind of glue in our body

Leaves and Flowers

that holds everything together. It can become inflamed if you do not move enough; it can lead to your body retaining toxins.

Appearance

The yellow dandelion is the only flower that appears to represent the three celestial bodies of the sun, moon, and stars. The entire flower looks like the sun, the white ball with its dried seeds like the moon, and the dispersing seeds resemble the stars. This flower has one of the longest flowering seasons of any plant. The plant's seeds, which look like mini parachutes, are carried by the wind for a distance of five kilometers (about 3 miles).

Dandelions open in the morning and close at night. If you mow them down on your lawn, the flower will become smaller, but it will survive—the dandelion will simply not let its flowers rise as high above ground level and will sit just below mowing height.

The root of the dandelion can grow from 30 centimeters (1 foot) to 1 meter (3.3 feet) deep. When you dig them out, the roots are blackish-brown on the outside and white-loamy on the inside. The stems of the flowers are hollow and produce a white milky sap when you break them. The leaves of the dandelion are serrated and lie on the ground like a rosette, sometimes growing diagonally upwards around the stems of the flowers.

Extracting and Dosing

To make dandelion tea, dry the plant and then pour hot water over it. You can use the milky sap from the leaves and stems to treat warts, corns, and eczema. Pick the flower when it is still yellow. Rub it on the spot that you want to treat. Squeeze as much milk sap from it as possible; damaging the plant releases the sap. You can apply this directly onto the relevant spot until your problem has been resolved. If you break a stem, you will see the milky sap appear. The sap contains most of the active ingredients. Repeat twice a day.

If you want to use a dandelion tincture, it is best to do so for at least 1 month, but no longer than 6 weeks.

In the spring, you can use the leaves in salads. You can make your own alcohol tincture from the root. Verhelst suggests taking 40 drops, 3 times a day, for 4 to 6 weeks (no longer).

A powerful herbal tonic is easily made from the plant itself, by infusing the root in an alcohol substance for a few weeks (see p. 26). This macerate needs filtering.

Bitter-Wood Extraction

Earlier, I talked about another bitter substance (see p. 119), which I would like to return to here, in conjunction with the bitter dandelion. In Suriname, I learned how to make a cold-water extraction, or bitter drink, from the extremely bitter wood of the bitter-wood (*Quassia amara*). This plant is used as medicine for many different conditions. The bitter water stimulates digestion, kills parasites, purifies the blood, and has expectorant properties. In Suriname, I was told that your blood turns bitter because of this extract, which also makes mosquitoes less likely to bite you. In addition, it is said to restore your body's hormonal balance. *Quassia amara* has been used for centuries by the Indians in South America to suppress fever. The plant also combats malaria symptoms due to it bitter substances, which effectively stop malaria parasites from multiplying.

Cut small cups from the white wood of the plant, and fill with water (see photo page 19). Leave overnight, then drink the bitter extract the following morning on an empty stomach. A course of treatment usually last 3 weeks. The first week you drink this bitter-wood extract every day, the second week every other day, and the last week once every 3 days. Pregnant women are advised not to take this drink.

Once the bitter substance from the cup has "finished," you can put the wooden cup in a glass of water and weigh it down with a spoon to keep the wood submerged. This is how you extract the outside of the wood as well. Only use bitter-wood for a short period of time; you can repeat the course after about 3 months.

Leaves and Flowers

BITTER SALAD LEAVES, DANDELION, AND ROASTED GRAPEFRUIT

serves 4 people

FOR THE SALAD
- 1 head Castelfranco (a pale, milder-tasting Italian heirloom variety of radicchio)
- 1 head Rossa di Treviso radicchio (an endive-shaped Italian heirloom variety of radicchio)
- 1 bunch (approx. 200 g/7 oz weight, unwashed) mole's salad* (young dandelion leaves)
- 2 dandelion leaves
- 1 grapefruit

FOR THE GINGER VINAIGRETTE
- 15 ml/0.5 fl oz (1 T) sushi vinegar
- juice of ½ lime
- 30 ml/1 fl oz (2 T) sunflower oil
- 15 ml/0.5 fl oz (1 T) ginger syrup

EQUIPMENT
- chef burner

method

*Mole's salad is a type of dandelion grown in the dark, just like chicory, which keeps its whitish-yellow color by also being grown buried in the soil. Mole's salad gets its name from "molehill." If the dandelion continues to grow underneath it, it stays a pale yellow and is more edible.

Remove the leaves from the Castelfranco and Rossa di Treviso radicchio, along with the mole's salad and dandelion leaves. Wash and dry the salad leaves.

Peel the grapefruit, including the white membranes of the segments, and carefully cut out each individual segment. Roast with a chef burner until the grapefruit segments are black.

In a bowl or jam jar, mix together the ingredients for the ginger vinaigrette until homogeneous. In a larger bowl, dress the salad with the vinaigrette, and garnish with the roasted grapefruit.

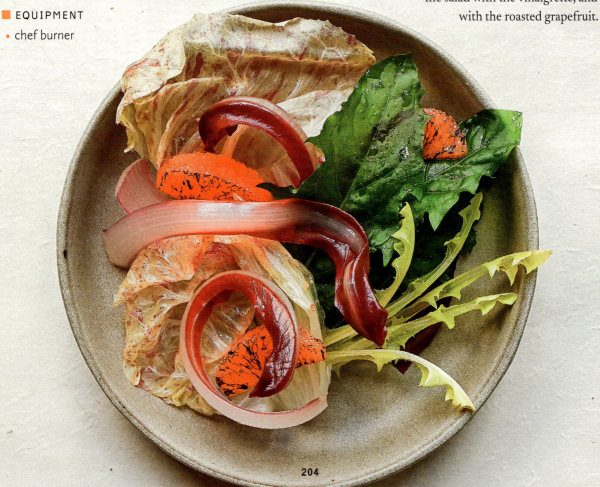

SALSA VERDE WITH DANDELION AND ZUCCHINI

serves 4 people

■ FOR THE SALSA VERDE
- 2 bunches (approx. 160 g/5.6 oz) leaf parsley
- 100 g/3.5 oz dandelion leaves
- 3 garlic cloves
- 42.5 g/1.5 oz (3 T) capers
- 14 g/0.5 oz (1 T) fine Dijon mustard
- fine sea salt
- 400 ml/13.5 fl oz olive oil
- 44 ml/1.5 fl oz (3 T) red wine vinegar

■ FOR THE SALAD
- 1 yellow zucchini
- 1 green zucchini
- 4 baby zucchinis

■ EQUIPMENT
- mandolin (optional)

method

Finely chop the parsley, dandelion leaves, garlic, and capers in a food processor. Add the mustard and a pinch of salt. With the food processor running add the olive oil, a few drops at a time. Add the red wine vinegar last; whizz for a few more minutes.

Thinly slice the yellow and green zucchini lengthways, preferably on the mandolin, and blanch briefly in a pan of salted boiling water. Char-grill the baby zucchini on a barbecue or in a grill pan *al dente*, which takes about 5 minutes.

Arrange the blanched zucchini slices in a wave pattern over 4 plates, and top each plate with a grilled baby zucchini. Sprinkle with salt to taste. Spoon the salsa verde around it.

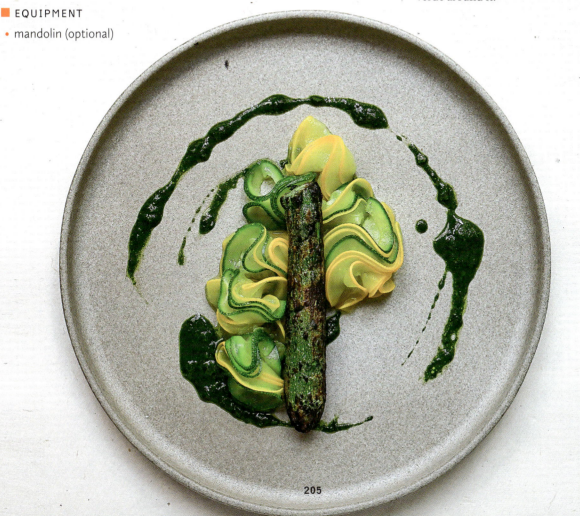

FURTHER PLANT JOURNEYS

COCA

*Erythroxylum coca /
Erythroxylum novogranatense*

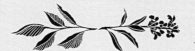

Teacher Plant

The sacred coca plant has been used by the traditional cultures in the Andes and the Amazon for its healing and energy-boosting properties for no fewer than 8,000 years. The plant has potent alkaloids and is regarded as a so-called "teacher" or "master" plant, because it arouses a devotional alertness. The plant is also widely used in rituals and is considered sacred. Coca has concentration-, endurance-, and meditation-improving properties. Indigenous people chew the leaves together with an alkaline substance such as lime or ash in a ratio of 1:10. By combining a base (ash, lime, or sodium bicarbonate), the leaf, and saliva, the plant's substances can be taken up through the mucous membranes of the mouth. The leaves are occasionally smoked to induce a trance, but this has no stimulating effect. In some places, the dried leaves are powdered and mixed with ashes before they are placed between the cheek and gums. They call this mixture *ipadu* in Bolivia.

Harvard University researchers found that coca leaf contains large amounts of lime, iron, and vitamins, including very high levels of vitamin A. Also present in the leaves is 0.2–1 percent cocaine. The leaves also contain vitamins C, E, and B2 and minerals such as magnesium, barium, copper, zinc, aluminum, and phosphate. They additionally contain proteins, fats, carbohydrates, and essential oils.

In the Netherlands, most people associate two things with the word coca: Coca-Cola and cocaine. Currently, Coca-Cola is by far the largest company to buy coca leaves—by the ton-load—from Peru. Research has been conducted for some time on the role Coca-Cola has played in bringing about a ban on coca leaf, which is now on the international Single Convention on Narcotic Drugs' list of narcotics. Coca has been used for millenia by Andean people as a ritual and medicinal plant. There, coca is accepted as a normal part of life like coffee, tea, and alcohol. In Peru and Bolivia, many people are convinced that the Coca-Cola lobby is the cause of the global ban on the plant. The former president of Bolivia, Evo Morales (2006–2019), who was originally a coca farmer himself, initiated a new strategy when he took office: "Yes to Coca, No to Cocaine." Bolivia is trying to correct the historical error at the United Nations by having the traditional uses of the coca plant recognized through legal procedures.

The increasing popularity of cocaine in the 1980s led to a drugs war. In fact, the so-called "war on

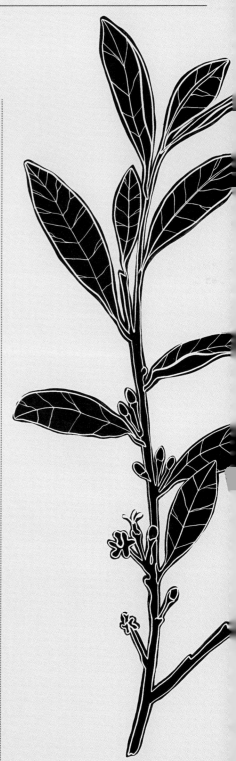

Leaves and Flowers

COCA

FURTHER PLANT JOURNEYS

*Erythroxylum coca /
Erythroxylum novogranatense*

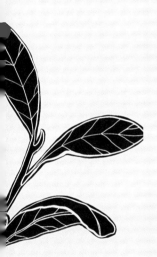

drugs" began with a battle against Mexican marijuana and peyote. Later, coca plantations were dug over or, in Colombia, sprayed with pesticides. Nevertheless, every country can import cocaine for medical and scientific purposes; there is no secret about that.

At the beginning of the 20th century, the Netherlands was an important trader in coca leaf and produced its own cocaine from this. The Netherlands East Indies became the largest grower of coca plants during that period, and in Amsterdam, in particular, the proceeds were traded. The factory that processed the raw material into cocaine was the Nederlandsche Cocaïne Fabriek (Dutch Cocaine Factory) in the Amsterdam Schinkelstraat. The Dutch Cocaine Factory was taken over by KZO, which was later to become Akzo Nobel.

In 1878, the first coca bushes were brought from South America to the Botanic Garden in Buitenzorg on Java. Shortly thereafter, a start was made with growing the crop for commercial purposes on Java, Madura, and Sumatra. The Colonial Bank of Amsterdam, in particular, played an important role in coca production and trade. The annual reports of this bank show that, by 1891, nearly 20 tons of leaves had been traded. During the following years until the turn of the century, the Colonial Bank traded between 34 and 81 tons of coca leaves. The consignments were initially exported to Germany, but due to the growing demand for cocaine and rising production on Java, introducing domestic cocaine manufacture was seen as a profitable proposition.

The Dutch Cocaine Factory was established by the Colonial Bank for this purpose on March 12, 1900.

Coca plants imported from Bolivia were raised on Java. These were then processed into cocaine in Amsterdam. The product was used as a remedy for neck, chest, and lung complaints. However, it was an open secret that it was also traded as a stimulant.

Coca leaves are used in the popular beverage Coca-Cola once most of the cocaine has been eliminated by heating the leaves a little. Yet Coca-Cola still contains cocaine—albeit in very small quantities—as has been demonstrated by students at the University of Deventer. An exception is made for the Coca-Cola Company on the UN trade ban on the cultivation, use, and trade of coca leaves as a flavoring agent, under the condition that the final product does not contain any cocaine alkaloids. Coca-Cola mentions the presence of decocainized coca extract on its website.

Until 1905, the leaves were not decocainized, and Coca-Cola thus contained a considerable amount of cocaine. Cocaine's bad name has led to many beneficial effects of coca receding into the background, and to the native culture of the coca-consuming peoples coming under pressure. The dried leaves chewed in the right way have super-tonic properties and are seen as a superfood by many people.

Leaves and Flowers

FURTHER PLANT JOURNEYS

BLUE LOTUS

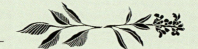

Nymphaea nouchali var. caerulea

Holy Flower

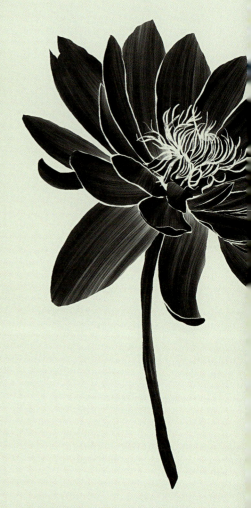

In ancient Egypt, blue lotus—known to us as blue water lily—was a sacred flower. Together with papyrus, the flower was the most important medicinal plant. Both plants symbolized Upper and Lower Egypt, respectively. Depicted together, they symbolized the union of the two parts of the country. Evidence has been found of blue lotus having been cultivated as early as 3,000 BCE, in square, evenly ordered areas. The blue lotus has meanwhile become the national flower of Egypt and continues to feature regularly in architectural decorations. Except as decoration, very little knowledge now exists about the use of this special Egyptian flower.

To the ancient Egyptians, the flower called *seshen* was a symbol of birth and rebirth and the River Nile. Seen from above, the Nile and its delta has the shape of a lotus. The Egyptians associated the blue lotus with the sun, which would disappear in the night and come back in the morning, just as the lily closed and opened again.

But the flower was also associated with death and rebirth. The famous *Egyptian Book of the Dead* mentions spells through which a person could be changed into a blue lotus. On a number of sarcophagus paintings, I saw an image of a blue lotus where the third eye should be, in between the eyes of the person interred in the sarcophagus.

The flowers were widely used as offerings at religious festivals and consumed during mind-expanding rituals. Blue lotus was used by ancient Egyptian priests for more than 3,000 years for its medicinal properties, and as a spiritual sacrament in the form of psychedelic wine from the death and rebirth cult; the flower's constituents are alcohol soluble.

It was often combined with *Peganum harmala*, the plant of the god Bes. Today, blue lotus has become very rare, and in Egypt grows almost nowhere in the wild (it is being cultivated in Thailand nowadays). This is because of the construction of the Aswan Dam on the Nile, preventing the river from seasonally overflowing and depositing mud on its banks. Some Egyptologists doubt that blue lotus was used for consumption. I disagree. It is clear that ancient Egyptians consumed blue lotus, as it is pictured in ancient hieroglyphics, including in the Tomb of Idut in Sakkara, among other foods offered to the pharaoh and the gods—I have seen this with my own eyes.

Likewise, during my travels to many other places in Egypt, I saw blue lotus representations among other foods. We have also found drinking cups in the form of a blue lotus.

In fact, I believe that the secret and the consumption of the blue lotus by ancient Egyptian priests is one of the keys to the consciousness of that time. In ancient Egypt, blue lotus was often pictured with mandrake and poppy, both plants with psychoactive properties.

Leaves and Flowers

FURTHER PLANT JOURNEYS

BLUE LOTUS

Nymphaea nouchali var. caerulea

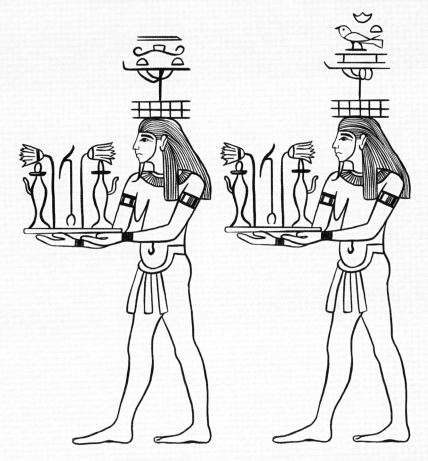

According to biology professor William Embodem, the Egyptians used blue lotus for its narcotic properties, and it was used by the elite of priests to induce shamanic ecstasy. Blue lotus causes mild hallucinogenic effects that were believed to be celestial in origin.

The effects I myself have observed are mildly euphoric and soothing, comparable to MDMA and opium. It is a very subtle effect. During the First World War, blue lotus was used in Europe as an anesthetic. The flower further contains a number of antioxidants that help remove free radicals.

In November 2014, I was in Egypt for six weeks working with botanist Madam Sohar in a botanical garden in the heart of Cairo. There, I collected, cut up, and soaked 50 blue lotus flowers in strong alcohol for three weeks. We then allowed the alcohol to evaporate using a *bain-marie* and drank the extract. The effects were mild but certainly noticeable.

I experienced a similar shift in consciousness with stronger extracts that I found in the Netherlands. Several independent studies have shown that blue lotus has psychoactive and stimulating properties.

Blue lotus was used to treat the liver, as a remedy for constipation, to regulate urine, and as an antidote to summer heat. Both the tubers and the flowers were used internally as well as externally. Lotus is commonly consumed medicinally throughout the world. It is reputed to enhance the libido and relieve adrenaline-induced stress. Like ginseng, lotus is an adaptogen, and improves the production and circulation of body fluids. Blue lotus has long been used to make perfume, and in aromatherapy. The fragrance is unique and soft and has a calming effect on the mind.

BLUE LOTUS – In ancient Egypt, blue lotus was used, along with other psychedelics such as mushrooms, opium, and mandrake, in psychedelic concoctions that were consumed in the mystery schools as a sacrament and often in offerings to the gods and pharaohs. The Egyptian priests seen here used blue lotus to induce a shamanic trance. They are carrying blue lotus on sacrificial platters. (Based on a drawing from *Ornamented Design Encyclopedia*, 2001.)

Leaves and Flowers

FURTHER PLANT JOURNEYS

HUACHUMA CACTUS

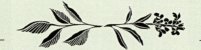

Trichocereus macrogonus var. pachanoi

Fountain of Knowledge

Huachuma is one of South America's oldest magic plants and has been used for more than 3,000 years. The plant is seen as one of the most important "teacher plants." In Peru, mescaline-containing cactus—following the arrival of the Spaniards and thus Christianity— was also called San Pedro cactus, after the Christian saint Peter. St. Peter, like the cactus, was believed to have the keys to heaven. When important decisions had to be made, huachuma was consulted as an advisor. In Bolivia, the cactus is often planted in or near the house to protect it and is kept as an "antenna" nearby.

People continue to work with the power plant in their healing ceremonies. The plant is used in fortune-telling. As a folk medicine, it is used "to reset the brain" and in microdoses as a brain tonic. Psychotherapeutic ceremonies, during which more substantial amounts of cactus juice are drunk, can last 24 hours. From experience, I know that the effects of the cactus at a high dose can be perceptible for up to 18 hours.

During the experience, which begins about one hour after you have taken it, your perception of the world as you know it changes, and it appears as though you can travel in other dimensions. Time and space as you know it in a normal waking state is transformed. Western scientists thus regard the cactus as hallucinogenic. Scientists would designate mescaline as an enabler of visions and spiritual experiences; the shaman would say, "It's God." It's that simple; it all depends on your perspective.[116] Most people in the West have a linear and reductionist materialistic worldview and can barely comprehend and understand what happens to their consciousness until they have tried it out for themselves. The cactus allows the user, independent of third parties, to come into direct contact with "heaven"–without the intervention of saints, priests, or a church, and while they are still on Earth.

Some artists and writers use the mescaline from huachuma for inspiration. One of the most famous was Aldous Huxley, who experimented with mescaline and therefore experienced higher forms of consciousness. Many people are familiar with his book on the subject, *The Doors of Perception*. In concrete terms, Huxley argues that we live in a narrow perceptual field, and opening up our mind to a greater diversity of perceptual experiences will improve our lives. He believed that psychedelic experiences can be useful for everyone and argued that mescaline

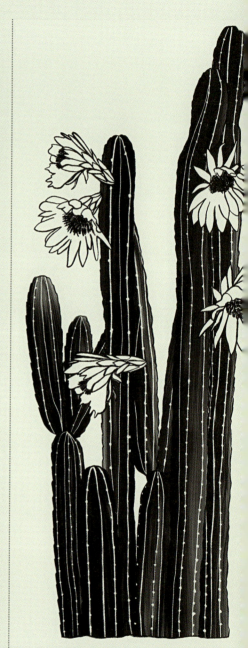

is a much more beneficial medicine for changing our consciousness. It is more spiritual and offers many more benefits than other drugs, such as alcohol and tobacco.

Leaves and Flowers

HUACHUMA CACTUS

FURTHER PLANT JOURNEYS

Trichocereus macrogonus var. pachanoi

Mescaline helps break down social conventions so that we can observe the world around us in our own unique way.

During ceremonies where the huachuma sacrament is taken— usually at night—a *curandero* (medicine man or ritual specialist) takes the lead. Participants sit in a circle around a fire, and the curandero tends to be accompanied by two assistants.[117] During ceremonies I have witnessed, the medicine man told us what properties the spirit of the cactus had and what to expect. A cleansing ritual follows, using burning palo santo (sacred incense from the Bursera graveolens tree that grows in the Yucatan and South America) or other aromatic smoke. Everyone is asked to think about their wishes or share them. The huachuma extract is drunk from clay bowls. The facilitators sing songs and play instruments to accompany the participants. During the ceremony, more rounds of sacrament are handed out, if desired. If you up the dosage of the drug, the visual visions and lucid dreams become stronger. With closed eyes, you then perceive beautiful geometric patterns and (fluidizing) colors. The extract does not give you a hangover, as with alcohol. The drug also continues to make itself felt in subtle ways days and weeks after the ceremony. In addition to the healing character of a huachuma ceremony, the cactus is believed to have properties to make prayers and wishes come true.

In San Pedro ceremonies, tobacco often plays an important role as well. During ceremonies, tobacco snuff (*rapé*) is used to "open the gates." The tobacco powder, mixed with ash and sometimes other plants, is blown into the nostrils through a special bamboo or bone pipe or tube. Sometimes tobacco is smoked. Before the tobacco is used, the medicine man usually sings a song to invite the spirit of tobacco, which activates its medicinal effect.

Should you ever have the opportunity to witness a San Pedro ceremony, to be on the safe side, please indicate that you do not want Brugmansia (Angel's Trumpet).

CHAVÍN CIVILIZATION – A hieroglyph from the non-violent Chavín civilization from Peru depicts a creature with a huachuma cactus (800 BCE). The original is located in Peru.

Brugmansia is sometimes added in ayahuasca potions. I had the plant on my roof terrace, until my dog ate some of it and trembled with anxiety for five days. Be well informed as to what you must do prior to the ceremony; you should usually abstain from certain foods or activities.

The magic cactus has helped the residents of South America for thousands of years to experience subtle energies, to obtain information, and to bring healing. More and more Westerners are discovering the cactus now as well. Not only as entertainment but in order to gain deep consciousness-altering experiences and visions, and as a key for opening the gate to wisdom.

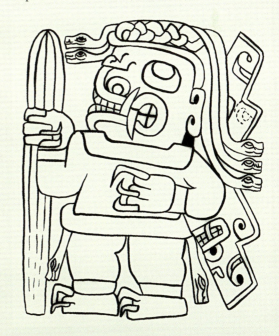

Leaves and Flowers

FURTHER PLANT JOURNEYS

PEYOTE CACTUS

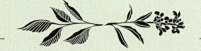

Lophoforia wiliamsii

Plant of the Heart

Peyote cactus, as most people know this power plant, originally comes from Mexico and southern North America and can still be found there in the wild. The cactus contains the powerful alkaloid mescaline. In the Indigenous Mexican language Nayuatl, which was also spoken by the Aztecs, *peyotl* means "radiant, shining, or brilliant heart." In the Aztec *Florentine Codex*, peyote is described as a medicine for fever and protection. According to the Wixárika (the oldest still active indigenous civilization, who live near the desert where the peyote grows), *peyotl* translates to "hearth of the earth" and is considered very *hu hu* (sacred).

The cactus is used medicinally for joint pain, paralysis, and to heal wounds. The cactus is a sacred plant. For the original Indigenous inhabitants of the Americas, peyote plays a central role in their perception of the world and is used as a therapeutic, and in ritual settings, as a sacrament. Many people have a sacred relationship with this "teacher plant."[118] The plant can now be found all over the world because travelers took the cacti with them and spread the seeds via botanical gardens, and because people have started breeding the cactus at home. To some Huichol Indians, this is blasphemy; they believe peyote's only true home is their sacred motherland. Huichol Indians meet annually and maintain a tradition that goes back many thousands of years. During these gatherings, they consume the cactus in a special sacred location, the *Wirikuta*. By going on peyote pilgrimages, the Huichol can accumulate "spirit power," regain their equilibrium, and "complete themselves as human beings." The ceremonial pilgrimages allow the *peyoteros* to undergo a metamorphosis, and after a number of trips they can transform into shamans. According to medicine man Kuathtli Vasquez, whom I met in 2014, the Huichol are the most powerful energetic healers in the world. For this they use bird feathers, with which they can clean the human energy field, as if with a lightning shaft, and remove ballast.

Sacred peyote is also discussed in the 1959 book *The Indian Dies* by Ernst Löhndorff, which describes the ruthless intrusion of Western "civilization," the deprivation of Indigenous lands, and the demise of Mexico's Yaqui Indians. During the First World War, the author lived for four years among the Yaqui in the vast Sierra Madre, the high mountains of northern Mexico, and describes the customs of the last descendants of this tribe. To the Yaqui, peyote was an important sacrament to induce visions. Löhndorff writes that under the influence of mescaline, it is as if his luminous eyes themselves project the images that come to his mind, like a magic lantern.[119] Peyote occupied a central role in the ceremonies and ritual customs of the Maya and the Aztecs. The Indigenous tribes of Mexico experience peyote as enabling them to connect with the spirit realm, their ancestors, and the gods of the earth and nature. Peyote was, and still is, being used for healing personal problems and traumas, to reinforce connection with nature, and to enable people to grow as individual human beings, and collectively. In most states of the USA, the use of peyote is restricted to religious ceremonies of the Native American Church, whose members primarily consist of descendants from Native American tribes. As peyote is used as a sacred sacrament, it falls under freedom of religion.

I have participated in several ceremonies, some as long as 20 hours, in which the cactus was distributed as a sacrament. I was invited to do a magic show at 8 o'clock in the morning for a group of people who had just experienced an all-night initiation and ceremony. Flowers arranged in a big red heart served as an altar in the middle of the room. People dressed in white sat around this in a circle. During my surprise appearance I was dressed in magical black. After concluding my show by making a table float through space, I took my seat in the circle and was given the medicine in exchange for my performance.

Leaves and Flowers

PEYOTE CACTUS

Lophoforia wiliamsii

I first received a very small amount of dried peyote powder to eat and, after about three-quarters of an hour, felt that it was a friendly plant. I say this, because I know that some plants can give you a mental beating. The medicine man told me that he did not want to overwhelm me with the experience the cactus can induce. It is safer to build up doses steadily to see what it does to you. Then I was given a larger amount of powder. Everything became crystal clear, and my observations sharpened. When I closed my eyes, I started to see geometric patterns, similar to the patterns on the mask I had bought in Mexico City during that trip. The art of the Huichol Indians is symbolic, geometric, organic, radiatingly colorful, and powerful; often beads glued with beeswax in geometric patterns onto anthropomorphic and animal figures.

Most Indigenous inhabitants of the Americas live by the grace of visions and live their lives from their visions. I learned this from the important book *Lame Deer: Seeker of Visions* and talks with Indigenous people. This kind of ritual and therapeutic use of entheogenic plants and mushrooms has been part of the free way of living of many countries' Indigenous inhabitants for thousands of years. They have contributed to the great American civilizations, to which the temple ruins in the jungles of the Yucatan Peninsula in Mexico and the handed-down writings on advanced astronomy and medicine masters attest. Various methods can be used to induce a vision. Sioux Indians induced visions by spending four days on a mountain, digging a pit in which they would stay crouched while fasting, and during that time would beg for a vision. Fasting is used in this way as a source of concentrating power. So-called "vision quests" occupy a central place in the lives of many American Indians. If, during such a session, they are blessed with a vision, they know from their soul what they have to do in their life. For a number of tribes, the sacrament to induce visions is the sacred mescaline-containing peyote cactus.

We should not confuse a vision with a hallucination. In a vision, everything becomes crystal clear and is accompanied by deep insights that later tend to be implemented. All cultures on Earth see visions. To us, the most well-known ones are the visions described in the Bible. A vision comes to us through the inner eye; the spiritual eye that is also called the "third eye" in some cultures. A hallucination is an impression that presents itself as a real perception but has no objective reality; it is an illusion. I believe that reality as we perceive it, is an agreement between hallucinations, as it were, and that reality is shaped by assumptions and previously agreed-upon outcomes, allowing the brain to see hallucinations as reality. This is what we call reality: controlled hallucinations interpreted by the brain in order to survive.

Do the predictive perceptions of the brain form our consciousness, or are we consciousness? Visions are meaningful, curious, but natural experiences in which profound, symbolic, and significant scenes are seen in the mind in multiple dimensions. From visionary experiences, people have been able to make great things happen. Not only in ancient traditions and rituals, but also both Steve Jobs (founder of Apple) and very likely Bill Gates (co-founder of Microsoft) received their visions under the influence of LSD, where they were shown clearly in their minds what they had to do. LSD resembles mescaline and psilocybin.

These kinds of stories, the use of psychedelics by academics, and so-called "microdosing" (in which small amounts of psychedelics are used to boost creativity and become smarter) are very popular in Silicon Valley. Correctly applied psychedelics simply provide humans with an advantage over other humans and animals because through the use of these prehistoric and magical agents more connections are made in the brain. Psychedelics also make you aware of the fact that everything is interconnected. The doors of perception open more widely.

BULBS AND ROOTS

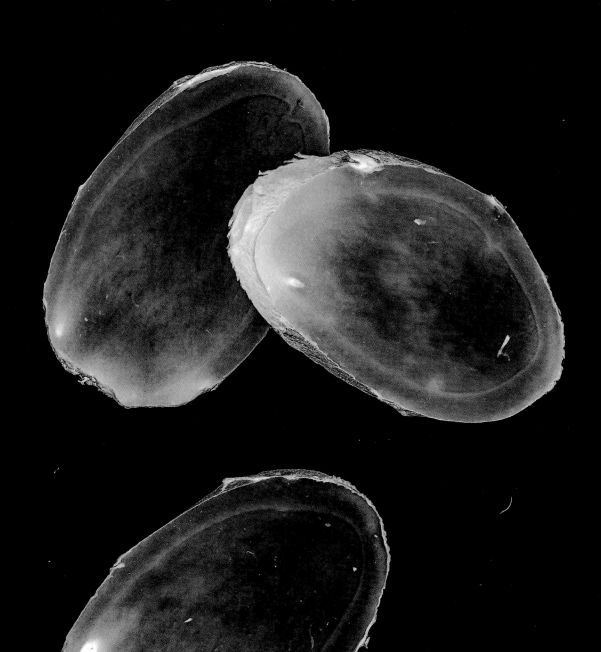

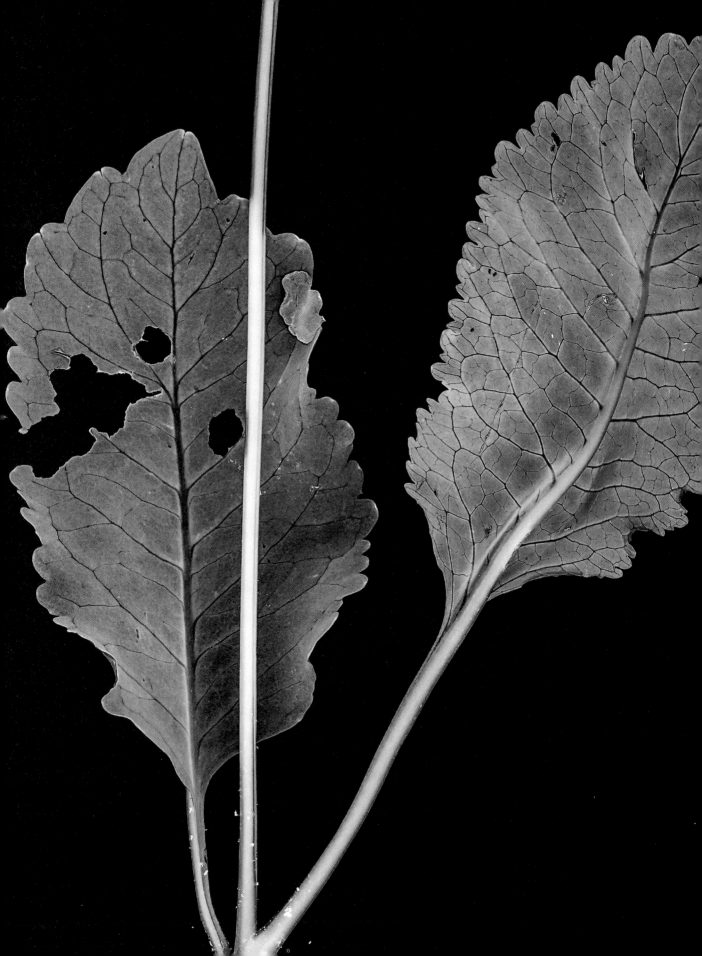

JORIS "Tubers and bulbs tend to have an important place in my dishes. They are a key ingredient in soups and sauces. Millefeuille of beet is one of my signature dishes, as is roast celeriac. In the restaurant, we often roast a celeriac on the spit for three hours. The outside turns a beautiful golden-brown, the inside well cooked and totally delicious."

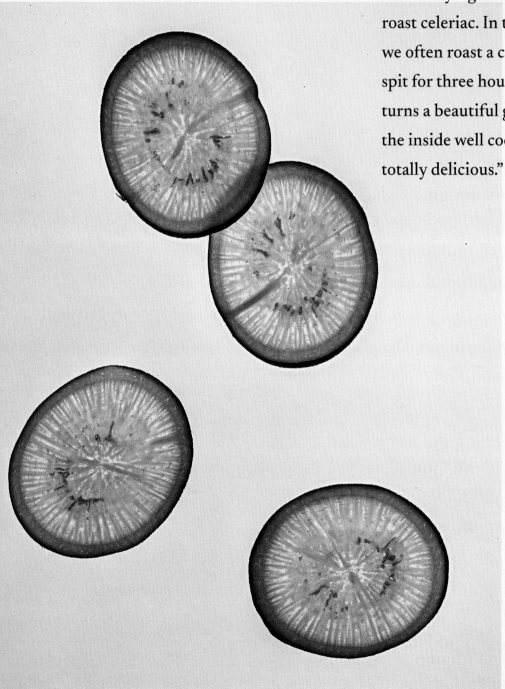

"And how about onion? I can't imagine a kitchen without onions. They occupy such an important place in almost every dish I make. Cooked, raw, or marinated; chopped alongside an oyster; minced with chives in a tartare; nicely caramelized with French beans—roots and bulbs are a mainstay in my kitchen. This is also because they are so deliciously sweet. These vegetables need to stand up to the cold in winter so that they don't disintegrate when there's a frost. Sugar, like salt and alcohol, has a freezing point–lowering effect."

W "True, plants have developed special methods to protect themselves. Crops cannot defend themselves like we do as animals, with sharp teeth, muscles, and claws. So they have developed different survival strategies."

J "Are those kinds of defenses or defense substances in plants actually bad for you?"

W "It varies. The bioactive substances in plants that have a positive effect on the human body are called *phytonutrients* and can be categorized in different classes. Also, plants sometimes contain *antinutrients*, which generally have negative effects on health. Antinutrients are natural substances that are found in some foods. They can inhibit the absorption of nutrients or are toxic. Known antinutrients are oxalic acid, phytic acid, and lectin. Oxalic acid is found in some fruits and vegetables and is used, among other things, to remove stains in wood. In small amounts, oxalic acid does little or no harm to human beings. Phytic acid is found in some grains and contributes to your body losing minerals, among other things. You can remove phytic acid by fermenting flour. For example, pancake flour used to be soaked overnight in buttermilk to reduce phytic acids and make it easier to digest."

J "How funny, now that you say that, I am reminded of oxalis, a kind of sorrel that grows in the forests and which we like to use for the delicious acidity that it adds to dishes. We know that we always have to use it in small quantities, but too much isn't particularly tasty anyway."

W "Do you ever ferment foods, albeit without the explicit aim of removing phytic acid from the product?"

J "Fermentation is actually a process of controlled decay, and I love it. It is one way through which ingredients will keep longer and is often delicious. A lot of our food has gone through a fermentation process. Just think about sourdough bread, beer, real butter, yogurt, cheese, and dried sausages—all kinds of everyday products, in fact. Sauerkraut would not be sour without fermentation. Sauerkraut, pickles, and kimchi are all prepared through *lactofermentation*. We often use that technique in my kitchen. We add a small amount of salt, usually around 2 percent, which kills the bad bacteria. The lactic acid bacteria already present on products can withstand this and can multiply unhindered, making the vegetables nice and sour. Water, salt, and the product that needs to be fermented—that's all it takes. Just enough salt kills the harmful bacteria. The good bacteria stay alive and convert the sugars into lactic acid. In this acid, the product keeps well and safe. I also find it interesting to experiment with fermented drinks like ginger ale."

GINGER | ZINGIBER OFFICINALE

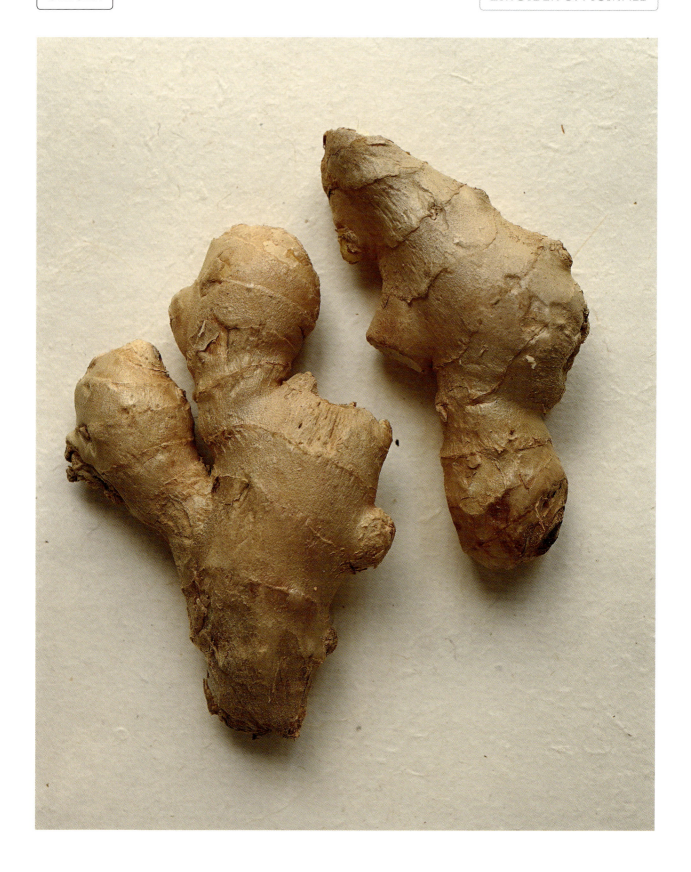

Stomach Strengthener

Ginger originally comes from Asia (presumably from tropical India), but it is now being grown in other subtropical climates. In India, where ginger has been used since Vedic times (1500 BCE), it is called *vishwabhenesaj*, "the universal medicine."[120] During the 13th and 14th centuries, ginger, together with black pepper, was one of the most traded spices. In the southwestern Indian province of Kerala, where I lived for six months, the spice is still widely traded. The ginger in the supermarket comes mostly from China, Brazil, and Peru these days, where it is grown. Ginger root hardly exists in the wild now.

Ginger belongs to the family *Zingiberaceae*, which also includes turmeric. The name *Zingiber* has its origin in Sanskrit and is derived from the word *srngavera*, meaning "deer antlers," a reference to its root. *Officinale* refers to the fact that the root has been in long use pharmaceutically, including in Western medicine. Ginger is a sweet, pungent, and aromatic spice that is widely used in cooking.

Use

In specialist medical literature, much has been written about ginger. Ginger supports various processes in the body such as digestion, combats nausea, is anti-inflammatory, antimicrobial, helps with high blood pressure, and is warming.[121] The root contains several vitamins and minerals, such as vitamins B1, B2, B6, and C, calcium, magnesium, iron, and zinc.

The Chinese sage Confucius (551–479 BCE) is known to have eaten fresh ginger with every meal to stimulate digestion and as a carminative (to reduce intestinal formation of gas). Chinese sailors chewed on ginger to help with seasickness.[122] Ginger strengthens the stomach and is an anti-emetic. Greek, Roman, and Arabic doctors used it for digestive complaints and stomach disorders.

Ginger is seen by herbalists in ayurveda and traditional Chinese medicine as a general stimulant, antispasmodic, stomach strengthener, carminative, and menstrual stimulant. In Western herbalism and ayurveda ginger is often used as a bio-enhancer. Like piperine from black pepper it enhances the bioavailability and effectiveness of other compounds. It is packed with antioxidants. Some studies show that ginger is effective in reducing the symptoms of osteoarthritis, especially in the knees.

Appearance

Ginger roots look a bit like deer antlers. The main root is branched into several fingers. The root has a matte light-brown surface and is pale yellow inside. Above ground, the plant is reed-like, with spear-shaped, alternate, grassy leaves. The plant grows 30 centimeters–1.5 meters (1–5 feet) high and likes well-drained humus-rich, alkaline soil in partial shade. Ginger does not grow in arid areas, and in the Netherlands and many other places can only be grown in greenhouses or indoors.

PROPERTIES
- Strengthens the stomach
- Anti-emetic
- Stimulates digestion
- Bio enhancer
- Improves appetite
- Vessel-dilating and stimulates the circulation, especially that of the skin
- Anti-inflammatory
- Antioxidant
- Warming

SOURCING

Ginger is widely available in supermarkets and at greengrocers and health food stores in fresh, dried, and powder form. You can also grow ginger yourself at home. It is a tropical plant, and thus needs heat to grow. During hot summer months the plant can be left outside, but conditions are generally more stable indoors. Before planting, soak the rhizome for several hours in water, then plant it just below the surface in potting compost, eyes facing up.

CAUTION

*Ginger interacts with some medications, including the anticoagulant warfarin and the cardiovascular drug nifedipine. If you have much inner heat or according to traditional Chinese medicine a lot of **yang**, take care with ginger. Do not take ginger if you have a high fever.*

Bulbs and Roots

Once the plant has matured (which, in the tropics, is 9–10 months after planting), the rhizome is harvested, cleaned, and dried. Ginger is best kept in cool, well-ventilated areas. In order to make ginger powder, the dried root is pulverized.

Extracting and Dosing

Just 1–1.5 grams (0.03–0.05 ounces) of ginger can help prevent various types of nausea, including nausea from chemotherapy, post-surgery, and travel and morning sickness. Just 1 gram (0.03 ounces) of fresh ginger or a glass of ginger tea is enough. To make ginger tea, slice a piece of ginger, and pour hot boiling water over this.

Ginger, along with black tea leaves, cinnamon, cloves, and cardamom pods, forms an integral part of the Indian spicy milk-tea known as *chai*. In Suriname, alcohol-free ginger beer (with cloves) is a popular thirst quencher.

In winter, drinking ginger as a tea and using it a little more often in cooking helps the body stay warm. As a basis of much Chinese food, a piece of ginger along with a few garlic cloves is pounded in a mortar and briefly fried in oil. This is an easy way to incorporate it into your cooking. Grating a piece of ginger into pumpkin soup adds delicious flavor and promotes digestion.

If you consume 1 teaspoon (5 grams/0.16 ounces) of ground ginger a few times a week, you lower the risk of inflammation in your body. It removes fat from the liver, thereby improving the functioning of this crucial detoxification organ.

Ginger can also be applied externally and, as an oil, improves blood flow locally.

CANDIED STEM GINGER WITH CREAM

serves 4 people

Use as much as you like of the following:

■ INGREDIENTS
- 250 g/8.8 oz young ginger
- Approx. 250 g/8.8 oz granulated sugar
- 100 ml/3.4 fl oz whipped cream

method

This is a dessert my mother loves. It's very simple, but because of the powerful flavor of the stem ginger, you do not need anything else with this except whipped cream.

Take a few good, fresh pieces of ginger. It's important that it's young ginger, otherwise it will be too stringy. Peel the ginger. This is easier to do if you first cut it into rough pieces. You can divide the peeled ginger into balls or cubes or leave it whole. Whole looks pretty, I think, but it's a little less practical to store.

Fill a pan with cold water, add the ginger, and bring to a boil. Simmer gently for 1 hour. Make sure the ginger is always covered in water. Drain, and put the ginger back in the pan, again just submerged under cold water. Note: Weigh how much water you added, and add the same weight in sugar.

Bring to a boil again and simmer gently for 30 minutes. Remove from the heat, allow to cool, and put the ginger, including the syrup, in the refrigerator overnight, or until it has cooled completely.

Then cook the ginger again for 10 minutes in the syrup, set aside to cool, and boil one last time for 10 minutes. If the syrup has evaporated too much, keep adding a little water when needed. The ginger should now be soft.

You can keep the ginger in the syrup for 2 weeks in the refrigerator, and if have you preserved it, in airtight jars for months. Or eat immediately with a spoon of half-beaten, unsweetened whipping cream.

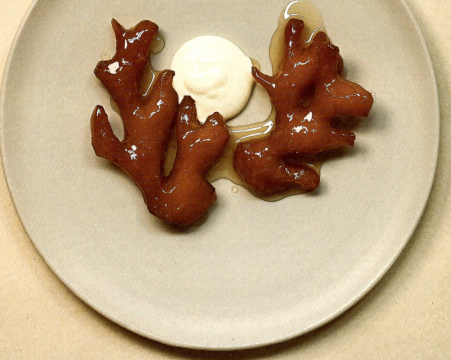

GINGER BEER WITH STRAWBERRIES

for about 1½ liters/51 fluid ounces

■ **FOR THE GINGER BEER STARTER**
- 1 L/34 fl oz water
- 30 g/1 oz granulated sugar (per day, for 7 days)
- 20 g/0.7 oz of grated ginger (per day, for 7 days)

■ **FOR THE SYRUP**
- 1 kg/2.2 lbs strawberries
- 1 L/34 fl oz water
- ½ bunch (approx. 45 g/1.5 oz) basil
- 100 g/3.5 oz granulated sugar

■ **EQUIPMENT**
- approx. 1-liter (34-fl-oz) capacity sterilized preserving jar
- cheesecloth
- elastic band
- approx. 1.5-liter (51-fl-oz) capacity sterilized, pressure-resistant bottle with cap (or several smaller ones); a strong plastic mineral water bottle is ideal

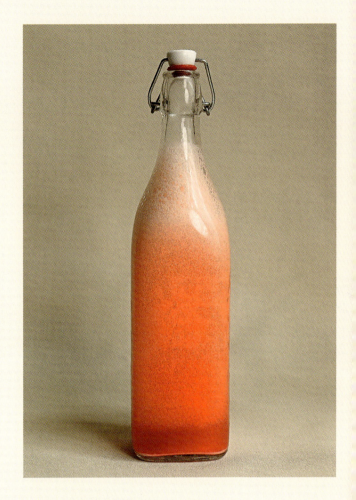

method

Start with the ginger beer starter, as it needs a week to settle. Pour the water into a large, sterilized preserving jar and, while stirring, dissolve the sugar into this—do not heat the water. Stir in the grated ginger. Store the preserving jar, without a lid but covered with some cheesecloth secured with an elastic band, outside the refrigerator in a dark warm place, ideally with a temperature of about 30°C (86°F). Feed the ginger beer starter every day for 7 days with 30 grams (1 ounce) sugar and 20 grams (0.7 ounce) grated ginger. If you see bubbles at the end of the week, it is ready.

Make the syrup. De-stem the strawberries, and slice thinly. Pour the water into a saucepan, add the strawberries, and bring gently to a boil. Simmer for 30 minutes and then add the basil. Strain into a bowl through the cheesecloth. Squeeze the cloth well (watch out, it will be hot!), so that the last of the juice is also extracted.

All being well, you will now have about 1.5 liters (51 fluid ounces) of liquid. Stir in the sugar until dissolved, and allow the syrup to cool completely.

Weigh the liquid, then weigh the amount of ginger beer starter needed; that is, 10 percent of the weight of the syrup—so, if you have 1.5 liters (51 fluid ounces) of syrup, add 150 grams (5.3 ounces) of ginger starter to the liquid. Add the weighed amount of starter to the syrup. Stir well, and divide the drink over the bottle(s). Store outside the refrigerator for 2 days in a warm, dark place, ideally at a temperature of about 30°C (86°F). Squeeze the bottle occasionally, which will become increasingly firm due to the building pressure of the starter. When you can hardly squeeze the bottle, put it in the refrigerator, where the drink will keep for a week.

Bulbs and Roots

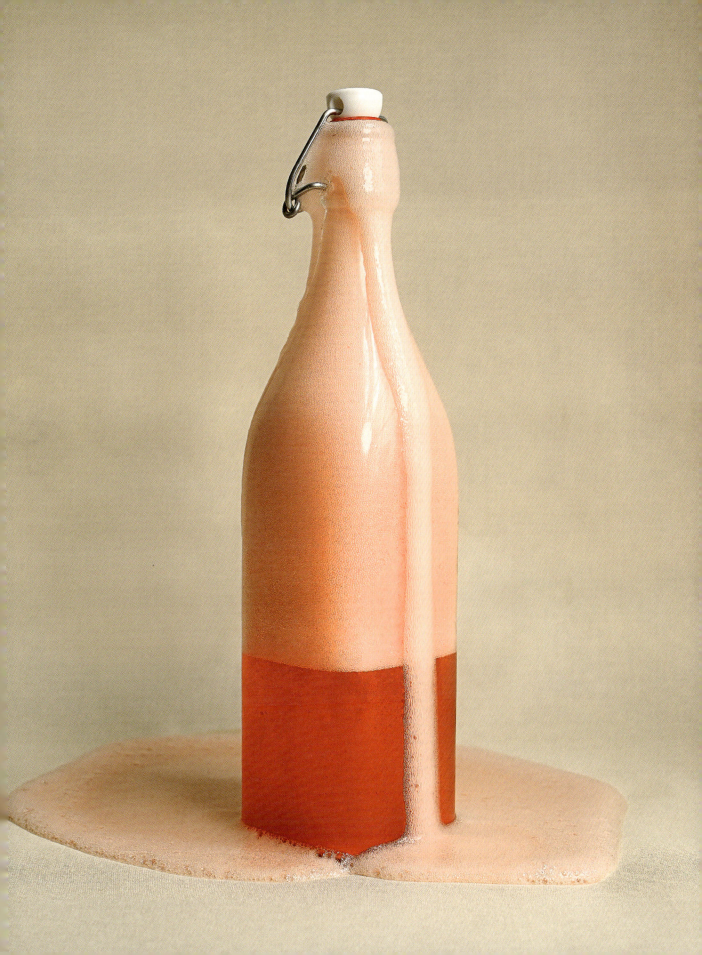

GINSENG

PANAX GINSENG

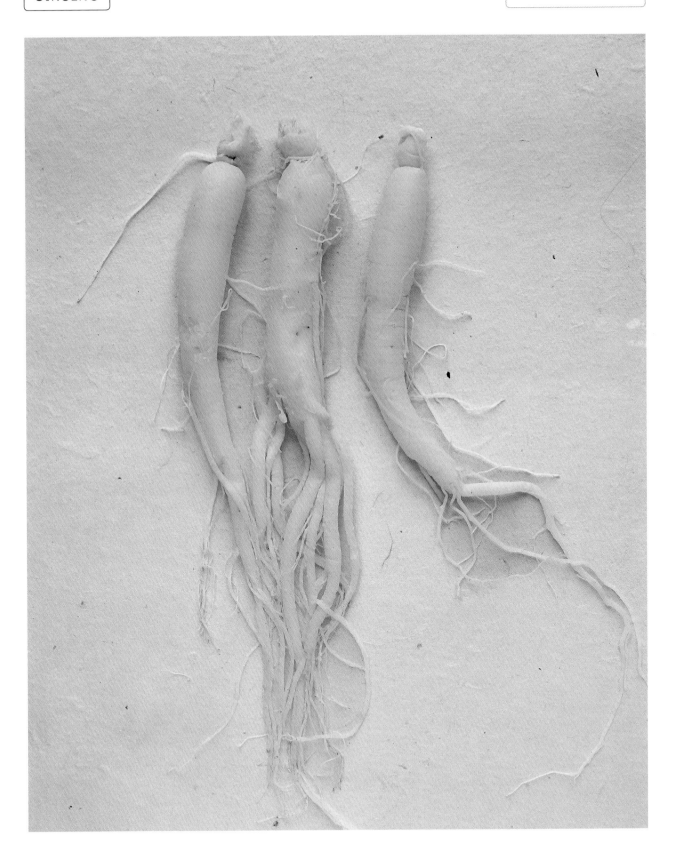

Spirit of the Earth

There are various species of ginseng. The best known is *Panax ginseng*, which grows in Korea, China, and eastern Russia. In addition, there is *Panax japonicus* in Japan (which is originally from Korea); Siberian ginseng, or taiga root, the Latin name of which is *Eleutherococcus senticosus*; and *Panax quinquefolium*, which grows in the United States and is therefore called American ginseng.

Ginseng is *the* symbol of Asian medicine and phytotherapy and has been used for millennia. There is almost no other plant that appears in as many myths and magical tales as ginseng. It is one of the few plants that has been designated a *panacea*, a remedy for all ills. When I was 12, I told my pharmacist uncle that I had read about ginseng's special effects. He dismissed it with a laugh. Years later, he backtracked about it after publications had revealed that ginseng was used by astronauts from the International Space Station (ISS) to reduce stress symptoms.

Wild ginseng used to be "hunted." During the nighttime ginseng hunt, the hunters used a unique sign language so as not to wake up the nature spirits. Under special circumstances, the ginseng leaves were believed to give off a kind of light glow. Bows and arrows were used to shoot the plants, so that the next day they could be found in daylight through the arrow markings.

Use

One of ginseng's active ingredients (ginsenosides) contributes to the root's adaptogenic and tonic effects that improve energy, stamina, and concentration. The root also helps during recovery after illness. Ginseng is often used in combination with ginkgo extract (see page 174), which enhances the blood flow in the small capillaries. Ginseng is traditionally used in Chinese medicine to treat dementia and improve cognitive skills and memory.[123] Ginseng helps strengthen the *chi*, or vital life force, and warms up the body.

According to traditional Chinese medicine, ginseng produces *yang* energy. In some cases, this can have too strong an effect for certain people, in which case it is recommended to use ginger instead of ginseng.

Ginseng is a fortifying agent that does not negatively affect sleep. It also helps with relaxation. It thus has multiple properties you might think were opposites.

In animal experiments, pharmacologist Israel Brekhman from Vladivostok demonstrated that ginseng boosted endurance significantly. Mice were put in water and taken out just before they had reached the point of exhaustion. Mice that had been given ginseng in advance were able to keep going almost twice as long during a second round.[124]

PROPERTIES

- Panacea
- Energy generator
- Warming
- Adaptogen
- Tonic effect
- Fortifies vitality
- Anti-stress
- Helps break down alcohol
- Protective effect against radiation

SOURCING

Ginseng is usually available in powder form in capsules or as a paste (extract) at drugstores. Fresh ginseng can sometimes be found in Chinese supermarkets.

CAUTION

Do not use ginseng in combination with certain medications, such as blood sugar reducers, blood thinners, and those for heart function; there may be interactions. If you are taking any medication, discuss with your doctor whether it is wise to use ginseng. Ginseng is discouraged when you have flu or a cold, or for those young in age. Avoid caffeinated drinks when using ginseng. Do not take before bedtime, but during the day or in the morning. In normal doses, ginseng does not cause any side effects.

Furthermore, a 2005 study by Korean professor Tung-Kwang Lee demonstrated a protective effect against radiation toxicity.

Bulbs and Roots

The study showed that ginseng protects against DNA damage and mutations.[125] Ginseng helps break down alcohol in the body. Siberian ginseng is a traditional adaptogen and liver tonic.

Appearance

Ginseng is very rare in the wild, so if you pick the plant in the wilderness always replant the seeds! If you want to grow ginseng, do so on the northern side of a mountain or slightly in the shade. You need patience as it takes two years for the seed to germinate, then the root will have to grow for at least six years.

The plant grows to 25–50 centimeters (9.8–19.7 inches) high and can be recognized by its white flowers and small red berries; it has 5 partial leaves. The root looks a little like a human body with many root-hairs. In Korea, cultivation is accompanied by various rituals.

In South Korea, ginseng is a very important source of income and cultivation is state-controlled. In China, astronomical sums are paid for ancient wild ginseng *roots*. Greater powers are often attributed to these specimens, especially *roots* that are more than 20 years old. Most ginseng available in the West has been cultivated.

Extracting and Dosing

One Chinese recipe I found is as follows: Simmer an approximately 10-gram (0.35-ounce) piece of fresh ginseng root for 5 hours in about 2 liters (68 fluid onces) of water with a chicken carcass, making sure the carcass is covered in water. Then strain the stock through a sieve into a bowl. Drink one bowl of fresh stock daily for at least 3 weeks. This powerful stock is also prescribed to enhance potency.

You can also chew on a piece of fresh root. Dosages range from chunks of root the size of a peanut to a walnut. Up to 2–5g (0.07–0.18 ounces) per day is appropriate for an extended period of time. Should you react strongly to plants, then you can start with 0.5–1g (0.018–0.035 ounces) per day.

Another possibility is dried ginseng. The *roots* are dried in a special manner. Red variants are dried in a different way, preserving all their medicinal properties. They are often rock hard. In Hong Kong, I witnessed them being softened under high steam pressure with some kind of small stove-looking devices. The *roots* were then thinly sliced so that they would be easier to consume.

Finally, extracts are also available. I find the syrupy Korean ginseng extract the best, which you can buy in good Chinese stores.

If you really want to benefit from ginseng, you have to use it for some time; it's what's known as a "course." Keep up the ginseng course for at least 1 month, but preferably 2 months. It's a plant that works better the longer you use it; you will only notice its effect after 3 weeks. According to some Chinese doctors, everyone should do a ginseng course annually.

Once you have built up experience with ginseng and want to use it at an advanced age to improve your health and support your vitality, you can consume 1 gram (0.035 ounces) in the desired form every day.

I recommend that you also get advice on the use of ginseng from a Chinese herbalist. According to Chinese herb theory, you have to have breaks in using any herb.

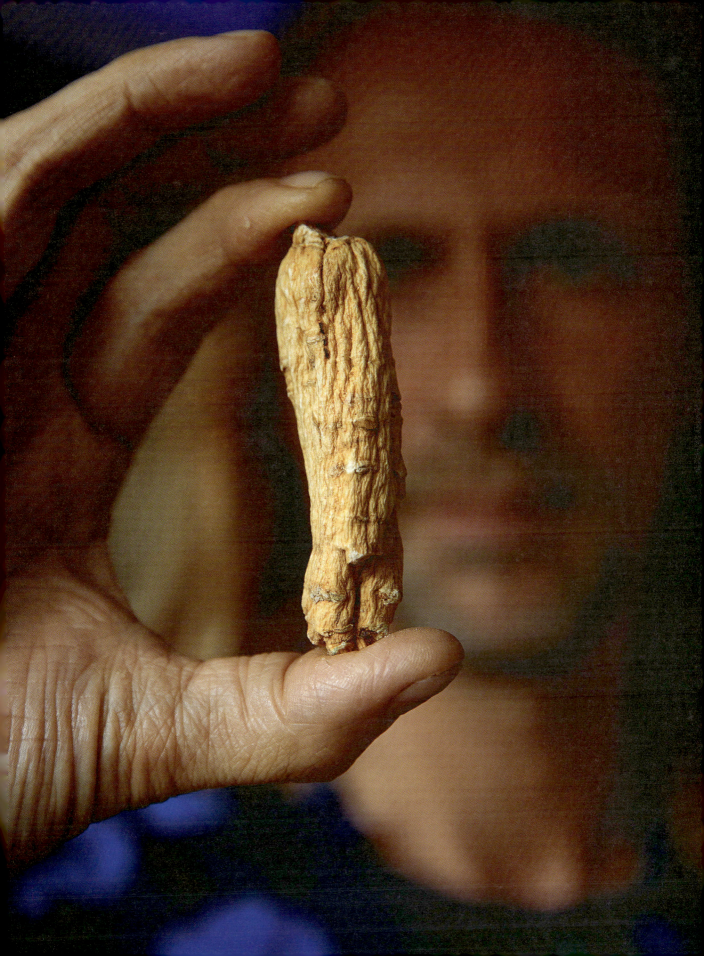

CHAWANMUSHI – SAVORY GINSENG CUSTARD

serves 4 people

■ **FOR THE CHAWANMUSHI**
- 500 ml/17 fl oz vegetable stock
- 2 dried ginseng roots (approx. 20 g/0.7 oz)
- 4 eggs
- 5 g/0.16 oz (1 tsp) fine sea salt
- 15 ml/0.5 fl oz (1 T) mirin (sweet rice wine, Asian supermarket)
- 15 ml/0.5 fl oz (1 T) light soy sauce

■ **AS WELL AS**
- 20 g/0.7 oz enoki mushroom, cut into pieces
- 1 red onion, in strips
- ½ bunch (approx. 40 g/1.4 oz) cilantro (coriander), leaves only

■ **EQUIPMENT**
- 4 heat-resistant bowls
- oven dish

method

Lightly heat the vegetable stock in a pan. Thinly slice the ginseng roots, and simmer in the stock for 1 hour, allowing it to infuse.

Meanwhile, in a bowl, beat the eggs without allowing air to get in and the mixture starting to foam. Add the salt, the mirin, and soy sauce, and whisk again.

Preheat the oven to 150°C (300°F).

Strain the stock with the ginseng slices into a bowl. Do not discard the ginseng!

Whisk the egg mixture into the still-lukewarm stock, again making sure that no air gets in. Pour the custard into the heatproof bowls, and cover with plastic wrap (clingfilm). Put them in an oven dish or container with water; make sure that the water comes up to three-quarters of the bowls. Bake the *chawanmushi* for 30 minutes in the oven.

You can serve the *chawanmushi* cold or warm. Place the slices of ginseng on the custard, followed by the enoki mushroom and red onion. Garnish with cilantro.

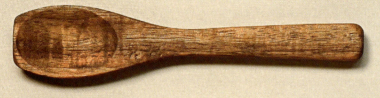

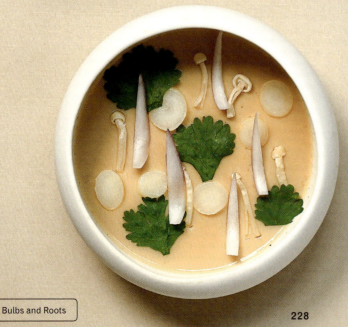

Bulbs and Roots

STRAWBERRIES WITH GINSENG MOUSSE

serves 8–10 people

■ **FOR THE MOUSSE**
- 3 dried ginseng roots (approx. 30 g/1 oz)
- 250 ml/8.5 fl oz water
- 85 g/3 oz granulated sugar
- 2 gelatin leaves
- 200 ml/7 fl oz whipped cream
- 1 egg white

■ **AS WELL AS**
- 200 g/7 oz strawberries
- 40 g/1.4 oz nasturtium flowers

■ **EQUIPMENT**
- piping bag

method

Start with the mousse. Thinly slice the ginseng roots. Put them in a pan with the water and 50 grams (1.8 ounces) sugar, and bring to the boil. Turn off the heat, and leave to infuse for 30 minutes.

Strain the water through a sieve into a bowl, pour back into the pan, and heat one more time. Do not throw away the ginseng slices!

Soak the gelatin leaves for 5 minutes in a bowl of cold water. Squeeze them, and add to the warm ginseng syrup. Stir until they are completely dissolved. Remove the pan from the heat.

Whip the cream until it has the thickness of yogurt.

In a second, sterilized bowl, beat in the egg whites with the rest of the sugar until peaks form. Fold the ginseng syrup into this, followed by 3 servings of the whipped cream until you have a stiff mousse. Spoon this into a piping bag.

Pipe the mousse into the center of deep plates. De-stem and halve the strawberries. Arrange on the mousse, along with the saved slices of ginseng root. If a little residual moisture starts to run, that's not a big deal. Garnish with the nasturtium flowers.

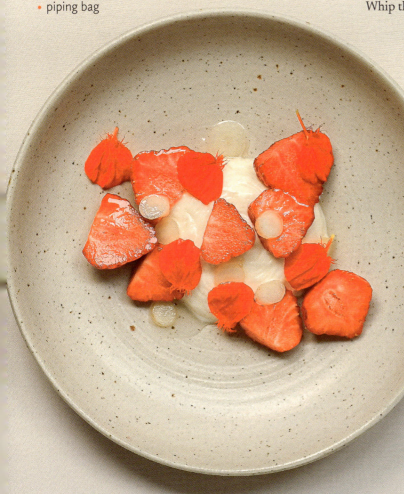

Bulbs and Roots

| GARLIC |

| ALLIUM SATIVUM |

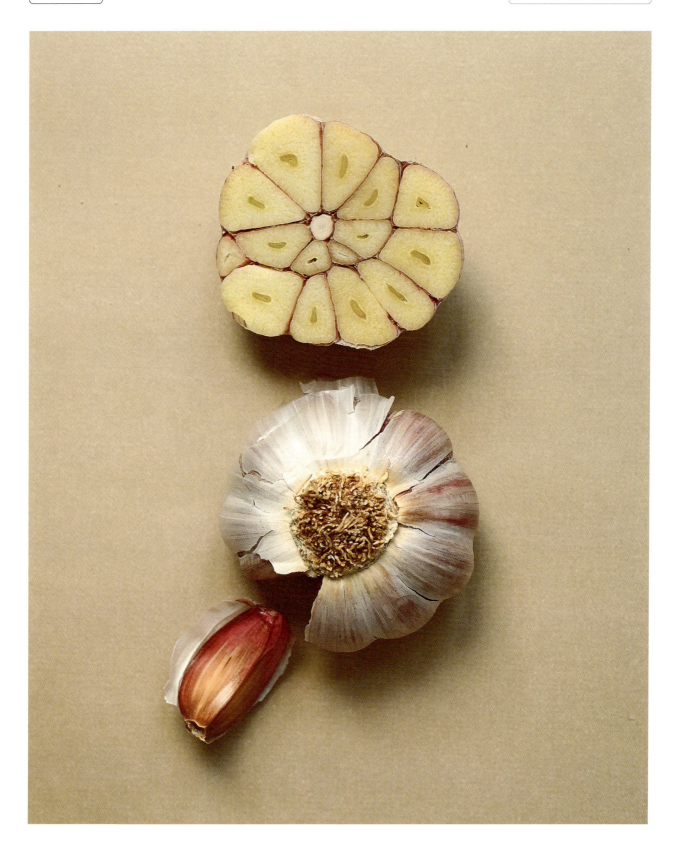

Blood Tonic

Garlic is a herb and medicine and not a food like onions, even though it is a member of the onion family, which include leeks, chives, and shallots. The use of garlic as a medicine goes back many millennia and seems to be as old as humankind itself. Garlic is indigenous to Central Asia and northeastern Persia, where it grows wild on the steppes, the way wood garlic grows naturally in shady spots in the countryside in the Low Countries, United Kingdom, and eastern and central United States.

The oldest known descriptions of garlic can be found on ancient Sumerian clay tablets dating back more than 4,000 years, which were found in the 1930s. The Sumerians lived around 2600 BCE in the area between the Euphrates and the Tigris rivers, today's Iraq.

Garlic was sacred among the ancient Egyptians, who took their oaths holding a bulb of garlic. Three and a half thousand years ago, the *Ebers papyrus* were written in Egypt, which is seen as one of the most important Egyptian sources of medical information.

Garlic has traditionally been used to strengthen the heart. Egyptians, like other peoples at the time, used garlic and onion as a heart tonic. Egyptians consumed raw garlic to boost their perseverance and willpower and to cure asthma. It is also known that Egyptian slaves were fed garlic to make them work harder.

Greek athletes used garlic to perform better during the Olympics. Pythagoras, himself educated at the Egyptian mystery schools, called garlic the "king of spices." Yet the Greek philosopher and mathematician forbade his own students and priests from eating garlic. This was probably because of its aphrodisiac effect; in classical antiquity, garlic was drunk with wine and coriander as an aphrodisiac.

Garlic was also mentioned in the *Edda* (the sacred Icelandic and Norwegian poems from the 10th century). In 11th-century Norway, garlic was used to medically diagnose the depth of warriors' wounds. They were given garlic to eat and if their abdominal wounds smelled of garlic, it meant the abdominal wall was completely penetrated. The female herbalist then knew what she had to do in order to cure him.

In China, garlic was first described as a medicine 2000 years BCE, as a remedy for poisoning.

Almost everywhere in the world, garlic is associated with magic, especially as a protective and repellent.

Use

Throughout the millennia, this agent has been almost universally regarded as one of the most important medicinal plants. All the doctors in antiquity saw garlic as a panacea, or miracle drug. In his writing, the Roman naturalist Pliny the Elder (AD 23–79) noted that garlic opens up arteries and dilates the veins. Recent scientific studies confirm that garlic lowers cholesterol levels in the blood and can thus reduce the risk of cardiovascular disease.

PROPERTIES
- Tonic for the cardiovascular system
- Antibiotic (against viruses, bacteria, and fungi)
- Helps with detoxification (including chronic lead poisoning)
- Dissolves blood clots
- Improves circulation of the blood
- Protects the heart muscle from oxygen deficiency
- Immunostimulatory
- Blood pressure–lowering
- Effective against fungal infections
- Improves the elasticity of the aorta
- Helps against acne

SOURCING

Garlic is available year round in fresh or dried form at the supermarket or greengrocers. You can also grow it in your own vegetable garden. Garlic is usually planted in November. It tolerates very alkaline (calcareous) soil. Harvest the garlic when it starts to "talk"; that is, it is so dry that the outer leaves are crisp and crinkle when you touch the bulb.

Bulbs and Roots

Garlic is one of the most widely used medicinal plants in three of the world's most important traditional medicinal systems: Indian Ayurvedic, traditional Chinese, and traditional European medicine. This universal natural healing agent has also been highly regarded as a flavoring for centuries.

In modern herbal medicine, garlic is prescribed as a cardiovascular tonic. In daily use, it has a proven beneficial effect on the intestines and cardiovascular system.

The body detoxifies itself through the sulfur compounds found in garlic. Garlic not only activates all the glands, and thereby the body's life forces, but also restores the intestinal microbiome and dispels what's not required.[126]

CAUTION
Because of its blood-thinning effect, do not eat garlic before surgery. If you go out at night or have to speak in close proximity to a lot of people for work, bear in mind that your breath may start to smell of garlic. Eating some raw parsley helps counter this. If you prefer not to eat any garlic because of its smell or flavor, then garlic pills are available as an alternative.

Laboratory tests have revealed that garlic can kill a number of species of bacteria.

An English herbal book from the ninth century, *Bald's Leechbook*, gives a prescription for an eye ointment made from garlic, onion, wine, and cow bile. When this mixture was tested for the superbacterium *Staphylococcus aureus*, which is resistant to methicillin, 90 percent of the bacteria were killed. An impressive result, as the bacterium is resistant to almost every antibiotic.[127]

In this context, it may also be interesting to note that Russian soldiers during the Second World War always carried a few cloves of garlic for disinfecting wounds, hence the name "Russian penicillin."

The French chemist and microbiologist Louis Pasteur, known for his discoveries of the principles of vaccination, microbial fermentation, and pasteurization, discovered garlic's bactericidal action during his laboratory studies in the 19th century.[128] The medicinal effects of garlic are therefore primarily anti-inflammatory and antibiotic. Garlic is said to work preventatively against blood clot formation and too many fats in the blood.

The juice of garlic has been used in toxic bites from snakes, scorpions, and insects for centuries. Garlic was also used to help the body detoxify in cases of lead poisoning.

Appearance
The appearance of garlic is not unlike that of the leek. Garlic leaves are grassy and pointed and are connected to each other just above the bulb around the stem. It usually grows upright and quite tall, up to 50 centimeters (19.7 inches). The bulbs are usually white, but there are also pink and red varieties. The bulb is made up of several cloves. The cloves are closely packed together and are separated by a parchment-like membranous leaf. Garlic grows only in the sun, not in the shade.

Extracting and Dosing
Eat one clove every day, and sometimes take a break. Preparing a dish with garlic once a week offers a good maintenance dosage. Raw squeezed garlic is delicious in a salad with vinaigrette. Most of garlic's medicinal effects are broken down through heating; in order to utilize its medicinal benefits to the maximum, it's therefore best to eat garlic raw.

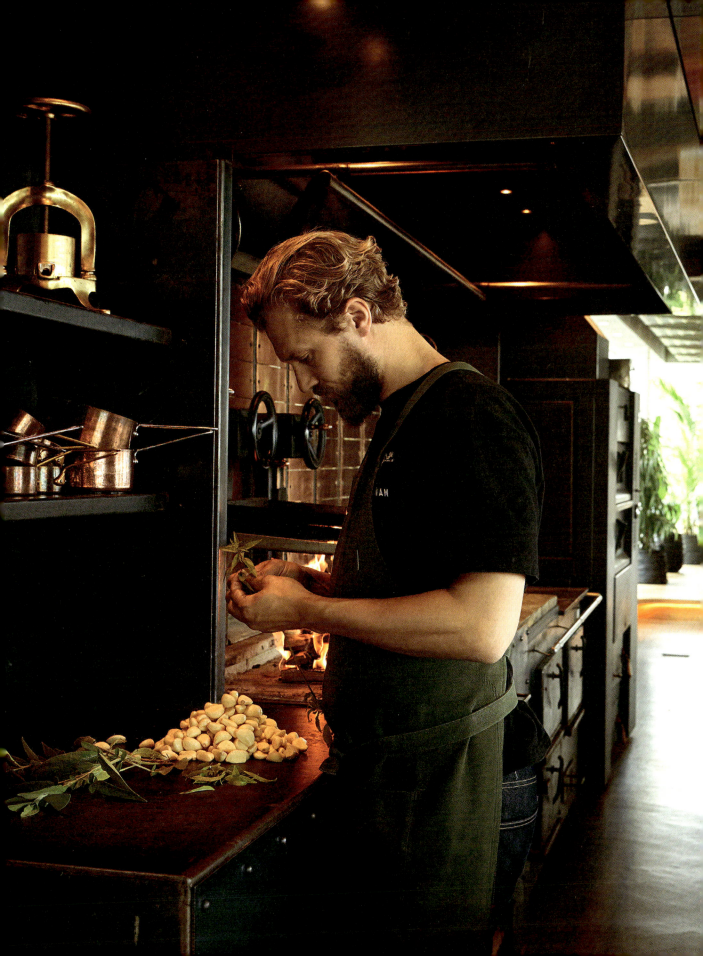

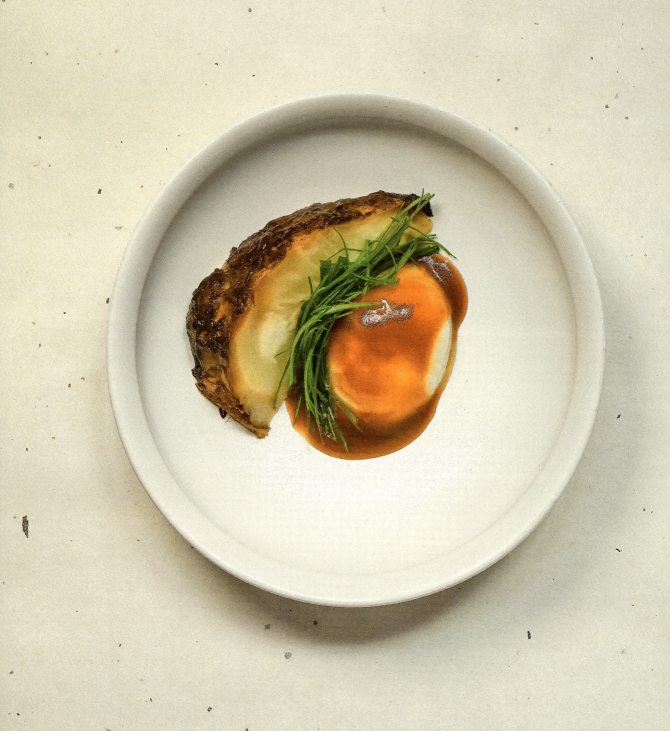

CARAMELIZED CELERIAC WITH GARLIC, MIRIN, SOY, AND SOFT-BOILED EGG

serves 8 people

■ **FOR THE CANDIED GARLIC**
- 1 garlic bulb
- 200 ml /6.8 fl oz olive oil

■ **FOR THE GARLIC GLAZE**
- 45 ml/1.5 fl oz (3 T) dark soy sauce
- 45 ml/1.5 fl oz (3 T) sake (Asian supermarket)
- 45 ml/1.5 fl oz (3 T) mirin (sweet rice wine, Asian supermarket)
- 15 ml/0.5 fl oz (1 T) maple syrup

■ **FOR THE CARAMELIZED CELERIAC**
- 1 celeriac weighing up to 1 kilogram (2.2 lbs)
- olive oil
- fine sea salt and freshly ground black pepper

■ **AS WELL AS**
- 30 g/1 oz fine sea salt
- 20 ml/0.7 fl oz natural vinegar
- 8 eggs
- 3 spring onions, just the green part

method

Peel the garlic cloves, and put them in a pan with the cold olive oil on as low a heat as possible. Leave the garlic to confit very gently without coloring; this takes about 20 minutes. Turn off the heat once the cloves are soft, and allow them to cool down in the oil. You can use the confited garlic for all kinds of things. This technique makes the garlic a little sweeter and more caramelized. In the refrigerator, the confited garlic cloves will keep for about 5 days. The garlic oil (remove the cloves to avoid the risk of botulism!) can be kept for a long time and is delicious as a drizzle over all kinds of food, such as pasta or pizza.

Put all the ingredients for the garlic glaze in a saucepan and bring to a brief boil. Mix in all the confited garlic cloves with a hand blender until you have a smooth sauce. Set aside to cool.

Preheat the oven to 170°C (338°F).

Coat the celeriac in a small amount of olive oil, and sprinkle with salt and pepper. Transfer to a parchment-lined baking tray, and place in the oven, where it will definitely need 2 hours to cook. Use a skewer to test if the celeriac still offers resistance. The vegetable should be well cooked on the inside and nicely golden-brown on the outside. Coat the cooked celeriac in half of the garlic glaze, and bake for another 5–10 minutes. Remove from oven, and cut it into 8 wedges. In our professional kitchen, we cook eggs beautifully soft by gently steaming them for 35 minutes at 65°C (150°F). We then tap them open and have a perfectly boiled egg with a soft yolk and soft egg white. Delicious. At home, poaching an egg comes the closest to this, or an egg boiled for 7 minutes and then peeled.

Fill a pan with 2 liters (68 fluid ounces) of water, and stir in the salt and vinegar. Salt and vinegar ensure that the outer layer of the egg solidifies faster. Bring the water almost to a boil. Using a whisk, create a small vortex in the hot water. Break an egg in a cup, and slowly pour this into the water. Repeat with several more eggs in the same pan. In my experience, 4 eggs at a time fit perfectly comfortably in one pan. It may take some practice.

Some broken-off egg white will probably rise to the surface; you can remove this from the water with a skimmer and discard. To avoid this, and in order to create more beautifully shaped poached eggs, immediately discarding the thin egg white in its raw state works even better; this can be done by breaking the egg into a fine sieve. The fresher the egg, the better the result.

After 3–5 minutes, the eggs are sufficiently cooked. Remove them from the pan with a skimmer, and pat dry with some kitchen paper. Repeat with the rest of the eggs.
Cut the green part of the spring onions into long, thin strips. Serve the poached eggs in deep dishes, with the chopped spring onion and wedges of celeriac placed alongside. Pour over the rest of the garlic glaze.

Bulbs and Roots

GARLIC VELOUTÉ WITH ROASTED CARROTS AND ONION

serves 4–6 people

FOR THE VELOUTÉ
- 30 ml/1 fl oz (2 T) sunflower oil
- 1 onion, chopped
- 200 g/7 oz fresh young garlic, finely chopped
- 200 g/7 oz celeriac, in small cubes
- 30 g/1.5 fl oz (2 T) garlic puree
- 2 sprigs of thyme
- 25 g/0.9 oz kombu (Asian supermarket)
- 500 ml/17 fl oz vegetable stock
- 500 ml/17 fl oz whipped cream
- 500 ml/17 fl oz whole milk
- 2.8 g/0.87 oz (½ tsp) black peppercorns
- 125 g/4.4 oz cold butter, in small cubes
- fine sea salt

AS WELL AS
- 1 yellow carrot
- 1 purple carrot
- 1 orange carrot
- 100 g/3.5 oz fresh pearl onions
- 60 g/2 oz (4 T) butter
- 2 sprigs of thyme, leaves only
- 4 garlic cloves, confited
- fine sea salt

EQUIPMENT
- mortar or cook's knife
- sieve

method

For the *velouté* (rich savory creamy soup), heat the sunflower oil in a soup pan over medium-high heat, and sauté the onion and young garlic without coloring. Add the celeriac, garlic puree, thyme, and kombu, and sauté for a moment longer. Then add the vegetable stock, whipping cream, and milk. Bring to the boil, and cook the celeriac for about 15 minutes until tender. Crush the peppercorns in a mortar or with the side of a chef's knife, and add to the pan. Cook for another 5 minutes. Strain the *velouté* through a sieve into a bowl, pressing everything well into the sieve's sides and bottom with the back of a spoon. Mix in the butter with a hand blender, and season with salt.

Meanwhile, peel and slice the carrots. Peel the pearl onions, and leave whole. Heat the butter in a large saucepan over medium-high heat until bubbly, and add the carrot slices, pearl onions, thyme leaves, and garlic at the same time. Roast the vegetables for about 15 minutes, until everything is cooked. Season to taste with salt.

Place the roasted vegetables into deep dishes, and add the *velouté*.

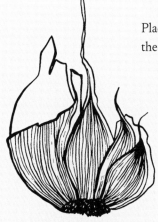
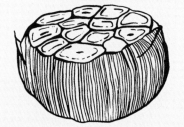

Bulbs and Roots

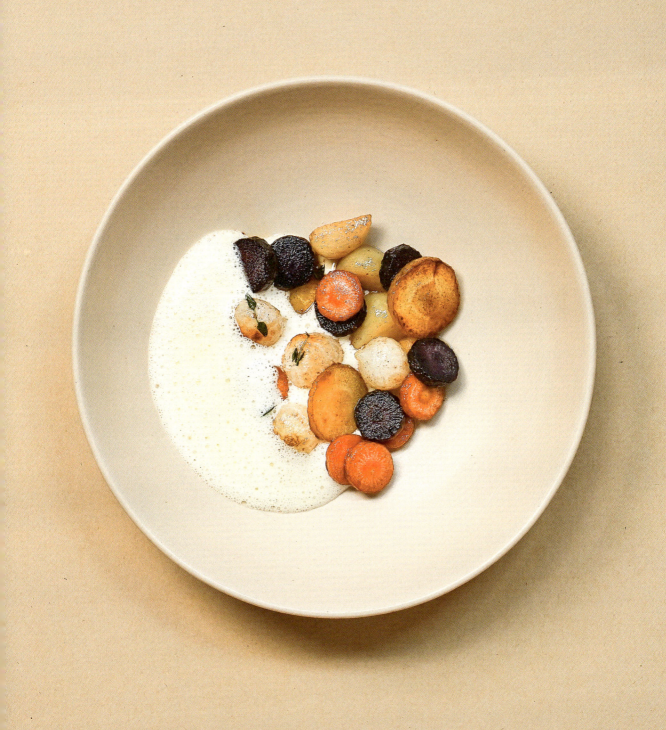

| TURMERIC | CURCUMA LONGA & CURCUMA ZANTHORRHIZA |

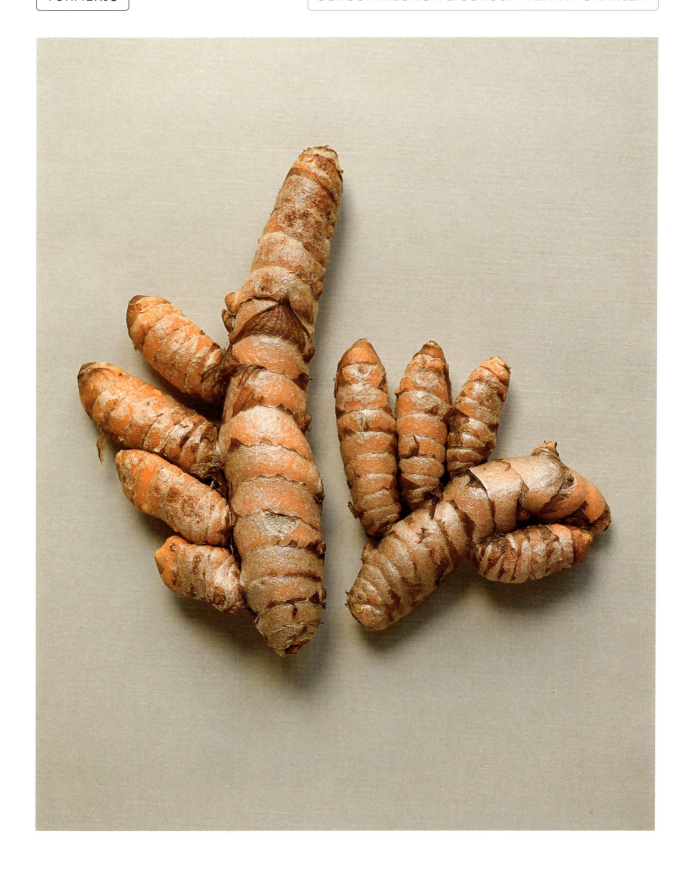

Anti-Inflammatory

Turmeric is related to ginger; more than 100 species are known. The origins of curcuma (turmeric) lie in India and Indonesia, where, following the doctrine of signature, it was used in bile disorders. Turmeric has been used for medical purposes in India since ancient times; this country is turmeric's largest producer—and consumer. The South Indian city of Erode, where most of the world's turmeric is produced, has therefore been nicknamed "The Yellow city."

Now, the plant is cultivated all over the tropics, and in some countries even grows in the wild in the jungle. I have seen them being picked for lunch on the spot in a Jamaican forest, some of which I then planted in The New Ark LSP Paradise Garden. In 2022, I spent three months there, having been invited to help create a paradise garden, following legendary dub and reggae producer and musician Lee "Scratch" Perry's vision. As we stood in the paradise garden, Auckland Morris from Dandepen (Lucea), Jamaica, told me that, according to Rasta philosophy, "Roots are the foundation, and the foundation is the roots."

Most people probably know turmeric as an ingredient in curry powder or as a spice that is used to color dishes yellow. In the Middle Ages, people called turmeric "Indian saffron" because it was a cheaper alternative to the extremely expensive saffron. In ayurveda, one of India's traditional systems of medicine, turmeric is one of the most-used medicinal plants for inflammation and in medicinal ointments and balms. It is furthermore known for its beneficial effect on the skin. Near Mahabalipuram in South India, where I stayed for a while in 1999, I saw women rubbing their entire faces with the powder in the morning, leaving them with a bright yellow face.

During Indian marriages, turmeric paste is applied to the bodies of the bride and groom, mainly on their faces and arms. This ceremony is called *haldi* and takes place at the parents' home the morning before the wedding to give a glow to their bodies and faces. The colors yellow and orange are sacred and symbolize prosperity in a number of Asian cultures. The yellow dye colors fabrics permanently and is used for that purpose in Asia.

Use

Turmeric is a spice that has been long known for its various medicinal properties, and over the years has become the subject of much interest from both the medical world and culinary enthusiasts, because it is the most important source of the antioxidant curcumin. Turmeric is anti-inflammatory, bile forming, liver protecting, and detoxifying, and an antimutagen (it prevents genetic mutation by chemicals); it can furthermore be used to prevent symptoms of ageing from developing; is antiviral, antibacterial, and fungicidal, and protects our nervous system.

PROPERTIES
- Anti-inflammatory
- Skin tonic (external)
- Bile-forming
- Liver protective and detoxifying
- Antioxidant
- Antimutagen (prevents genetic mutation by chemicals)
- Prevents symptoms of ageing
- Antiviral
- Antibacterial
- Antifungal
- Neuroprotective (protects the nervous system)

SOURCING

Ground turmeric is available from supermarkets and health food stores. Supplements containing curcumin can be purchased at most drugstores. Make sure that they also contain pepper or peperine for optimal effect. Fresh turmeric can be bought in health food stores and in (Asian) supermarkets. Wrap the fresh roots in kitchen paper, and store airtight in the refrigerator, where they will keep for a few weeks. Most people use turmeric in powder form, which has a shelf life of up to 3 years.

CAUTION

Low doses are recommended for seniors. When used externally, sitting in the sun for extended periods of time is not advised.

Bulbs and Roots

Neurologists at the University of California established that, among septuagenarians, in countries where curcumin is much used, there were approximately four and a half times fewer cases of dementia and Alzheimer's disease.

Turmeric cream is available from many Indian pharmacies. It is good for the skin, leaving it soft, refreshed, and glowing. It also helps with pimples and redness, and the antioxidants in turmeric cream prevent acne and arrest the development of post-acne scarring. Another action is that it can bring down facial swelling and, in time, can even seem to make small wrinkles disappear or fade.

Appearance

Curcuma longa is a perennial herb with pointed broad leaves and funnel-shaped yellow flowers. The root of the plant is the part we use; they form in small bunches and are light brown with a red hue on the outside. When you open the roots, they are bright yellow on the inside, almost orange. If you touch it, your skin will turn yellow. This color lasts for a few days.

Extracting and Dosing

Taking curcumin has no direct health benefits, because it is poorly absorbed and will be excreted quickly by your body. Turmeric is best taken with some oil and is up to 2,000 percent more absorbable when combined with black pepper (peperine).[129] 1.5–2 grams (0.05 –0.07 ounces) of turmeric per day is an average dosage.

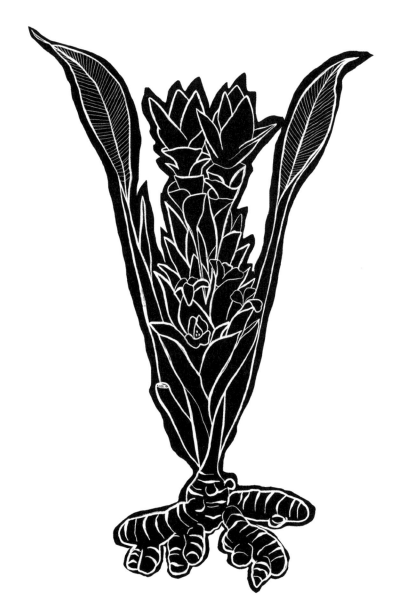

Bulbs and Roots

TURMERIC PANCAKES WITH ENOKI MUSHROOM, CILANTRO, AND SPANISH PEPPER

serves 4 people

■ FOR THE BATTER
- 250 ml /8.5 fl oz water
- 100 g/3.5 oz rice flour
- 1 banana
- 15 ml/0.5 fl oz (1 T) coconut milk
- 4 spring onions, just the green part
- 5 g/0.17 oz (1 tsp) turmeric powder
- 30 ml/1fl oz (2 T) sunflower oil

■ AS WELL AS
- 4 spring onions, white part only
- juice of 1 lime
- 15 g/0.5 oz (1 T) granulated sugar
- 100 g/3.5 oz enoki mushrooms (Asian supermarket)
- 3 cilantro sprigs
- 1 red chili pepper

method

Start by making the batter. In a bowl, stir the water with the rice flour into a smooth batter. In a second bowl, mash the banana in the coconut milk. Finely chop the spring onion leaves. Fold the banana–coconut mixture, spring onion leaves, and the turmeric powder into the batter.

Heat the sunflower oil in a skillet to a very high heat. Pour the batter into the pan. Fry the pancake for a few minutes until golden-brown on both sides. Slide onto a plate and, with a glass, cut out 4 small discs, or tear the pancake into 4 pieces.

In the skillet, sauté the white parts of the spring onions, remove the pan from the heat, and cut the spring onions into small pieces. In a small bowl, mix the lime juice with the sugar. Cut the base of the enoki mushrooms, and cut them into pieces, as well as the cilantro sprigs. Cut the red chili pepper into rings. Mix the spring onions, enoki mushrooms, cilantro, chili pepper, and the lime-sugar mixture, and arrange on top of the turmeric pancakes.

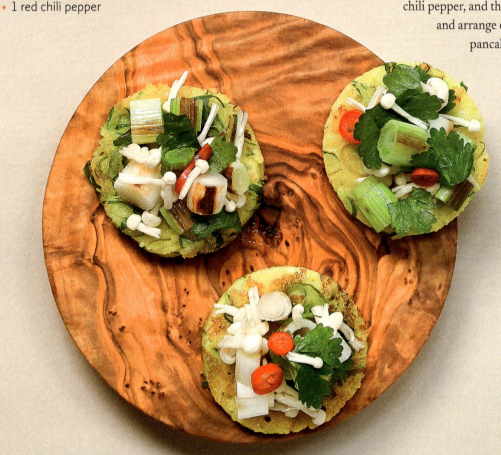

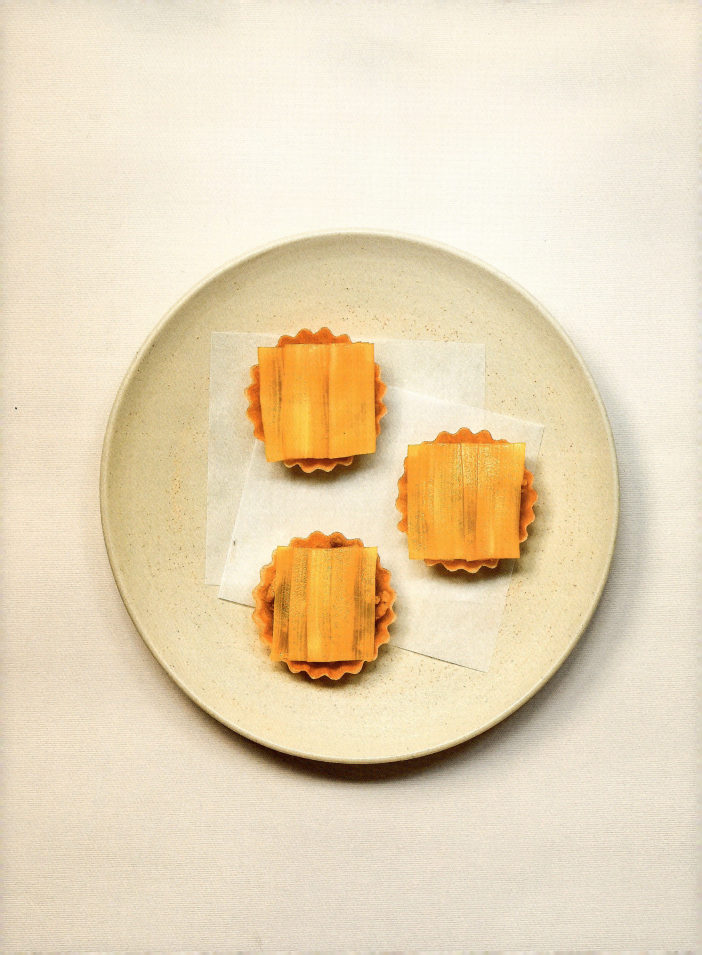

TARTLET WITH VEGETARIAN RENDANG AND WHITE ASPARAGUS PICKLE

serves 4 people

■ **FOR THE TARTLET**
- 2 sheets of North-African brick dough (available at Moroccan supermarkets); filo dough may be substituted
- splash of sunflower oil

■ **FOR THE VEGETARIAN RENDANG**
- 500 g/17 oz firm tofu
- 30 ml/1 fl oz (2 T) sunflower oil
- 1 vegetable stock cube, crumbled
- 1 tub Koningsvogel bumbu besengeh (mild Indonesian spice mix)
- 1 garlic clove
- 15 g/0.5 oz (1 T) coriander powder
- 15 g/0.5 oz (1 T) laos powder
- 1 cm/0.4 in turmeric root
- 50 g/1.8 oz creamed coconut
- 15 g/0.5 oz (1 T) sambal ulek (Indonesian spice made from hot chili, salt, oil, and vinegar)
- 1 stalk lemongrass, bruised

■ **FOR THE WHITE ASPARAGUS PICKLE (ACAR)**
- 250 ml/8.5 fl oz white wine vinegar
- 85 g/3 oz granulated sugar
- 25 g/0.9 oz ginger
- 2 garlic cloves
- 2.5 g/0.07 oz (½ tsp) turmeric powder
- 40 ml /1.35 fl oz water
- 4 spears white asparagus

■ **EQUIPMENT**
- 4 tartlet molds with a diameter of approx. 4 cm (1.5 in)
- mandolin (optional)

method

Preheat the oven to 170°C (338°F).

Cut 8 discs from the brick (filo) dough that are just slightly larger than your tartlet molds. Place them briefly in some sunflower oil and then press down 2 exactly on top of each other. Place the double sheet in a tartlet mold, and press another mold on top. Bake for 10 minutes in the oven, and allow to cool. Repeat for the rest of the tartlets.

For the vegetarian *rendang*, cut the tofu into small cubes. Heat the sunflower oil in a skillet on medium-high heat, and fry the tofu for a few minutes until golden-brown. Add enough water to submerge the tofu, and add the vegetable stock cube. Add the other ingredients for the *rendang*, and simmer gently for 1 hour. It is ready when it all comes together after cooking down. If necessary, simmer for a little longer, or add a little water if it is in danger of drying out.

While the *rendang* is simmering, make the *atjar* (white asparagus pickle). Put the white wine vinegar, sugar, ginger, garlic, turmeric powder, and water in a saucepan, and bring to a boil. Remove from the heat. This is your *atjar* base.

Cut each of the white asparagus spears into 3 equal pieces. Slice lengthways as thinly as possible, or use the mandolin for uniform slices. Place them in a bowl, pour over the hot *atjar* base, and refrigerate for 1 hour.

Spoon the *rendang* into the tartlets, and top with the *atjar* of white asparagus.

Bulbs and Roots

| HORSERADISH | ARMORACIA RUSTICANA |

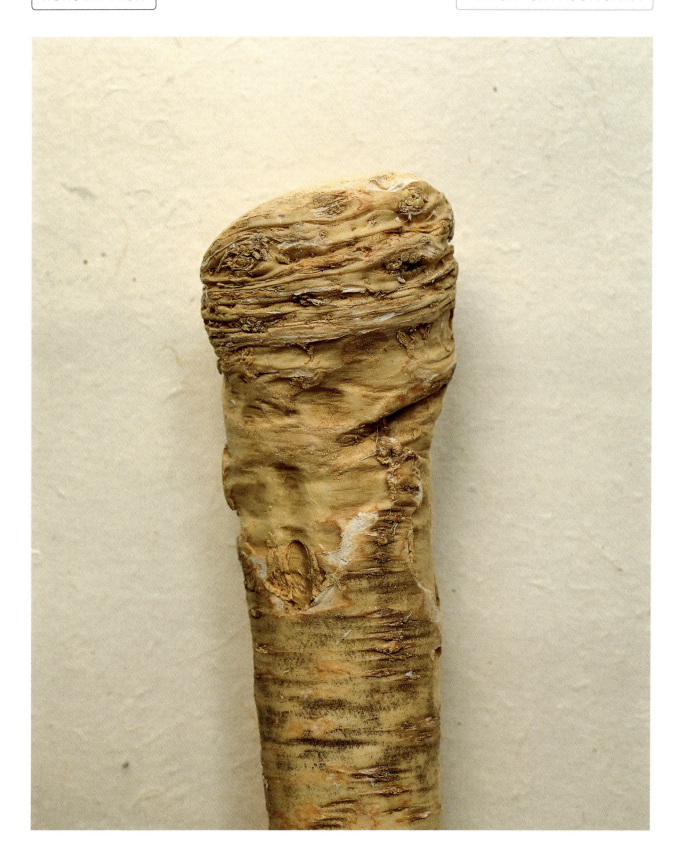

Expectorant

Horseradish is a root that has a sharp mustard-like taste and is used as a flavoring for various dishes. The root comes from Southeast Europe. The Japanese kitchen has an even stronger species of horseradish, *Eutrema japonicum*, better known as *wasabi*. Jewish cuisine uses horseradish in fish dishes, and the plant is known in Hebrew as *maror*, the bitter herb consumed during Passover. The plant symbolizes the bitter times the Jews experienced as slaves in ancient Egypt. The plant has been around for more than 3,000 years, although the Jews only came into contact with it in Eastern Europe, and it was a relatively late addition to their kitchen. Horseradish is a member of the same family as broccoli, cabbage, and mustard.

Use

The root contains the volatile compound allyl isothiocyanate, which is also found in mustard and gives it its sharp taste. Vinegar can stabilize this sharpness, but the compound is retained to some extent. An enzyme released through bruising of the root's cell structure creates this compound. According to Ben-Erik van Wyk, a professor of Indigenous botany, and Michael Wink, a professor of pharmaceutical biology, isothiocyanates can form chemical bonds with proteins and thus change their activity.

Horseradish has antimicrobial, antispasmodic, and cell-killing properties. Applied externally, the root acts as a rubefacient, which means that it enhances local blood flow in the skin and drains waste products faster.[130] Herbalist Mellie Uyldert also believes that you can draw out rheumatic pain by placing some grated horseradish on the sore spot.[131]

The root has diuretic, expectorant, and cough-suppressing properties. This white root vegetable helps remove inflammation in the pharynx and oral cavities. In lozenge form, horseradish is occasionally used for acute benign lung disease.[132]

As a diuretic, the root can help expel water-soluble toxins faster from the body. Diuretics are additionally used in medicine for heart failure, when the body retains more water than desired; for cosmetic reasons; to reduce swelling in feet and legs; and for high blood pressure.

Horseradish acts as an appetite stimulant and promotes digestion. The root is rich in vitamin C and contains large amounts of the minerals zinc, manganese, copper, calcium, potassium, iron, and phosphorus.

Appearance

Horseradish can grow to 15–60 centimeters (5.9–24 inches) tall and up to 5 centimeters (2 inches) wide. The taproot has horizontal lateral roots with root nodules on the sides. The outside of the root is yellow-brown and is creamy white on the inside. The above-ground leaves are oval shaped with an undulate edge and can grow to a size of 30 centimeters to 1 meter (1–3.3 feet). If you have horseradish in the garden and want to get rid of it, you need to remove the entire root, or it will come back up again. The plant is extremely invasive. The root is brittle and breaks easily.

PROPERTIES
- Diuretic
- Expectorant
- Stimulates appetite
- Externally – encourages blood flow
- Antibiotic
- Source of vitamin C, B1, B2, and B3 and various minerals

SOURCING

Available fresh from greengrocers and in jars at the supermarket. You can also grow the roots yourself by sowing them after mid-May or by putting a rhizome in the ground. The roots are usually harvested between November and March.

CAUTION

Horseradish is unsuitable for people who have stomach problems, such as heartburn and stomach ulcers, or who have low thyroid function. Horseradish should be used in small quantities and only sporadically.

Bulbs and Roots

Extracting and Dosing

Horseradish is usually incorporated into dishes. You can get the fresh roots at some greengrocers, or you can grow it yourself in the garden. People who grow vegetables or have an allotment often grow it. You might find a fresh root by asking around on an allotment site. Soak the fresh roots in hot water for 2 minutes before grating them.

In order to stimulate your metabolism, and when you have a cold or flu, for a short time, you can ingest 2 teaspoons (11.4 grams/0.3 ounces) freshly grated horseradish daily. Preserved horseradish from a jar is also suitable for this purpose.

You can make a cough medicine with horseradish. To do this, grate some horseradish into a sterilized jar, and pour some honey over it. Leave overnight, and strain into a bowl the next day. When you have a cough, you can use 1 teaspoon (5 milliliters/0.17 fluid ounces) daily until it disappears.

It is generally recommended not to take too much horseradish; only use sporadically.

Bulbs and Roots

FENNEL SALAD WITH HORSERADISH BUTTERMILK DRESSING

serves 4 people

■ **FOR THE FENNEL SALAD**
- 4 fennel bulbs
- 20 g/0.7 oz nasturtiums flowers and leaves
- (freshly) grated horseradish
- 30 g/1 oz mizuna
- 30 ml/1 fl oz (2 T) parsley oil (see page 62)

■ **FOR THE HORSERADISH-BUTTERMILK DRESSING**
- 5 g/0.17 oz (1 tsp) fine sea salt
- juice of 1 lemon
- 3 garlic cloves
- 5 g/0.17 oz (1 tsp) freshly grated horseradish
- 250 ml/8.5 fl oz buttermilk

■ **EQUIPMENT**
- mandolin (optional)

method

Preheat the oven to 200°C (395°F).

Halve 2 fennel bulbs lengthways, then, starting from the center, cut rounds as thinly as possible. It is best to use a mandolin. Place the slices in ice water. Halve the other fennel bulbs lengthways.

Cut each half into 4 wedges, starting at the center. Place the wedges on a parchment-lined baking tray, and bake in the oven for 10–15 minutes until cooked and golden-brown.

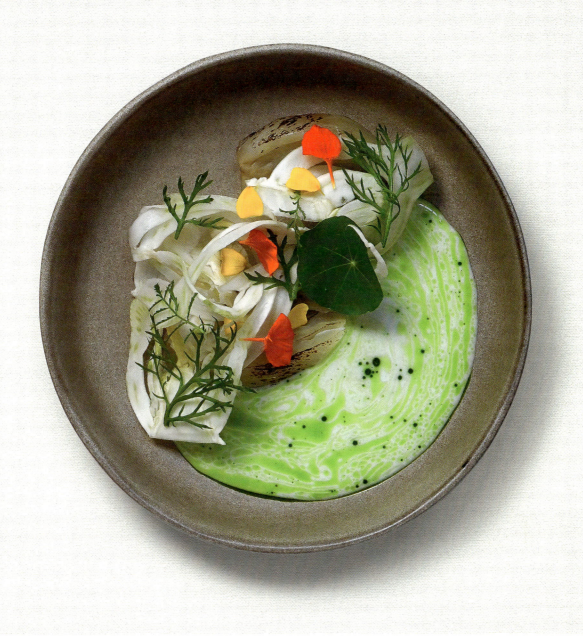

Meanwhile, in a saucepan, bring the salt, lemon juice, garlic, horseradish, and 50 milliliters (1.7 fluid ounces) of the buttermilk to a boil. Turn off the heat, and let the mixture steep for 30 minutes. Add the rest of the buttermilk, and either using a hand blender in the pan or transfer everything into a blender, whizz into a dressing, and strain through a fine sieve into a bowl.

Arrange the wedges of roasted fennel on the plates and cover with thin slices of raw fennel. Garnish with the flowers and nasturtium and mizuna leaves. If you like, you can grate some more horseradish over the salad. Mix the horseradish-buttermilk dressing with the parsley oil, and spoon this onto the plates alongside the fennel salad.

Bulbs and Roots

GLAZED EGGPLANT WITH HORSERADISH CREAM AND SEAWEED

serves 4 people, small portions

■ FOR THE GLAZED EGGPLANT
- 1 eggplant
- 59 ml/2 fl oz (4 T) light soy sauce (Asian supermarket)
- 59 ml/2 fl oz (4 T) tbsp dark soy sauce
- 30 ml/1 fl oz (2 T) Shaoxing rice wine (Asian supermarket)
- 30 g/1 oz (2 T) granulated sugar
- 5.7 g/0.17 oz (1 tsp) cornstarch

■ FOR THE HORSERADISH SWEET AND SOUR DRESSING
- 30 g/1 oz (2 T) freshly grated horseradish
- 59 ml/2fl oz (4 T) sushi vinegar

■ FOR THE HORSERADISH CREAM
- 15 g/0.5 oz (1 T) freshly grated horseradish
- 125 g/4.4 oz crème fraîche
- grated zest of ½ organic lemon
- fine sea salt and freshly ground black pepper

■ AS WELL AS
- 100 g (3.5 oz) fresh wakame, sea spaghetti, beach bananas, and kombu (Asian supermarket)
- grated zest of 1 organic lemon

■ EQUIPMENT
- pan for deep frying
- kitchen thermometer
- skimmer

method

Heat the sunflower oil in a thick-bottomed pan to 180°C (350°F). Cut the eggplant into finger-thick slices, and fry them in small portions for 3 minutes until golden-brown. Drain on kitchen towels.

Meanwhile, in a saucepan, bring the two kinds of soy sauce, Shaoxing rice wine, sugar, and cornstarch to a boil. Turn off the heat, and dip the slices of fried eggplant in the sauce.

In a small bowl, mix the horseradish with the sushi vinegar into a sweet and sour dressing.

In another bowl, mix together the ingredients for the horseradish cream, and season with salt and pepper.

Spoon the horseradish cream onto the plates, and arrange the eggplant slices on top of this. Top with the various types of seaweed and the horseradish sweet and sour dressing. Sprinkle with the lemon zest.

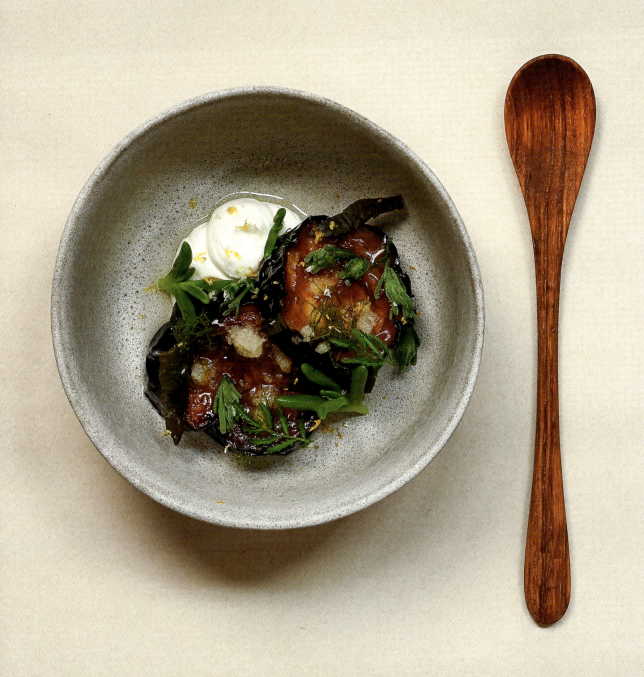

BLACK RADISH

RAPHANUS SATIVUS SUBSP. NIGER

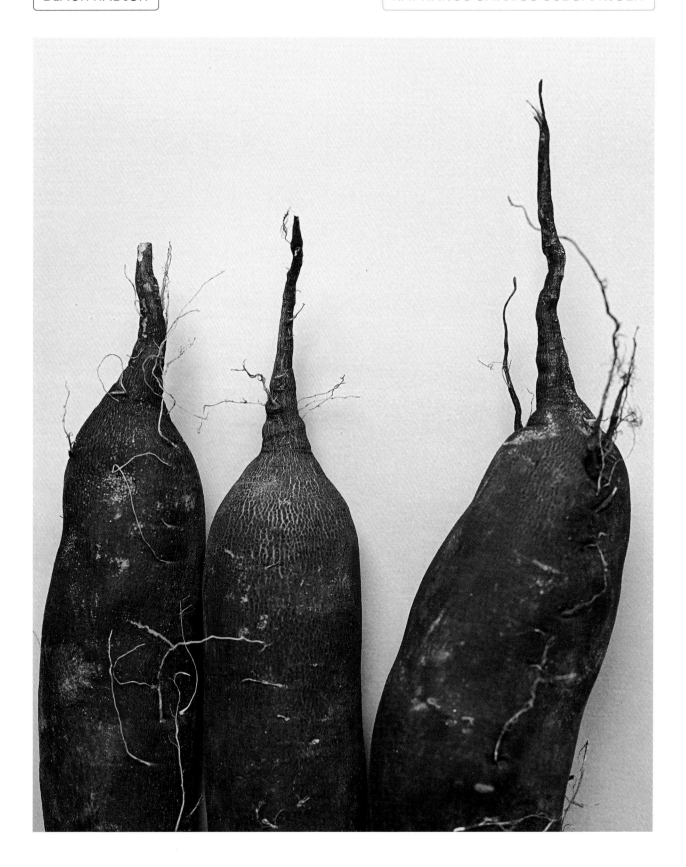

Tonic for the Bile Ducts

Black radish is related to the radish and belongs to the Brassicaceae family known for its many edible species, such as kale, radishes, Brussel's sprouts, cabbage, cauliflower, and kohlrabi. If you come across the word *sativus* in a Latin plant name, it means "cultivated." The common name of "radish" is derived from the Latin for carrot, *radix*. Radishes originated thousands of years ago in China and gradually spread westward. Black radish is usually elongated in form and, in ancient Egypt, was grown as far back as 4,500 years ago. It was eaten alongside garlic as a stimulant for the body and the mind.

Joris and I were given black radish as children, thinly sliced and sprinkled with some salt on bread. I have continued to eat the root and now grow it in my vegetable garden, just like our parents did in the Belgian Ardennes. You do need to have some patience. Geralt Joren, director of the Botanical Garden of VU Amsterdam, now the Zuidas Botanical Garden, and master botanist Hans Vissers taught me that "the most important tool for gardeners is patience." Black radish is planted in late spring and harvested in September and October. Thanks to the black radish in the vegetable garden, our parents taught us to think long term and wait patiently until a crop could be harvested or reseeded.

Use

According to ancient tradition, black radish's medicinal effects are greatest when there is an "r" in the month.[133]

Black radish is usually eaten raw, in salads or on bread, and is milder in flavor than the pink and white round radish. Phytotherapy black radish tinctures are available for medicinal use.

According to herbalist Mellie Uyldert, black radish is an effective remedy for asthma, because the root has a disinfectant effect, loosens mucus and stimulates the digestive organs and kidneys.[134] Black radish's expectorant properties were already described by the Greeks and Romans.

In phytotherapy, black radish is known to stimulate bile, thus playing a role in digestion, which it improves. Bile enables you to digest fats better. Eating black radish also helps prevent gallstones from developing. The root contains strong, health-promoting antioxidants. Black radish stimulates the appetite and can therefore be an active support in therapy for anorexia patients. Black radish promotes the secretion of gastric juices and is therefore seen as a fortifying agent.

It is also a natural disinfectant. The antibacterial and antifungal properties are also applied externally at times; the juice or root slices are rubbed on the skin against fungal infections.

Black radish is a good source of the minerals calcium, potassium, and phosphorus, and hosts countless other medicinal nutrients, including sulfur compounds. This type of radish contains raphanusine and vitamins A, B, C, and D. These substances, along with the many sulfur compounds, are responsible for the majority of the medicinal effects listed above. Black radish has a stronger effect than other types of radishes.

Appearance

The root exists in several colors, but the best-known is the variety with a pitch-black skin and bright white inside.

PROPERTIES
- Stimulates the appetite
- Expectorant
- Source of vitamins and minerals
- Prevents gallstones
- Fortifying agent (in small doses)
- Antidiabetic
- Antibacterial and antifungal properties
- Thins and liquidizes bile

SOURCING

You can grow the root yourself in your vegetable garden or buy it at health food stores or greengrocers.

CAUTION

Overuse can be harmful—do not do a black radish course for longer than 1 month. Swiss physician Alfred Vogel recommends using no more than 1 teaspoon (5 milliliters/0.17 fluid ounces) of juice daily.[135]

Bulbs and Roots

Black radish can grow to a height of 30 centimeters (1 foot) and vary in thickness from 4 to 10 centimeters (1.6–3.9 inches). The plants' leaves are tough, bristly, and irregular deeply serrate. The plant likes to grow in a sunny spot in soil in which the root can grow comfortably to a good depth.

Extracting and Dosing

Black radish is safe to eat raw. Start with a little bit, and slowly build up. Always remove the black skin. Herbalist Mellie Uyldert prescribes hollowing out black radish for conditions of the respiratory tract and filling it with brown sugar or honey. Make a hole in the bottom, and put it in a glass to allow the juice to drip out. Take up to 1 teaspoon (5 milliliters/0.17 fluid ounces) of juice per day.

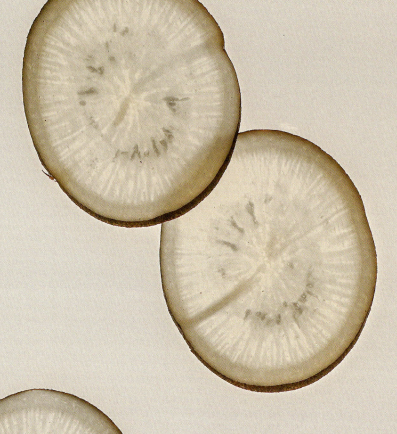

Bulbs and Roots

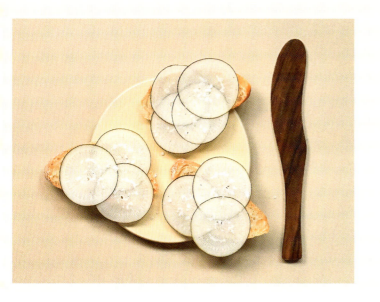

RADISH WITH BREAD AND BUTTER

Spread a good layer of (flower) butter (page 152) onto slices of sourdough bread. Slice a radish as thinly as possible with a mandolin. In a bowl, sprinkle with some fine sea salt, and mix well. Arrange the black radish on the slices of bread.

PICKLED BLACK RADISH

for 300 g/10.6 oz

■ FOR THE PICKLING LIQUID
- 500 ml/16.9 fl oz white wine vinegar
- 500 ml/16 fl oz water
- 500 g/17 oz granulated sugar
- 1 bay leaf
- 15 g/0.5 oz (1 T) coriander seeds
- 15 g/0.5 oz (1 T) fennel seeds
- 15 g/0.5 oz (1 T) mustard seed

■ AS WELL AS
- 2 black radishes (approx. 250 g/8.8 oz)
- 1 shallot
- 1 bunch (approx. 250 g/8.8 oz) radishes

■ EQUIPMENT
- approximately 2.5 L (85 fl oz) sterilized preserving jar

method

Put all the ingredients for the pickling liquid in a saucepan, and bring to a boil. Wash all the vegetables. Cut the black radishes in equal slices and the shallot in thin rings. Cut the leaves off the radishes.

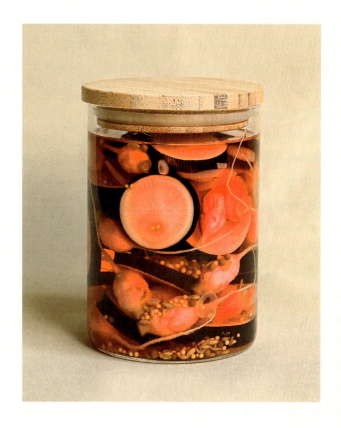

Put the vegetables in a hot, sterilized pot, and pour over the hot pickling liquid. Allow to cool.

These pickles can be kept in the refrigerator for about 3 months and are delicious with spicy food and on bread with cheese or cold cuts.

Bulbs and Roots

FURTHER PLANT JOURNEYS

MACA

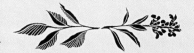

Lepidium meyenii

Legendary Strengthening Agent

South America is the continent of the tubers: the potato, Jerusalem artichoke, as well as lesser-known tubers such as maca all have their roots in the Andes Mountains. The tubers grow in Peru and Bolivia at an altitude of over 4,000 meters (over 13,000 feet) above sea level, making it the highest cultivated crop in the world.

Maca is tolerant of extreme weather conditions, such as cold, strong winds and bright sun, and grows on poor, rocky soil. As with ginseng, after maca has been harvested, the soil can no longer be used to grow crops for 10 years, as the maca will have completely exhausted it. Both before and after the Spanish presence in South America, maca was used as currency, especially for collecting taxes.

Following the introduction of rice, grain-based foods, white sugar, and canned foods in South America, maca was considered "poor people's fare" and was cultivated less and less—so little, in fact, that around the 1980s, it almost disappeared. Today it is known as the superfood of the Incas and is widely available.

Maca is a source of many minerals and vitamins and, like coca leaves, was a form of natural doping

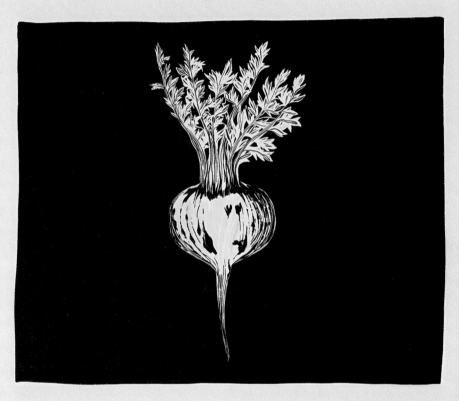

for Incan messengers, who ran through the high Andes covering immense distances.[136] Various studies with animals have shown that maca increases fertility and sexual activity. In South America, maca has consequently been used for centuries to improve the fertility of both humans and animals. Maca boosts both the endurance and libido of men and women and resets the body's (menstrual) hormone balance. The tuber is also used as a preventive for osteoporosis. Moreover, like ginseng and reishi mushrooms, it is a strong adaptogen. This means that it helps the body adapt to changing environments and living conditions. It strengthens resistance to various stressors (physical, as well as chemical and biological), helps transport oxygen around the body, boosts energy and physical strength, and supports neurotransmitter production and the glandular endocrine system. In short, it is an immune stimulant and helps strengthen our resistance.

Maca is typically sold as a powder in Dutch, Belgian, British, and American health food stores. Do not use continuously for too long, and do not take more than 2 scoops per day. Your body needs time to get used to maca.

Bulbs and Roots

FURTHER PLANT JOURNEYS

KAVA KAVA

Piper methysticum

Anxiety Reducer from Paradise

In every country in the world, people use stimulants, relaxants, and recreational substances. Among the people living on the island groups in the Pacific Ocean (Micronesia, Polynesia, and Melanesia) that lie roughly between the Easter Islands in the east and the large islands group of New Guinea, the root of the kava plant tops the list. The kava plant is related to the pepper and the *anijsblad wiri* (Surinamese Dutch), also known as *Piper marginatum* plant and is consumed for its calming effect.

The first Westerners to consume kava were Captain James Cook (1728–1779) and his fellow travelers. We know the plant has been used for more than 2,000 years. I have some experience with drinking kava extract, thanks to our Belgian relatives, who lived in the Kingdom of Tonga for years and brought the ground roots with them. During enjoyable get-togethers, we drank the kava extract, prepared in a traditional wooden bowl called the *kumete*.

Kava is an earth crop with strong anxiety-reducing properties. The islanders make cold-water extracts or chew the roots. The roots' fibers are not swallowed. The cold-water extract (see page 28) contains the psychoactive chemicals kavalactones or kavapyrones. The three different kavalactones in the plant work together synergistically. The customs and rituals around the plant and its cultivation methods vary from island to island, but kava's symbolic role is almost the same everywhere. Kava symbolizes the connection between the world of people and the world of spirits, and functions as a medium or conduit to other worlds. Kava is a tool for remembering the past and the ancestors who have come and gone before us.

Almost no one who drinks kava enjoys its flavor. As with tobacco and coffee, kava is an acquired taste. It tastes a bit like mud or earth with a typical fresh kava tone. Kava is classified as a hypnotic by ethnobotanists. Kavalactones bind to different neuroreceptors and thus provide narcotic, muscle-relaxing, analgesic, tranquilizing, and anticonvulsant properties.[137] Anthropologist James W. Turner calls kava "the water of life."[138] The drink has great symbolic and social significance for the people who have been traditionally using it.

Kava tends to be used in ritual settings associated with ceremonial acts, as in the Kingdom of Tonga, where the preparation and use of roots even plays a central role in royal ceremonies. In the Fijian Islands, after drinking a bowl of kava, people clap their hands in a specific way. Many people in Oceania use kava daily, in the same way that coffee and tea are consumed elsewhere.

When drinking kava, your mouth feels numb, just as with coca leaves, which also have anesthetic properties. It is comparable to the feeling of a

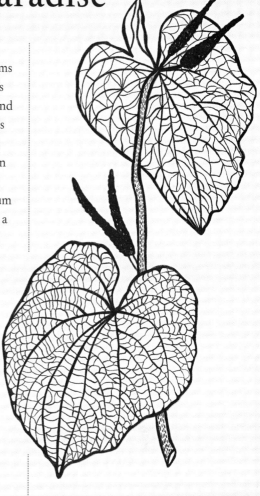

Bulbs and Roots

FURTHER PLANT JOURNEYS

KAVA KAVA

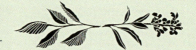

Piper methysticum

local anesthetic at the dentist. Half an hour after drinking the kava extract, it begins to take effect, which lasts about two hours. After that, the effects wear off; about seven hours after ingestion, they will have disappeared completely.

The sleep that follows kava use is considered invigorating. When waking up, there is no hangover. You can feel the effect as soon as you drink your first cup, but its action becomes particularly noticeable after consuming six to seven bowls. After the numb feeling, you often experience a need to talk, you feel euphoric, calm, and your anxiety is muted. You feel good and can think clearly, your muscles relax, and eventually you start to feel sleepy.

In recent years there have been reports of liver damage from the use of the plant among Westerners who used commercially manufactured root products. In many countries, including the Netherlands, this led to a ban on the root. This ban should, in fact, be lifted, because by now it is known what caused the liver damage: commercial oil and hot-water extracts that were admittedly stronger than the traditional cold-water extracts and proved to be harmful. Supplements that included kava extract were also linked to severe liver problems. Through oil extraction, other substances are released that remain present in the

carrier oil. Many of both types of commercial extracts turned out to contain parts of the plant that were traditionally not used. Although these green parts do contain psychoactive substances, they also contain toxic ones. Traditionally, kava is only extracted with cold water and sometimes with coconut milk, and this does not lead to any liver problems.

From this, we can learn that ancient extraction and usage methods are often the best and safest, even though, as always, there are exceptions. Some Western herbalists say you can extract the plant also in 65–90 percent alcohol because the kavalactones don't dissolve easily in water.

I believe you should lower the dose in this case, because the extract is much stronger. I don't know what kind of risk this involves, so I would go traditional. Traditional methods have been tested by people and time through years and years of use.

The wisely intended but incorrect use of plants can occasionally lead to harm or death, but to most people this tends to be solely through ignorance. Therefore, when working with and using medicinal and ritual plants, it is also important to involve an experienced shaman, herbalist, experienced expert, or trained phytotherapist.

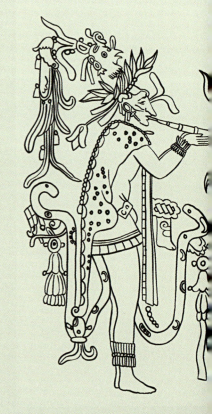

MAYAN RELIEF—A relief (ca. AD 690) in the Temple of the Cross in the Mayan city of Palenque. God L is smoking a cigar. These cigars are still smoked by the Lacandón Maya in hiapas as I have seen in Palenque. Tobacco used in South American countries has a very different effect to the industrial cigarettes and rolling tobacco sold in the West. Unprocessed *Nicotiana rustica* and *Nicotiana tabacum* is many times stronger than the flavored tobacco we know. Read about tobacco in the book *Plant Teachers: Ayahuasca, Tobacco, and the Pursuit of Knowledge* by anthropologist Jeremy Narby and Rafael Chanchari Pizuri.

Tobacco is used as a source of strength and knowledge, in order to detect diseases and get in touch with the spirit world. In the Amazon, they speak of the *maninkari*, those who are invisible to the naked eye like our DNA and inhabit living organisms. Through the use of pure tobacco, *maninkari* can become visible. (After drawings by Castaneda.)

Bulbs and Roots

FURTHER PLANT JOURNEYS

TEPEZCOHUITE

Mimosa tenuiflora

Spirit Molecule

Tepezcohuite, the root bark of the *Mimosa tenuiflora* tree, is smoked to induce a visionary trance. The plant is native to Central and South America. The name tepezcohuite is derived from the Aztec term *tepus-cuahuitl,* which means "metal tree," because of its extremely hard wood. The root bark of this tree contains approximately 1 percent N, N-dimethyltryptamine (DMT). As with many magical substances, some South American Indian tribes have known about DMT for an extremely long time.[139]

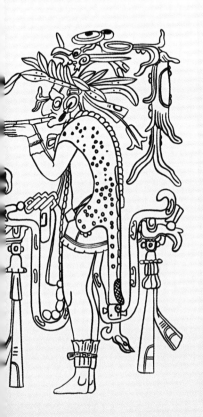

DMT is an entheogen, otherwise known as a tryptamine medicine, which occurs naturally in many plants and animals. It is even found in broccoli. In fact, everything that lives contains DMT; however, in some plants it occurs in higher concentrations. Substances containing DMT form part of the sacraments consumed during the ceremonies of many South American Indigenous people. DMT-containing powders are sometimes blown into the nose or drunk via sacred brews or smoked.

When DMT is smoked, it goes directly into the bloodstream via the lungs and enters the brain. Because it is a substance that occurs naturally in the body, after smoking, it is quickly broken down and the extremely powerful trip is short. Smoking DMT is also called "the businessman's trip," because you can use it during your lunch break at a quarter past twelve and be back in the office fully sober at half past one, as it were. But what you have experienced in the meantime is extraordinary. DMT is among the most powerful entheogenic substances, so the experience tends to be intense. People who have had it, including myself, speak of a mystical experience, other dimensions, seeing so-called electric elves, and multidimensional geometric patterns. After a DMT journey, most people feel a great clarity of mind.

Because of the intense psychedelic experience, DMT is also called the "*spirit molecule*" (see the book of the same name by Rick Strassman, M.D.). The same substance is also released during an intense REM sleep, lovemaking, at birth, and when you die. It allows us to be immersed entirely consciously in the sphere of ideas (perhaps the subconscious).

In 2018, in the Yucatan jungle in Mexico, I took part in a ceremony in which we smoked tepezcohuite, and one male and one female medicine supervisor made music and sang songs in a 9,000-year-old primal language. The songs were love songs for our souls. Everyone was asked to think about what they wanted to achieve with the ceremony. Before we smoked the substance, it was explained to us that we should focus on the seven cardinal points of the cosmos: north, east, south, west, above, below, and the center within ourselves. From all these points of the compass, we were to summon ancestor spirits to help us. We also were to allow in all our demons and fears so that we could transform them into love.

We had to spit out any mucus that would be released. Subsequently, tobacco powder (*rapé*) was blown into our nose to open "channels." During the ceremony, the sacred incense copal smoldered on glowing embers.

Bulbs and Roots

FURTHER PLANT JOURNEYS

TEPEZCOHUITE

Mimosa tenuiflora

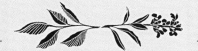

Copal is a tree resin that was used by the ancient Maya as an incense to appease the spirits and gods. The medicine supervisor had set up an altar with, among other things, an extraordinarily painted feather.

Using a pipe, we could take some draws of the tepezcohuite substance. We then lay on the ground and, guided by music, the visions would commence, lasting about 15 minutes. The medicine man himself also took a few puffs. During the ceremony, a kind of strange mucus did indeed come up that I spat out. It felt like it had come from deep within my body. While the male accompanist made music and sang, I began to see very structured geometric patterns. When the woman began to sing, the images instead became extremely organic. After the ceremony, I felt clear and full of vitality.

In Brazil, a drink is also made of the root bark, which is drunk together with passion fruit juice. This beverage is called *vinho de jurema*. You can also make an ayahuasca analogue with it.[140] In addition to DMT, new substances have been discovered in the root bark that have been called kukulkanins, after the Mayan god Kukulcan (the Plumed Serpent). The powder from the bark is used externally as an anesthesizing and analgesic remedy for burns. In addition, tepezcohuite is incorporated into various skin creams because of its beneficial effect on the skin. In Mexico, preparations of the root bark are sold in drugstores and on markets as a tonic.

In addition to ibogaine (see opposite), DMT is the most powerful psychedelic that exists, and by using it, you will discover many other dimensions you could not even have imagined, yet are so real that, after the DMT experience, the whole of life becomes relative.

At the same time, life becomes more meaningful. One small chemical change in our brain and body and our whole perception of the world changes within a few minutes. By working with entheogenic sacraments, you learn that the reality that we see as the real world, that we experience during our normal waking consciousness, is just one of several realities. Only a few among us can even imagine that there are other dimensions of reality.

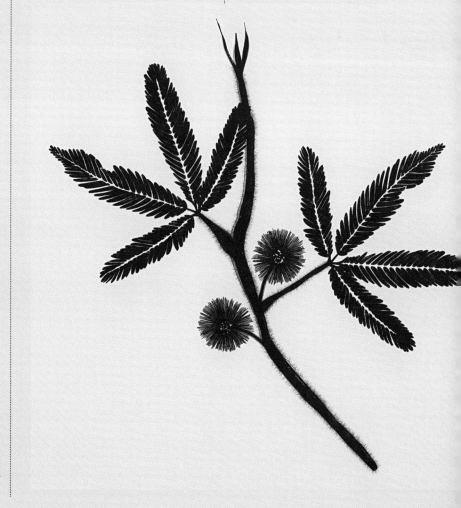

Bulbs and Roots

FURTHER PLANT JOURNEYS

IBOGA *Tabernanthe iboga*

Sacrament and Symbol of the Forest

The African cult of trees (*ombwiri* and *bwiti*) is part of a living Indigenous tradition that seems to have its origins in prehistoric times, and iboga, one of the strongest entheogens in the world, takes center stage. In West Africa, the plant is used as a sacrament in initiation rituals. It grows in the tropical rainforests of Gabon, Congo, Cameroon, and Guinea. There, iboga is a symbol of the power of the forest. The bwiti cult sprung up in the 19th century, but its origin stretches back thousands of years. Iboga is seen as the true Tree of Knowledge that came directly from the Garden of Eden, so that people could get to know God and the world.

Since the 1970s, the plant has also been used in the West to help people kick serious addictions. Iboga's anti-addictive properties were accidentally discovered by Howard Lotsof, who grew up in the Bronx, New York. In 1962, Lotsof and five friends—all heroin addicts— noticed that their cravings and withdrawal symptoms subjectively reduced when they took iboga. During the 1980s, Lotsof managed to persuade a Belgian company to produce ibogaine from iboga in capsule form and conducted successful trials in the Netherlands. He wrote numerous scientific articles and was granted patents in North America for the treatment of various chemical dependencies with ibogaine. These days, there are ibogaine clinics in Afghanistan, New Zealand, the Netherlands, and Israel.

According to experts by experience, an iboga initiation is comparable to 10 years of psychotherapy, but takes place in a pressure cooker. During the initiation, a mirror is sometimes placed in front of adepts (*banzis*) who are thus confronted with themselves. Then the introspective psychological journey can begin.

A traditional initiation takes place in the jungle and in temples, in a ritual setting with trance-inducing music. In the songs, the soul of the banzi is being accompanied. The initiation aims to take the banzi back to the origins of time. The ceremonies take place during a midnight mass (*ngozé*) and continue into the morning. Participants are usually given a few low doses of iboga, which do not cause hallucinations.

The full initiation experience with higher doses is so intense that it can only be undergone once or twice in a human life. The effect of the high doses may persist for up to a week and are meant to "crack open the head" through hallucinations that are a form of contact with the ancestors and "offer an anticipatory vision of life in the other world."[141]

Preceding an initiation, emetic herbs are drunk to clean the body. During a full initiation, which may take up several days to a week, several visits are made to the jungle where preparatory herbal and purification baths are taken. The movement is deeply connected to the jungle.[142]

After I had planted iboga seeds for the first time and opened the fruits with my bare hands, I experienced a mild intoxication that lasted three days, so this plant is tremendously powerful. I have not yet experienced a complete iboga initiation in Gabon. Very few Westerners have gone through this, but all of the descriptions from those who were initiated feature powerful but peaceful visions. Contact with deceased family members and animals is also often mentioned.

Iboga grows naturally in only a few countries in the world. The price of iboga roots has rocketed in recent years by hundreds of percent, and the plant is in danger of disappearing in the wild. People also recklessly poach the plants and smuggle them abroad due to the huge demand for it as a therapeutic agent elsewhere in the world. The poaching of elephants additionally

Bulbs and Roots

FURTHER PLANT JOURNEYS

IBOGA

Tabernanthe iboga

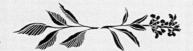

contributes to the disappearance of iboga in the wild. It is the elephants that disperse the seeds naturally through the jungle. One less elephant also means several fewer iboga plants.

As applies to many natural medicines, the pharmaceutical industry is not interested in turning this plant into medication, because not enough money can be made from it. Iboga is found in nature, after all, and anyone can grow the plant under the right conditions. In France, the plant's therapeutic value is not recognized, and it is considered a narcotic. Besides the fact that iboga is administered in high doses to kick addictions, many people are also experimenting with microdosing for the same purpose.

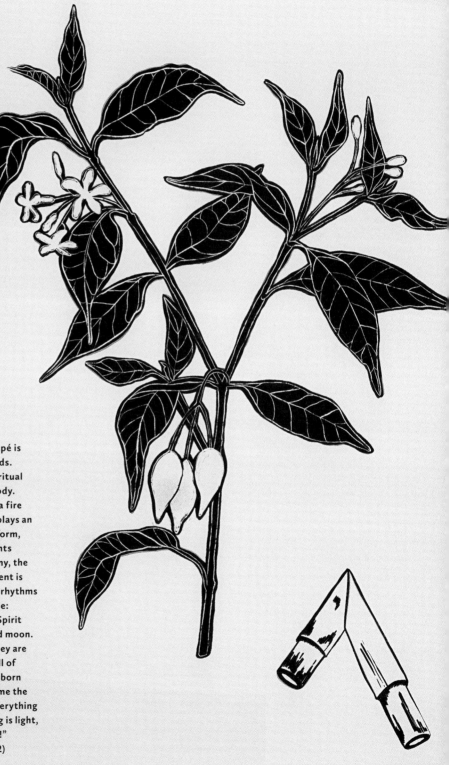

IBOGA PLANT with, below it, a *rapé* pipe—Rapé is a mixture of tobacco, ash, and sometimes seeds. This is blown into the nostrils to open the spiritual channels. The rapé seeks out disease in the body. Tobacco is also used in peyote ceremonies as a fire offering. Throughout the Americas, tobacco plays an important role during rituals and, in its pure form, is regarded a "teacher plant." Use of sacraments also occurs in Africa. Before an iboga ceremony, the body is cleansed with herbs. Then the sacrament is taken, while songs are sung, music made, and rhythms performed. Spoken words include, for example: "Thus was the beginning, Spirit of the earth, Spirit of the sky. (...) Lightning and thunder. Sun and moon. Heaven and Earth. They are life and death. They are all twins. (...) Joy, your ancestors greet you full of joy and hear the news. The anxious life of the born is at an end, at an end, at an end. And here come the disciples of death. I am going to death. (...) Everything is pure, pure. Everything new, new. Everything is light, light. I have seen the dead and I am not afraid!" (From Fernandez (1982) and Rätsch (2005:492)

Bulbs and Roots

AFTERWORD

This is a book about plants and mushrooms, but it is also about people—men and women who have conducted research over many thousands of years on the effects of plants and mushrooms, and who have discovered what kind of properties they possess. We come from nature and for a long time lived alongside her and gathered knowledge. Discovering that medicinal plant use was known as far back as 60,000 years ago tells us all we need to know about our primal connection with nature.

These teachings come back to us again, imparted orally or in writing, via Indigenous peoples, such as the Trio Indians in Suriname and the Sámi in Lapland, who are their living carriers. We ourselves can play a role in this transfer of knowledge. Pass your knowledge onto your children and grandchildren so that it is preserved for posterity. We are a young species with only about 10,000 generations behind us, and I hope that we will be able to coexist with all the other extraordinary organisms on this special planet for much longer.

The Western world is restoring its connection with nature, and we are slowly beginning to understand that we should cherish her, that she is part and parcel of ourselves, and we of her. You can take us out of the forest, but you cannot take the forest out of us. If, over the coming years, we begin to learn to think more circularly and develop a long-term vision for the conservation of biodiversity, rather than monocultures, great wonders will reveal themselves to us.

The key to planetary abundance is biodiversity. The wilderness harbors the strongest and most diverse natural remedies for body and mind. I would like to argue for rewilding certain areas of the Netherlands and other parts of the world. We can turn depleted farmland into forest again—forest that belongs to no one and to everyone; in the inspiring words of artist Aja Waalwijk, *iedersniemandsland* ("everyone's and no one's land").

Even though some of the best herbal medicines grow in the wilderness, it is important, however, not to blindly abuse wild-growing medicinal plants. We need to make sure areas of wilderness and biodiversity remain. Some medicinal plants should rather be organically cultivated.

I foresee a new bond with nature and a new appreciation for natural medicines, medicinal and ritual recipes rediscovered or reinvented, and everything dedicated toward healing universally and consciously to become interconnected with each other and nature.

The apothecary and seer Nostradamus said that you must return to the soil of your ancestors, the ground where you spent your early years, if you do not feel well. By eating and drinking products from that soil, you will get all the minerals and nutrients that once formed your body, and you will therefore regain your strength as a matter of course. Who knows? I, for one, believe in an omnipotent healing capability that can support you for a long time if you continue to take good care of yourself and the world.

A key question we could ask ourselves is inspired by the philosophy of the Iroquois, a Northern American Indian tribe: "Am I a good ancestor, and what is the impact of our actions now on the future?"

I have the impression that, among us, there is a psychospiritual desire to restore our connection with nature and "the divine" and "the essential" consciousness that can be found within it; to experience its vital force from the foundation, so that we can go back to the here and now. Together, we dance this eternal universal cosmic dance of implosion and explosion with occasional glimpses of enlightenment. I wish you strength on this wondrous journey.

Let your future flourish by planting seeds and trees at every opportunity, in full awareness and with joy. Let the inspiration from this book travel like a wave through the world. Pass it on, or donate a copy to your loved ones and, together, become the change you want to see on our planet!

GLOSSARY

Adaptogens. An adaptogen helps the body adapt to changing conditions and adverse states such as stress, heat, and cold.

Allopathy. The conventional form of medicine in which remedies are used to suppress symptoms or counter them.

Amino acids. Amino acids form the basic building blocks of all proteins in our body and are able to create tissue such as organs, muscles, skin, and hair and help the body to recover. There are 22 amino acids, 8 of which are essential. "Essential" means that you need them but your body is unable to make them, so you have to get them from food.

Anti-inflammatory. Reduces inflammation.

Antibacterial. Helps combat bacterial infections.

Antibiotic. Kills bacteria or inhibits development of bacteria.

Antidepressant. Uplifting.

Antidiabetic. Helps lower blood sugar levels.

Antimicrobial. Kills or weakens bacteria, fungi, or viruses and other organisms that cannot be seen with the naked eye.

Antioxidants. Antioxidants in your body neutralize free radicals (see page 263). Your body makes its own antioxidants, but you can also supplement them through diet and supplements. Powerful antioxidants are natural vitamin C, glutathione, and resveratrol. To prevent disease and slow down the aging process, it is important to ingest sufficient antioxidants. The body's own antioxidants work much more strongly than any external antioxidant.

Antiparasitic. Destroys and eliminates parasites.

Antirheumatic. Reduces rheumatic symptoms.

Antiseptic. Disinfects and suppresses infection or acts as a preservative.

Antitumor. Helps to prevent tumors from developing and inhibit them.

Antiviral. Fights viral infections.

Aphrodisiac. Has an arousing effect and stimulates sexual desire.

Astaxanthin. A carotenoid made by algae, plankton, and certain plant fungi and bacteria. Gives flamingos their pink color, among other things. It is active everywhere in the body and helps counteract aging processes due to oxidative stress and inflammation. Astaxanthin also supports and regulates the action of the immune system (particularly the humoral immune response). Astaxanthin is one of the most powerful antioxidants nature has to offer and affects both the inside and outside of cells in the body. Astaxanthin is available from drugstores.

Betulin. A substance found in birch trees and in the chagas fungus. Betulin is an anti-inflammatory and supports the healing of wounds. Betulin appears to destroy the engine room of tumor cells, killing off tumors, and is therefore being explored in cancer studies. Betulin has, among other things antioxidant, antiviral, and antitumor properties.

Bitter substances. The term "bitter substances" represents a comprehensive group of plants whose compounds share the common characteristic of a bitter flavor. They stimulate digestion and the secretion of digestive juices and ensure better absorption of nutrients. Their action works via the tongue's bitter receptors. Taking bitter substances in pill or capsule form is actually pointless in most cases, as you have to taste them. Bitter substances work better when you ingest them in small amounts. A well-known plant containing bitter substances is dandelion.

Carminative. Promotes digestion and reduces intestinal gas formation.

Chi. General life force. (term from traditional Chinese medicine).

Chitin. A kind of hard shell, similar to the material your hair and nails are made of.

Cholesterol. The best-known sterol is cholesterol that comes from animals. Plants and mushrooms also contain sterols. Cholesterol is important for the permeability of cell membranes. Plant and mushroom sterols can lower cholesterol in your blood. As a result of an unbalanced diet some people have too high or incorrect cholesterol levels for a long and healthy life. Sterols can help restore this balance.

Cultivar. A plant or group of plants that has been selected for desired properties and which can be preserved by means of cultivation methods. Examples are desired characteristics such as growth rate and presence of certain flower colors and substances.

Diuretic. Excretes water/moisture through the kidneys.

GLOSSARY

Entheogen. Term to describe psychoactive substances used in a religious or spiritual context to establish direct contact with the divine. Entheogenic literally means "the divine within yourself." Entheogenic sacraments are always made of power plants and mushrooms that have a demonstrable effect. These substances are often demonized. Entheogens function as keys to open the doors to the magical divine worlds and are omnipresent in nature. The term was introduced to us by classics professor Carl Ruck at Boston University and some of his colleagues in 1979.

Enzymes. An enzyme (Ancient Greek: ἐν and ζύμη zúme, yeast) is a type of protein and a catalyst that brings about a specific chemical reaction inside or outside a cell. Enzymes enable reactions or accelerate them, without being consumed themselves or by changing composition. Enzymes promote the metabolic process in the body and ensure that food disintegrates into small pieces so that it can be digested and absorbed by the body, among other things. Enzymes are also used in detergents to break up and break down dirt.

Essential oils. Fragrant substances that the plant uses to attract or repel insects and fungi. Ethereal oils are often volatile in nature. They are most commonly found in flowers and fruits but can be present in any plant part. Results with essential oils are primarily achieved via the nose and airways and through the skin. There are many well-regarded publications about essential oils and their chemical constituents that show their antimicrobial effects against a range of bacterial, fungal, and viral pathogens. The branch of phytotherapy in which essential oils are most used is aromatherapy. Volatile oils are diverse in composition.

Ethnobotany. The study of the relationship between plants and humans. Ethnobotany focuses on how plants work or are used in human societies and includes plants used for nutrition, medicine, architecture, tools, money, clothing, rituals, social life, and music.

Flavonoids. More than 5,000 different flavonoids are known, and they are very common in medicinal plants such as blueberries, green tea leaves, and *Ginkgo biloba*. Flavonoids are antioxidants (see page 262) and need sunlight in order to form. They are responsible for color in, for example, fruits and flowers. They feature most commonly in the outer parts of plants; for example, in fruit peel.

Free radicals. Cells in your body that damage other cells. An excess of damaged cells creates all kinds of diseases and accelerated aging. Antioxidants (see page 262) can eliminate free radicals.

Fruit body. Fruit bodies are parts of a plant or fungus or animal that bear the fruit and allow offspring to be created. A mushroom is the fruiting body of a fungus. A plum is a fruiting body from a tree that produces plums. All being well, the fruiting body contains seed or spores for the creation of offspring. In this way, life continues and can be passed on.

Glycosides. Dosed correctly, glycosides can play an important role in pharmacological applications. We know of several types of glycosides, some of which have a strong effect and are by no means harmless. One example is digitoxin from foxglove, which has the power to alter heart rhythm. Even in small doses, this substance can be lethal. In pharmacological microdoses, it is in fact used as a medication for cardiac arrhythmias.

Hallucinogen. Non-addictive narcotic substances that affect the mental processes in a such a way that they cause a temporarily changed state of consciousness.

Hypnotic. Induces sleep.

Immunomodulant. Improves function of the immune system.

Inulin. Inulin is primarily found in the root of the dandelion (*Taraxacum officinale*). The roots contain a high concentration of inulin, especially in the fall and early winter when the plant stores energy in the form of this soluble fiber. Plants highest in inulin include chicory root, Jerusalem artichoke, dandelion root, garlic, and leek. Inulin is a prebiotic fiber that supports gut health by feeding beneficial bacteria and helps regulate blood sugar levels by slowing digestion.

Laxative. Promotes bowel motion.

Macrophages. Macrophages are white blood cells that surround and destroy bacteria and microorganisms; they are part of your immune system. Macrophages also help remove old and damaged cells from your body.

Microbiome. Trillions of bacteria—more than 2 kilograms (4.4 pounds)—live in your gut and, together with viruses, yeasts, and fungi, form your microbiome. All those living micro beings have a major impact on your life, on how you feel, and how healthy you are. They work with your body; for example, helping to keep your intestinal wall healthy and to digest food. It also trains your immune system. This means that you are less likely to become unwell but if you do, you will recover faster. Make sure that you also feed your microbiome with fiber (prebiotics), like inulin from burdock root and Jerusalem artichoke, among other things. There are 10 times as many microorganisms present in and on us than human cells inside us.

Minerals, metals, and trace elements. Crystal-like substances, which, like vitamins, are essential nutrients we cannot live without. Minerals include calcium, phosphorus, bromine, iron, magnesium, sodium, chlorine, potassium, and sulfur. Trace elements include cobalt, copper, iodine, gold, chromium, selenium, silicon, fluorine, manganese, molybdenum, and zinc. **Calcium** is the prevalent mineral in our bodies. It makes our teeth and bones stronger. If you have a deficit, your body will consume the calcium from your bones, thereby weakening them. Calcium is especially important in childhood, when our bones grow the most, and in old age, when they can become thinner and brittle. Calcium is used for mood disorders and insomnia. Calcium depends on vitamin D for absorption and works together with phosphorus and magnesium. **Chlorine**, together with potassium and sodium, regulates the balance of fluids in the body. An excess of chlorine can be harmful to the brain. **Chromium** helps keep blood sugar levels stable, reduces hunger, and regulates cholesterol levels. It plays a role in the breakdown of fats. **Copper** is important for combatting cell damage and aging and reduces inflammation and the risk of arthritis. It helps our body convert iron into hemoglobin and pigment that transport oxygen to the blood through the act of breathing. It is also important for your nerves and increases resistance. Copper additionally has a role in the production of melanin, the pigment that gives skin and hair its color. Copper poisons sperm and is therefore incorporated into IUDs. Your body needs copper in order for vitamin C to be used properly. A great deal of copper is lost through food processing. **Iodine** is required for a proper working of the thyroid, which regulates metabolic functioning and rate, and thus energy levels; it also contributes to the mental and physical development of children. It plays an important role in the prevention of fatigue. Iodine deficiency during pregnancy can have serious consequences for brain function and the baby's development. Deficiency in adults causes concentration and memory problems. Our body needs potassium for energy storage and production of proteins. It helps regulate our fluid balance and blood pressure. **Iron** is essential for our immune system and helps destroy harmful bacteria and viruses. People with an iron deficiency are often tired, sick, and have a pale skin. We need this metal for the release and production of energy. A shortage of **magnesium** affects your whole body. It plays an important role in the release of insulin, which regulates blood sugar levels. Our nervous system needs magnesium because of its stress-reducing properties. It helps in the repair of body cells and relaxation of muscles. Insomnia, stress, depression, and fatigue are symptoms of a deficiency. **Manganese** helps keep our nervous system in good shape and ensures that our brain stays in working order. It is needed for the breakdown and utilization of food. It also helps with the production of red blood cells, which transport oxygen and nutrients around the body. Manganese is also important for strong bones. Manganese supports the production of sex hormones and activates a particular enzyme that can eliminate free radicals. **Molybdenum** is a trace element that is necessary for our metabolism. It is involved in the production and breakdown of proteins. It supports teeth and joints. It helps break down alcohol and sulfite that is added to many foods as a preservative. It also stimulates the production of red blood cells. **Phosphorus** helps activate vitamin B complex, which helps with energy production. It is essential for the repair and growth of your body and is part of your genetic material. Phosphorus needs vitamin D and calcium in order to work. Deficiencies are rare. **Potassium** allows nutrients to enter body cells and waste materials to be disposed of. It is an important mineral for our metabolism. Potassium deficiencies manifest themselves in irritability, low blood pressure, great thirst, and confusion. **Selenium** is mainly found in our liver, which it helps to function better. It also found in sperm. A deficiency can lead to infertility in men. It protects red blood cells and body cells from damage. It is a powerful antioxidant. It contributes to the detoxification of heavy metals that we occasionally ingest through food. Selenium has an important effect on our thyroid gland. Selenium works synergistically with vitamin E; both increase in strength if you ingest them at the same time. Selenium affects our eyesight and has a positive effect on skin and hair. A deficiency can lead to hair loss, lowered resistance, fatigue, and problems with fertility. It is an essential trace element. It has an anti-inflammatory effect and increases

GLOSSARY

resistance. The fluid levels in our body are strongly influenced by **sodium**. It is crucial for normal growth and helps with the proper functioning of our muscles and nerves. It allows muscles to contract properly. It is important that our body has the correct balance of potassium and sodium. Deficiencies can cause headaches, excessively low blood pressure, and dizziness. **Sulfur** is essential for the production of keratin, which is important for healthy skin, strong nails, and shiny hair. Without sulfur, the body is less able to produce glutathione. It is also important for your connective tissue, red blood cells, and muscles. **Zinc** plays a crucial role in the protection and repair of DNA and helps regulate hormone levels. Zinc is needed for enzyme activity. A lack of zinc can lead to infertility and poor growth. It is a powerful antioxidant and strengthens resistance. It also keeps your taste, smell, and vision senses in good working order. A side effect of too much zinc is that your sense of smell becomes too acute and powerful. Extra zinc accelerates wound healing.

Monograph. A scientific book or essay on one topic or one limited group of related topics.

Mycelial filaments. The system of mushroom threads that live mostly underground or in wood. Another term for mycelial threads is "fungal threads." Fungal threads form a network of connections with the roots of trees and plants and help them, for example, by clearing organic material. As a result of its mycelial threads from trees and plants, the fungus obtains other substances it cannot easily find itself in an exchange. Our brain and nervous system appear to have the same structure as mycelium.

Mycologist. Someone who studies fungi, including mushrooms.

Mystery schools. The word "mystery" comes from the Greek *muo*, which literally means "closing the eyes." Mystery schools were places or groups where the study of mysteries was examined and acquired. Well-known schools in antiquity were, among others, at Eleusis, near Athens, and in Egypt.

Neurodegenerative. Diseases of the nervous system and the brain in which nerve cells die over the years. Examples include Parkinson's disease and Alzheimer's.

Neurogenesis. Genesis comes from Greek, meaning "origin" or "coming into being"; neurogenesis means that "new nerve cells are being formed." Your brain is part of your nervous system and can thus also recover and regrow.

NGF. Nerve growth factor. Some plants and mushrooms, as well as some honey, contain substances that improve, stimulate, or restore the growth and recovery of nerve cells. In science, this is expressed as NGF.

Oxidative stress. This occurs when there is an imbalance between free radicals and the antioxidants that neutralize them. Alcohol intake, smoking, stress, too little sleep, synthetic make-up, air pollution, pesticides, too much UV radiation, and medications are factors that can increase the number of free radicals in our bodies. As a result, diseases can take hold more easily, our body cells become damaged, and we age faster.

Pathogen. Something—a bacterium, virus, or microorganism—that can cause disease.

Pharmacognosy. The study of drugs and entheogens from natural sources. It is a sub-field of pharmacy and focuses on the study of the physical, chemical, biochemical, and biological properties of drugs from natural sources. It also focuses on finding new drugs from these natural sources.

Pharmaka. Respectful word for "drugs" or etheogenic medicine. It's the plural of pharmakon and can also mean poison or remedy depending on the context.

Physiology. The scientific study of vital functions, such as metabolism of organisms, including humans.

Phytotherapy. Herbal medicine.

Plant breeding. Natural or artificial intervention in the natural selection of plants in order to achieve desired characteristics, such as substances, disease, heat resistance, color, et cetera. Breeding often involves applying pollen from male plants with a particular characteristic onto the female sexual organs (the pistils) of the plant with the desired characteristics. This is often done artificially with a brush. In nature, it is carried out by bees, other insects, and some bats. The wind can also work wonders in pollination. Some artificial growers think that by enhancing the natural characteristics and strengths achieved through breeding, they are able to patent plants for financial gain. This is called "biopiracy."

Polysaccharides. Also called carbohydrates or complex sugars. Examples of polysaccharides include starch, chitin (see page 262), and cellulose.

Psilocybin. A vision- and/or hallucination-inducing substance found in a number of fungi. Mushrooms containing psilocybin can be found virtually everywhere on the planet, and a number of species grow wild in the Netherlands and Belgium. Many consider psilocybin an entheogen. At present, about 200 species of psilocybin are known.

Rubefacient. Skin-stimulating and as a result blood flow-promoting. Because rubefacients promote blood flow, wounds can heal faster; they also help alleviate pain. Double-blind studies have demonstrated their versatile action and provided evidence of their efficacy.

Sacrament. Natural substances that are ingested by humans in order to come into contact with the divine dimensions and the realm of the dead. The Eucharist, or Holy Communion—the key moment in the celebration of Catholic mass and other Christian services—was originally psychedelic wine or beer that allowed people to directly experience the divine themselves. During the first 300 years of Christianity, Christians still used these wines, even in the necropolis underneath the Vatican. The church tried to ban the wines, which were made by women. Psychedelic wines were consumed in ancient Egypt, Persia, and Sumeria. Witch burnings were attempts to stop the old traditions and break lines of knowledge. To this day, the Catholic Church has been giving its followers a placebo, but the keys to Heaven and immortality have continued to exist—both in the New World (psilocybin mushrooms, peyote, ayahuasca, tepezcohuite and LSD) and in the ancient one (witches' salves, psilocybin mushrooms, blue lotus, fly agaric, and iboga).

Sedatives. Calming herbs.

Stimulant. A stimulating effect on the nervous system that removes fatigue and drowsiness.

Symbiosis. The coexistence of two different organisms whereby at least one of the organisms benefits from its habitat.

Tonic. Fortifying, vitalizing resource.

Vitamins. Organic substances, some of which are essential for metabolic processes and our body cannot make itself. We only need them in small quantities, but if they are lacking in our diet, we can become seriously ill or even die. **Vitamin A** is needed for healthy skin, growth, reproduction, and eyesight. It is an antioxidant. **Vitamin B1** (thiamine) is needed to convert carbohydrates and keep body and mind in good shape. **B2** (riboflavin) converts food into energy through the action of enzymes. This vitamin is rapidly lost in sunlight. **B3** (niacin/nicotinic acid) is essential for a healthy nervous system and the production of sex hormones. **B5** (pantothenic acid) increases resistance, replenishes energy, and reduces stress. **B6** (pyridoxine) helps convert food into energy, keeps the immune system healthy, and improves mood. **B12** (cobalamin) is essential for a healthy nervous system and necessary for our growth when we are young. It also plays a role in appetite. **Biotin** belongs to the B vitamins and is also called vitamin **H**. It is good for hair and skin and relieves eczema and skin inflammation. **Vitamin C** (ascorbic acid) is a strong antioxidant, increases our resistance, protects eyesight, and helps fight infections. **Choline** and **inositol** also belong to the vitamin B complex group; they help break down fat and improve our memory and mental capacity. **Vitamin D** is crucial for healthy bones and teeth. **Vitamin E** (tocopherol) is a strong antioxidant, important for a healthy heart and sufficient blood supply. It is also good for the skin. **Folic acid** belongs to the vitamin B-complex group; it prevents some congenital defects, helps against anemia, and keeps the body healthy. It can also lower the risk of heart problems. **Vitamin K** is essential for blood clotting.

Witch's salves. Both psychoactive and purely medicinal witch's salves were in use. The ingredients in the 15th-century Dutch recipe for witch's salve (flying ointment) are, in addition to the fat of a goat and the blood of a bat, the following plants: verbena, burning bush plant, mercurialis, house leeks, valerian, betony, marigold, henbane, deadly nightshade, and monkshood. Datura and/or saffron were occasionally added. This ointment was used by witches to fly (spiritually). It was applied under the armpits and on the back of the neck. The female herbalists had a high status and were not demonized by the church until after 1600. Unfortunately, the church was afraid of their immense power, which was directly connected to natural forces. All of a sudden, they were angry women who practiced black magic and were no longer associated with a goddess but with the devil. The witch burnings led to the loss of a huge wealth in plant knowledge, but there are secret places where this knowledge has been safeguarded.

NOTES

1. E.J. Carr et al, *The Cellular Composition of the Human Immune System Is Shaped by Age and Cohabition* (2016): 461–468.
2. J. Macciochi, *Immunity: The Science of Staying Well.* (2020).
3. G.A. Buijze et al, *The Effect of Cold Showering on Health and Work: A Randomized Controlled Trial* (2016).
4. Author fieldwork in Suriname.
5. *Vitamin Times: Werk aan de weerstand*, vol. 21, no. 3:6. Original source: healthcare.nu/wageningen.
6. Macciochi, *Immunity*, 47.
7. K. Verburgh, *Slowing Down Aging: The Longer Young Plan* (2016).
8. K. Verburgh, *The Longevity Code,* (2018).
9. J.R. Cameron, "Moderate Dose Rate Ionizing Radiation Increases Longevity," *Br.J.Radiol.* no. 78 (2005): 11–3; D.B. Panagiotakos et al, "Sociodemographic and Lifestyle Statistics of Oldest Old People (>80 years) Living in Ikaria Island: The Ikaria Study," *Cardiol. Res. Pract.* (2011): 679187; and C. Chrysohoou et al, "Exposure to Low Environmental Radiation and Longevity: Insights from the Ikaria Study," *Int .J. Cardiol.* no. 169 (2013): 97–98.
10. E. Burger, *Growing in the Art of Magic* (1996): 44.
11. K. Verburgh, *De voedselzandloper* (2006): 158.
12. Macciochi, *Immunity*, 146.
13. M. Walker, *Sleep: New Scientific Insights about Sleep and Dreams* (2018).
14. Macciochi, *Immunity*, 132.
15. Macciochi, *Immunity*, 106.
16. D. Servan-Schreiber, *Anticancer* (2008): 148, 150.
17. "Mushroom Consumption Delays Mild Cognitive Impairment," https://tekoafarms.co.il/wp-content/uploads/2020/05/mushroom-consumption-delays-mild-cognitive-impairment-1.pdf.
18. *Shen Nong Ben Jing* (written between 206 BCE and AD 220).
19. Among others, Suarez-Arroyo et al., *Anti-Tumor Effects of Ganoderma Lucidum (Reishi) in Inflammatory Breast Cancer in In Vivo and In Vitro Models* (2013).
20. H. L. Michiels, *Geneeskrachtige Paddenstoelen, De gezondheidsbevorderende effecten van paddenstoelen* (2014).
21. https://drugs.com/npp/reishi-mushroom.html.
22. Michiels, *Geneeskrachtige Paddenstoelen,*, 127.
23. Michiels, *Geneeskrachtige Paddenstoelen*, 128.
24. S. Elhuseinny et al, *Proteome Analysis and In Vitro Antiviral, Anticancer and Antioxidant Capacities of the Aqueous Extracts of Lentinula edodes and Pleurotus ostreatus Edible Mushrooms* (2021).
25. Ying Jianzhe et al. (1987).
26. P. Stamets, *Growing Gourmet and Medicinal Mushrooms* (2000): 268. See also https://www.youtube.com/watch?v=1Q0un2GPsSQ https://www.youtube.com/watch?v=7agK0nkiZpA
27. Michiels, *Geneeskrachtige Paddenstoelen*, 95.
28. J. Allegro, *The Sacred Mushroom and the Cross* (1970): 17.
29. C.A.P. Ruck, M.A. Hoffman, J.A.González Celdrán, *Mushrooms Myth & Mithras: The Drug Cult That Civilized Europe* (2011): 39.
30. Michiels, *Geneeskrachtige Paddenstoelen*, 32.
31. Allegro, *The Sacred Mushroom and the Cross*, 72.
32. D.E. Teeter, *Amanita Muscaria. Herb of Immortality* (2007): 55.
33. T. McKenna, *Food of the Gods: The Search for the Original Tree of Knowledge – A Radical History of Plants, Drugs, and Human Evolution* (1993).
34. L. Keller, *The Ritual Path of Initiation into The Eleusinian Mysteries* (2009).
35. A. Grey, *Net of Being* (2012): 114.
36. https://www.hopkinsmedicine.org/Press_releases/2006/07_11_06.html.
37. T. van Andel and S. Ruysschaert, *Medicinale en rituele planten van Suriname* (2011): 151.
38. M.C. Lejeune and M. De Cleene, *Compendium of Symbolic and Ritual Plants in Europe. Vol I Trees & Shrubs/Vol II Herbs* (2003): 279.
39. Lejeune and De Cleene, *Compendium of Symbolic and Ritual Plants in Europe*, 271.
40. A. Sizoo, *The Ancient World and the New Testament* (1946): 23.
41. B.C. Muraresku, *The Immortality Key: The Secret History of the Religion with No Name* (2020): 286.
42. J. Bruneton, *Pharmacognosy, Phytochemistry, Medicinal Plants*, 2008: 399.

43. L. Ganora, *Herbal Constituents: Foundations of Phytochemistry* (2009): 58.
44. R. Beiser, *Tee aus Kräutern & Früchten* (2020): 97.
45. S. Asgari et al, *Anti-Hyperglycemic and Anti-Hyperlipidemic Effects of Vaccinium Myrtillus Fruit in Experimentally Induced Diabetes (Antidiabetic Effect of Vaccinium Myrtillus Fruit)* (2016); and H. Khoo et al, *Anthocyanidins and Anthocyanins: Colored Pigments as Food, Pharmaceutical Ingredients, and the Potential Health Benefits* (2017).
46. W. Chu, S.C.M. Cheung, R.A.W. Lau, et al, *Bilberry (Vaccinium Myrtillus L.)* (2011).
47. M. De Cleene, M.C. Lejeune, *Compendium of Symbolic and Ritual Plants in Europe*, 497; and Al-Qayyim (2010): 322.
48. Verhelst, *Groot handboek geneeskrachtige planten* (2012): 395.
49. Bruneton, *Pharmacognosy, Phytochemistry, Medicinal Plants*, 603.
50. W. Sun, B. Frost, and J. Liu, *Oleuropein: Unexpected Benefits!* (2017).
51. M. Heinrich, J. Barnes, M. José, P. Garcuia, S. Gibbons, and E.M. Wiliamson, *Fundamentals of Pharmacognosy and Phytotherapy* (2018): 255–256.
52. M. Uyldert, *Lexicon der Geneeskruiden* (2nd ed.) (1977): 160.
53. Verhelst, *Groot handboek geneeskrachtige planten*, 396.
54. Bruneton, *Pharmacognosy, Phytochemistry, Medicinal Plants*, 144.
55. Verhelst, *Groot handboek geneeskrachtige planten*, 397.
56. Muraresku, *The Immortality Key*, 349.
57. Ibid.
58. https://pubmed.ncbi.nlm.nih.gov/18211023 and https://pubmed.ncbi.nlm.nih.gov/12830265.
59. B. Van Wyk and M. Wink, *Medicinal Plants of the World: An Illustrated Scientific Guide to Important Medicinal Plants and Their Uses* (1st ed. 2004/2019): 117.
60. Van Wyk, *Medicinal Plants of the World*, 117.
61. Van Andel et al. *Medicinale en rituele planten van Suriname*, 335.
62. M.C. Lejeune and M. De Cleene, *Compendium of Symbolic and Ritual Plants in Europe*, 88.
63. C. Rätsch, *Encyclopedia of Psychoactive Plants* (2005).
64. M. Farzaei et al, *Parsley: A Review of Ethnopharmacology, Phytochemistry, and Biological Activities* (2013).
65. Bruneton, *Pharmacognosy, Phytochemistry, Medicinal Plants*, 519.
66. https://mens-en-gezondheid.infonu.en/healthy-nutrition/148791-iron-rich-nutrition-list-with-all-iron-food.html and https://www.ommelanderziekenhuis.nl/wcm/connect/www/e0021586-88a3-49fa-8078accb38a1bd12/Document.pdf?MOD=AJPERES&CONVERT_TO=url&ContentCache=NONE&CACHE=NONE&CACHEID=ROOTWORKSPACE.Z18_HGC40802NGS070AVAVCPCV00C7-e0021586-88a3-49fa-8078-accb38a1bd12-nzUiqET.
67. D. Gadi et al, *Flavonoids Purified from Parsley Inhibit Human Blood Platelet Aggregation and Adhesion to Collagen. Under Flow* (2012); and *Verhelst* 2012: 423.
68. Verhelst, *Groot handboek geneeskrachtige planten*, 422; and J. Kloss, *Back to Eden: A Human Interest Story of Health and Restoration to Be Found in Herb, Root, and Bark* (1939/2009): 162.
69. M. De Cleene, *De Historia Naturalis: Geschiedenis van de kruidengeneeskunde* (2019): 333.
70. M. C. Lejeune and M. De Cleene, *Compendium of Symbolic and Ritual Plants in Europe Vol. 2* (2003): 529.
71. C. Müller Ebeling, C. Rätsch, and W.D. Storl, *Witchcraft Medicine* (2003): 14.
72. Ebeling et al (2003): 90.
73. De Cleene, *De Historia Naturalis: Geschiedenis van de kruidengeneeskunde* (2019): 333.
74. P. Kubica et al, *Verbena Officinalis (Common Vervain): A Review on the Investigations of This Medicinally Important Plant Species* (2020).
75. M.E. Grawish, M.M. Anees, H.M. Elsabaa, M.S. Abdel-Raziq, and W. Zedan, *Short-Term Effects of Verbena Officinalis Linn Decoction on Patients Suffering from Chronic Generalized Gingivitis: Double-Blind Randomized Controlled Multicenter Clinical Trial* (2006).
76. Kubica, *Verbena Officinalis (Common Vervain)*.
77. Gohari et al, *An Overview on Saffron, Phytochemicals, and Medicinal Properties* (2013); and L. Ganora, *Herbal Constituents: Foundations of Phytochemistry* (2009): 150.

78. M. Butnariu et al, *The Pharmacological Activities of Crocus Sativus L: A Review Based on the Mechanisms and Therapeutic Opportunities of Its Phytoconstituents* (2022); and J. Bian et al, *Neuroprotective Potency of Saffron against Neuropsychiatric Diseases, Neurodegenerative Diseases, and Other Brain Disorders: From Bench to Bedside* (2020).

79. A. Hosseini, et al, *Pharmacokinetic Properties of Saffron and Its Active Components* (2018).

80. Butnariu, *The Pharmacological Activities of Crocus Sativus L* (2022).

81. Uyldert, *Lexicon der Geneeskruiden* (1977): 176.

82. H. van Genderen, L.M. Schoonhoven, and A. Fuchs, *Chemical-Ecological Flora of Netherlands and Belgium* (1996): 229; and *Bruneton* (2008): 598.

83. Simmonds, Howes, Irving, *Botanisch Handboek Medicinale Planten* (2018): 206.

84. Verhelst, *Groot handboek geneeskrachtige planten*.

85. Ganora, *Herbal Constituents*, 48.

86. D. Pendell, *Pharmakopoeai: Power Plants, Poisons, & Herbcraft, 1st ed.* (1995/2010): 182–183.

87. R. Taylor, *Death and Resurrection Show: From Shaman to Superstar* (1985): 189–190.

88. B. Hughes, *Homo Sapiens Correctus Psychovitamins 1* (1964).

89. Bruneton, *Pharmacognosy, Phytochemistry, Medicinal Plants*, 453.

90. Ganora, *Herbal Constituents*, 127.

91. J. Suzman, *Work: A History of How We Spend Our Time* (2020): 193.

92. R. Redzepi and D. Zilber, *Noma's Handbook for Fermentation* (2019): 26.

93. S.H. Buhner, *Sacred and Herbal Healing Beers: The Secrets of Ancient Fermentation* (1998): 146.

94. J. Frazer, *The Golden Bough: A Study in Magic and Religion* (1922/1993): 219.

95. Buhner, *Herbal Antivirals*, 178.

96. S. Blankaart, *Den Nederlandschen Herbarius, 1st ed.* (1756/1980): 412.

97. D. Pendell, *Pharmakopeai: Power Plants, Poisons, & Herbcraft* (2010): 66.

98. Lejeune and De Cleene, *Compendium of Symbolic and Ritual Plants in Europe*, 417.

99. Verhelst, *Groot handboek geneeskrachtige planten*, 273.

100. Tapan Kumar Mohanta, Yasinalli Tamboli, P.K. Zobaidha, *Phytochemical and Medicinal Importance of Ginkgo biloba L.* (2014).

101. Hofferberth, *The Efficacy of EGb 761 in Patients with Senile Dementia of the Alzheimer's Type: A Double-Blind, Placebo-Controlled Study on Different Levels of Investigation* (1994).

102. Seligmann (1996): 115.

103. Ganora, *Herbal Constituents*, 140.

104. De Cleene, *Historia Naturalis*, 133.

105. M. Uyldert, *Lexicon der Geneeskruiden*, 141.

106. Simmonds, *Botanisch Handboek Medicinale Planten* (2018): 122.

107. Bruneton, *Pharmacognosy, Phytochemistry, Medicinal Plants*, 521.

108. Verhelst, *Groot handboek geneeskrachtige planten*, 365.

109. Ganora, *Herbal Constituents*, 107.

110. Verhelst, *Groot handboek geneeskrachtige planten*.

111. F. Bianchini, *Flora della regione veronese. Spermatofite* (1976): 36; or Lejeune and De Cleene (2003): 8.

112. J. McVicar, *Jekka's Complete Herb Book* (1994): 243.

113. Ganora, *Herbal Constituents*, 119.

114. A. Savich et al, *Analysis of Inulin And Fructans in Taraxacum Officilae.L. Roots: The Main Inulin-Containing Component of Antidiabetic Herbal Mixture* (2021): 527.

115. A.H.C. Vogel, *De Kleine Dokter, waardevolle raadgevingen, geput uit de rijke schat van aloude Zwitserse genezingsgebruiken* (1979, unchanged since 1967): 529.

116. R. Heaven, *San Pedro: The Gateway to Wisdom* (2016): 21.

117. D. Sharon, *The San Pedro Cactus in Peruvian Folk Healing* (1972): 128.

118. P. Furst, *Flesh of the Gods: The Ritual Use Of Hallucinogens* (1972): 137.

119. E.F. Löhndorff, *The Indian Dies: Struggle and Downfall of a People* (lst ed. 1933/1955): 135.

120. D. Frawley and V. Lad, *The Yoga of Herbs: An Ayurvedic Guide to Herbal Medicine* (2008): 122.

121. M.C.A. Tierra, *Planetary Herbology: An Integration of Western Herbs into the Traditional Chinese and Ayurvedic Systems* (1988): 244; and R.B. Semwal, D.K. Semwal, S. Combrinck, and A.M. Viljoen, *Gingerols and Shogaols: Important Nutraceutical Principles from Ginger* (2015).

122. Verhelst, *Groot handboek geneeskrachtige planten*, 606.
123. Ganora, *Herbal Constituents*, 143.
124. S. Fulder, *A Book on Ginseng, the Magic Herb of the East* (1976): 28; and Johannsen, (2006): 172.
125. Lee et al., *Radioprotective Potential of Ginseng* (2005): 237–243.
126. Uyldert, *Lexicon der Geneeskruiden*, 146.
127. Simmonds, Howes, Irving, *Botanisch Handboek Medicinale Planten* (2018): 20.
128. Verhelst, *Groot handboek geneeskrachtige planten*, 87.
129. Kalman Hennings, *Curcumin: A Review of Its Effects on Human Health* (2017).
130. Van Wyk and M. Wink, *Medicinal Plants of the World: An Illustrated Scientific Guide to Important Medicinal Plants and Their Uses* (1st ed. 2004/2019): 59.
131. Uyldert, *Lexicon der Geneeskruiden*, 157–158.
132. Bruneton, *Pharmacognosy, Phytochemistry, Medicinal Plants*, 203.
133. P. Neumayer, *Choosing Natural Antibiotics* (2001): 111.
134. Uyldert, *Lexicon der Geneeskruiden*, 157–158.
135. A.H.C. Vogel, *De Kleine Dokter, waardevolle raadgevingen, geput uit de rijke schat van aloude Zwitserse genezingsgebruiken* (1979, unchanged since 1967): 27. *The Nature Doctor: A Manual of Traditional and Complementary Medicine* (1994).
136. A. Dini, G. Migliuolo, L. Rastrelli, P. Saturnino, and O. Schettino, *Chemical Composition. or Lepidium Meyenii* (1994); and C.F. Quiros, A. Epperson, Jinguo Hu, and M. Holle, "Physiological Studies and Determination of Chromosome Number in Maca, Lepidium Meyenii (Brassicaceae)," *Economic Botany*, Vol. 50, No. 2 (Apr.-Jun., 1996): 216-223.
137. B. Van Wyk and M. Wink, *Medicinal Plants of the World*, 256.
138. J. Turner, *The Water of Life: Kava Ritual and the Logic of Sacrifice* (1986).
139. G. Hellinga and H. Plomp, *Uit Je Bol* (1st ed. 1994/2003).
140. Rätsch, *Encylopedia of Psychoactive Plants*, (2005): 362.
141. P. De Smet, *Herbs, Health, and Healers: Africa as Ethnopharmacological Treasury* (1999): 138.
142. Rätsch, *Encylopedia of Psychoactive Plants*, (2005): 489.

RESOURCES

Your Immune System

J. Enders, *The Inside Story of Your Body's Most Underrated Organ* (revised edition, 2018).

C. Hoffman, *Fit and Healthy with Antioxidants: Improve Your Natural Defense System* (2000).

https://bristol.ac.uk/Depts/Chemistry/ MOTM/taxol/taxol.htm.

https://cell.com/cell/fulltext/S0092- 8674(21)00072-6.

https://cell.com/trends/immunology/ fulltext/S1471-4906(21)00056-9?_returnURL=https%3A%2F%2Flinkinghub. elsevier.com%2Freve%2Fpii% 2FS1471490621000569%3Fshowall%3Dtrue.

https://energiekevrouwenacademie.nl/ immune system-where-is-that.

https://jamanetwork.com/journals/jama/ article-abstract/417085.

https://medicalnewstoday.com/articles/ human-microbiota-the-microorganisms- that-make-us-their-home.

https://mushroomreferences.com.

https://nos.nl/artikel/2357016-stiltegebiedsteeds- more-often-under-pressure.

https://pubmed.ncbi.nlm.nih.gov/12751781.

https://pubmed.ncbi.nlm.nih.gov/23733436.

https://pubmed.ncbi.nlm.nih.gov/27475233.

C. Janeway et al, *Immunobiology*, 6th edition (2005).

A. Khan et al, *Anticancer Activities of Nigella Sativa (Black Cumin)* (2011).

E. Spielman, *The Spiritual Journey of Joseph L. Greenstein, The Mighty Atom: World's Strongest Man* (1979).

T.S. Wiley and B. Formby, *Lights Out: Sleep, Sugar, and Survival* (2001).

D. Wolfe, *Superfoods* (2009).

MUSHROOMS

Chaga

P. van Ineveld, *Medicinal Mushrooms* (2020).

P. Stamets, *Mycelium Running* (2005).

M. Stengler, *Health Benefits of Medicinal Mushrooms* (2005).

D. Wolfe, *Chaga, King of Medicinal Mushrooms* (2012).

Button Mushroom

H. L. Michiels, *Geneeskrachtige Paddenstoelen, De gezondheidsbevorderende effecten van paddenstoelen* (2014).

Ying Jianzhe, Mao Xiaolan, Ma Qiming Zong Yichen, and Wen Huaan, *Icons of Medicinal Fungit from China* (1987).

Ink Cap

H. L. Michiels, *Geneeskrachtige Paddenstoelen, De gezondheidsbevorderende effecten van paddenstoelen* (2014).

Ying Jianzhe et al, https://pubmed.ncbi.nlm.nih.gov/32479019 (1987).

Reishi

https://pubmed.ncbi.nlm.nih. gov/23468988.

P. van Ineveld, *Medicinal Mushrooms* (2020).

P. Stamets, *Mycelium Running* (2005).

G. Verhelst, *Groot handboek geneeskrachtige planten* (2012).

Ying Jianzhe et al., https://pubmed.ncbi.nlm.nih.gov/32479019, 1987.

Shiitake

M. Stengler, *The Health Benefits of Medicinal Mushrooms* (2005).

Lion's Mane

van Ineveld, *Medicinale paddenstoelen: een nieuw perspectief op genezing*, 2020.

P. Stamets, *Mycelium Running* (2005).

Ying Jianzhe et al., https://pubmed.ncbi.nlm.nih.gov/32479019, 1987.

Fly Agaric

A. Alberts and P. Mullen, *Psychoactive Plants, Mushrooms and Animals: How Nature Can Affect Our Brains* (2001).

I. Al-Qayyim, *The Authenticity of the Medicine of the Prophet Based on Works by Shaykh Muhammad Nasir ad-Din-al-Albani* (2010).

K. Feeney, *Fly Agaric: A Compendium of History, Pharmacology, Mythology, and Exploration* (2020).

T. Hatsis, *Psychedelic Mystery Traditions: Spirit Plants, Magical Practices, and Estatic States* (2018).

G. Hellinga and H. Plomp, *Out of Your Mind* (1st ed. 1994/2003).

V.P. Lehtola, *The Sámi People: Traditions in Transition* (2002).

B. Masha, *Microdosing with Amanita Muscaria* (2022).

T. McKenna, *Food of the Gods: The Search for the Original Tree of Knowledge – A Radical History of Plants, Drugs, and Human Evolution* (1st ed. 1992/1998).

H. L. Michiels, *Geneeskrachtige Paddenstoelen, De gezondheidsbevorderende effecten van paddenstoelen* (2014).

B.C. Muraresku, *The Immortality Key: The Secret History of the Religion with No Name* (2020).

Psilocybin

A. Grey, *Net of Being* (2012).

https://ir.compasspathways.com/news-releases/news-release-details/compass-pathways-announces-positive-topline-results?fbclid=IwAR18AhqPXBNzkftiICpluCRE0jDipCdBqwFtEE7YqQ9mtVENT5DenzWsw6M.

https://news.nus.edu.sg/mushrooms-mayreduce-risk-of-cognitive-decline.

B.C. Muraresku, *The Immortality Key: The Secret History of the Religion with No Name* (2020).

P. Stamets, *Mycelium Running* (2005).

P. Stamets, *Psilocybin Mushrooms of the World* (1996).

FRUIT AND NUTS

Papaya

J. Bruneton, *Pharmacognosy, Phytochemistry, Medicinal Plants* (2008).

J.L. Slagveer, *Sranan Oso Dresi: Geneeskracht uit Surinaamse kruiden* (2009).

G. Verhelst, *Groot handboek geneeskrachtige planten* (2012).

https://www.medicalnewstoday.com/articles/275517#benefits.

Grape

Hatsis, *Psychedelic Mystery Traditions* (2018).

P. Ruck, "Entheogens in Ancient Times: Wine and the Rituals of Dionysus" (2019):

https://www.academia.edu/44299052/Entheogens_in_Ancient_Times_Wine_and_the_Rituals_of_Dionysus.

Bilberry

Bianchini, F. Corbetta, and M. Pistoia, *The Plant in Medicine: Standard Work for Application, History, and Flora of Medicinal Herbs with Pharmacompendium* (1976).

Bruneton, *Pharmacognosy, Phytochemistry, Medicinal Plants* (2008).

De Cleene and Lejeune, *Compendium of Symbolic and Ritual Plants in Europe* (2003).

K. Allgeier, *The Secret Physician Recipes of Nostradamus* (1994).

https://www.ncbi.nlm.nih.gov/pmc/articles/PMC2850944.

https://www.ncbi.nlm.nih.gov/pmc/articles/PMC5613902.

https://newswire.caes.uga.edu/story/866/healthberries.html.

https://pubmed.ncbi.nlm.nih.gov/17602170.

L. Wilms et al, *Impact of Multiple Genetic Polymorphisms on Effects of a Four-Week Blueberry Juice Intervention on Ex Vivo Induced Lymphocytic DNA Damage in Human Volunteers* (2007).

G. Verhelst, *Groot handboek geneeskrachtige planten* (2012).

Cloudberry

M. Jaakkola, V. Korpelainen, K. Hoppula, and V. Virtanen, *Chemical Composition of Ripe Fruits of Rubus Chamaemorus L. Grown in Different Habitats* (2012).

B. Thiem and V. Berge, *Cloudberry: An Important Source of Ellagic Acid, an Anti-Oxidant* (2003).

"A Guide to Cloudberries: All About the North's Most Sought-After Fruit, https://www.scandinaviastandard.com/aguide-to-cloudberries-all-about-thenorths-most-sought-after-fruit.

Kola Nut

Bruneton, *Pharmacognosy, Phytochemistry, Medicinal Plants* (2008).

P. de Smet, *Herbs, Health, and Healers: Africa as Ethnopharmacological Treasury* (1999).

C. Rätsch, *Encyclopedia of Psychoactive Plants* (2005).

B. Van Wyk and M. Wink, *Medicinal Plants of the World: An Illustrated Scientific Guide to Important Medicinal Plants and Their Uses* (1st ed. 2004/2019).

HERBS AND SPICES

Clove

Bruneton, *Pharmacognosy, Phytochemistry, Medicinal Plants*.

L. Ganora, *Herbal Constituents: Foundations of Phytochemistry* (2009).

J. Grünwald, *Plant Medicine from A to Z* (2008).

H. McGee, *On Food and Cooking* (2004).

https://pubmed.ncbi.nlm.nih.gov/34770801.

G. Verhelst, *Groot handboek geneeskrachtige planten* (2012).

Parsley

N. Aisani et al, *Anticancer Effect in Human Glioblastoma and Antioxidant Activity of Petroselinum crispum L. Methanol Extract* (2021).

E. Tang et al, *Petroselinum Crispum Has Antioxidant Properties, Protects Against DNA Damage, and Inhibits Proliferation and Migration of Cancer Cells* (2015).

https://stringfixer.com/nl/4,5-Methylenedioxyphenyl-3-methoxy-2-propene.

https://tegenkanker.nl/project/antikankerstoffen-in-groenten.

Sage

Ganora, *Herbal Constituents* (2009).

A. Ghorbani and M. Esmaeilizadeh, *Pharmacological Properties of Salvia officinalis and Its Components*, 2017.

https://pubmed.ncbi.nlm.nih.gov/29034191.

M. Simmonds, M. Howes, and J. Irving, *Botanisch Handboek Medicinale Planten* (2018).

Uyldert, *Lexicon der Geneeskruiden* (1977).

G. Verhelst, *Groot handboek geneeskrachtige planten* (2012).

Verbena

P. Kubica et al, *Production of Verbascoside, Isoverbascoside, and Phenolic Acids in Callus, Suspension, and Bioreactor Cultures of Verbena Officinalis and Biological Properties of Biomass Extracts, Molecules MDPI* (2020).

G. Verhelst, *Groot handboek geneeskrachtige planten* (2012).

Odon de Meung, *La Pharmacie des Moines: Macer Floridus Des Vertus des Plantes*, 9th century.

Saffron

Bruneton, *Pharmacognosy, Phytochemistry, Medicinal Plants*.

Lejeune and De Cleene, *Compendium of Symbolic and Ritual Plants in Europe*.

https://www.ncbi.nlm.nih.gov/pmc/articles/PMC8860555. Keller, 2009.

G. Verhelst, *Groot handboek geneeskrachtige planten* (2012).

Van Wyk and Wink, *Medicinal Plants of the World* (2019). Heinrich, 2018.

Cannabis

G. Verhelst, *Groot handboek geneeskrachtige planten*.

W. Bruining, *Eeenvoudig wietologisch handboek* (1991).

W. Bruining, *Mediwietolie: het ideale voksmedicijn* (2011).

B. Dariš et al, "Cannabinoids in Cancer Treatment: Therapeutic Potential and Legislation," in *Journal of the Association of Basic Medical Sciences* (2019).

M. Frank and E. Rosenthal, *Marijuana Growing Book* (1978/1986/2018).

https://trimbos.nl/docs/e084a515-84af-4f69-8ea5-1291641a1df3.pdf.

L. Manniche, *An Ancient Egyptian Herbal* (2006).

R. Niesink and M. van Laar, *THC and CBD and the Health Effects of Marijuana and Hashish* (2012).

F. Pellati et al, *Cannabis sativa L. and Nonpsychoactive Cannabinoids: Their Chemistry and Role against Oxidative Stress, Inflammation, and Cancer* (2018).

M. Guzman. *Cannabinoids: Potential Anticancer Agents* (2003).

Sweetgale

A. Doppagne, *Les Grand Feux* (1972).

M. Eliade, *The Sacred and The Profane: The Nature of Religion* (1st ed. 1957/1987).

De Cleene and Lejeune, *Compendium of Symbolic and Ritual Plants in Europe*.

A. Jongstra, *Ecologieën. Een album in de natuur* (2020).

F. Lardot (2019) https://blik-ardennen.luxembourg-belge.be/de-heksen-van-de-ardennen.

C. Rätsch, *Encyclopedia of Psychoactive Plants* (2005).

C. Rätsch and C. Müller-Ebeling, *Pagan Christmas: The Plants, Spirits, and Rituals at the Origins of Yuletide* (2006).

R. Vervoort, "Vrouwen op den besem and derghelijck ghespoock: Pieter Bruegel en de traditie van hekserijvoorstellingen in de Nederlanden tussen 1450 en 1700" (2011).

LEAVES AND FLOWERS

Matcha

Y. Guo et al, "Green Tea and the Risk of Prostate Cancer: A Systematic Review and Meta-Analysis" (2017) in *Medicine* 96.

X. Ba et al, *L-Theanine in Cancer Prevention and Treatment* (2006).

https://cebp.aacrjournals.org/content/15/12_Supplement/A157.

K. Matsumoto et al, *Effects of Green Tea, Catechins, and Theanine on Preventing Influenza Infection among Healthcare Workers: A Randomized Controlled Trial* (2011).

https://www.ncbi.nlm.nih.gov/pmc/articles/PMC3049752.

Meadowsweet

S. Zamardzic et al, *Antioxidant, Anti-Inflammatory and Gastroprotective Activity of Filipendula Ulmaria (L.) Maxim. and Filipendula vulgaris Moench* (2018).

Dandelion

De Cleene and Lejeune, *Compendium Of Symbolic and Ritual Plants in Europe*.

J. Green, *The Herbal Medicine Makers Handbook* (2002).

G. Verhelst, *Groot handboek geneeskrachtige planten* (2012).

A.C.H. Vogel, *The Little Doctor: Valuable Advice Drawn from the Rich Treasure of Time-Honored Swiss Healing Practices* (1979, unchanged since 1967).

Coca

A. Atonil, *Mama Coca* (1978).

A. de Lestrange, *Coca Wine, Angelo Mariani's Miraculous Elixir and the Birth of Modern Advertising* (2016).

C. Rätsch, *Encyclopedia of Psychoactive Plants* (2005).

Ganora, *Herbal Constituents* (2009).

Blue Lotus

L. Manniche, *An Ancient Egyptian Herbal* (2006).

C. Rätsch, *Encyclopedia of Psychoactive Plants* (2005).

Huachama Cactus

R. Schultes (1998), and R. Schultes, A. Hofmann, and C. Rätsch, *Plants of the Gods* (2001).

Furst, *The Flesh of the Gods: The Ritual Use of Hallucinogens* (1972).

C. Rätsch, *Encyclopedia of Psychoactive Plants* (2005).

A. Huxley, *The Doors of Perception* (1954).

Uyldert, *Lexicon der Geneeskruiden*.

Peyote Cactus

C. Castaneda, *Journey to Ixtlan: The Lessons of Don Juan* (1961).

John (Fire) Lame Deer and R. Erdoes, *Lame Deer, Seeker of Visions: The Life of a Sioux Medicine Man* (1970).

E. Löhndorff, *The Indian Dies* (1955).

C. Rätsch, *Encyclopedia of Psychoactive Plants* (2005).

Schultes et al. *Plants of the Gods* (2001).

De Waarheid newspaper (10-12-1955).

BULBS AND ROOTS

Ginger

McVicar, *Jekka's Complete Herb Book* (2007).

K.V. Zwelebil, *The Siddha Quest for Immortality* (2003).

Ginseng

Rätsch, C. and C. Müller-Ebeling, *The Encyclopedia of Aphrodisiacs* (2003).

G. Verhelst, *Groot handboek geneeskrachtige planten* (2012).

World Health Organization, *WHO Monographs on Selected Medicinal Plants, Vol. 1* (1999): 172.

RESOURCES

Garlic
Ganora, *Herbal Constituents* (2009).

Genderen, Schoonhoven, and Fuchs, *Chemisch Ecologische Flora Van Nederland en Belgie*.

Uyldert, *Lexicon der Geneeskruiden*.

Horseradish
Arumugam and A. Razis, *Apoptosis as a Mechanism of the Cancer Chemopreventive Activity of Glucosinolates: A Review* (2018) https://mdpi.com/2311-7524/7/7/167/pdf?version=1624958181.

https://tegenkanker.nl/project/antikankerstoffen-in-groenten.

K. Ku et al, *Correlation of Quinone Reductase Activity and Allyl Isothiocyanate Formation Among Different Genotypes and Grades of Horseradish Roots* (2015).

S. Manuguara et al, *The Antioxidant Power of Horseradish, Armoracia Rusticana, Underlies Antimicrobial and Antiradical Effects, Exerted In Vitro*, 2020.

G. Verhelst, *Groot handboek geneeskrachtige planten* (2012).

A. Walters, *Horseradish: A Neglected and Underutilized Plant Species for Improving Human Health* (2021).

Black Radish
G. Verhelst, *Groot handboek geneeskrachtige planten* (2012).

A. Manivannan, J. Kim, D. Kim, E. Lee, and H. Lee, *Deciphering the Nutraceutical Potential. Of Raphanus sativus-A Comprehensive Overview* (2019).

Maca
National Research Center, *Lost Crops of the Inca* (1989).

C. Rätsch, *Encyclopedia of Psychoactive Plants* (2005).

Wolfe, *Superfoods* (2009).

G. Verhelst, *Groot handboek geneeskrachtige planten* (2012).

Kava Kava
C. Kilham, *Kava Medicine Hunting in Paradise* (1996).

V. Lebot, M. Merlin, and L. Lindstrom, *Kava, The Pacific Elixir: The Definitive Guide to Its Ethnobotany, History, and Chemistry* (1997).

C. Rätsch, *Encyclopedia of Psychoactive Plants* (2005).

M. Sahlins, *How "Natives" Think: About Captain Cook, For Example* (1995).

Tepezcohuite
Hall, *The Secret Teachings of All Ages* (1928, 2003 reissue).

R. Schultes, *Plants of the Gods*.

Iboga
Buhner, *Sacred and Herbal Healing Beers: The Secrets of Ancient Fermentation* (1998).

ça s'explique IBOGA, Gabon TV (2014).

R. Schultes, *Plants of the Gods* (update by C. Rätsch, 2002).

RECIPE OVERVIEW

MUSHROOMS

Chagakombucha, 37

Mung Bean Soup with Chaga and Souffléd Naan, 39

Millefeuille of Raw Button Mushroom, Cocoa, Apple, and Avocado, 42

Champignon á la Grecque with Artichoke and Fennel Seeds, 44

Toast with Fried Ink Caps and Parsley Butter, 48

Vegetarian Pasta Carbonara with Ink Cap and Remeker Cheese, 49

Tiramisu with Reishi Coffee, 52

Reishi Chai Latte, 53

Avocado with Fermented Shiitake Powder, 56

Shiitake Dashi with Furikake Eggs, 58

Tempura of Lion's Mane with Garlic Powder and Parsley Aioli, 62

Poached Pom Pom Blanc with Ponzu and Ginger, 63

FRUIT AND NUTS

Papaya Sambal, 78

Green Papaya Salad, 78

Kiwi, Cucumber, Verbena, and Fried Grapes Salad, 86

Ajo Blanco with Melon, 86

Bilberry Candy, 91

Bilberry Pie, 93

Focaccia with Olives and Sage, 98

Pasta Aglio e Olio, 98

Fesenjān with "Chicken of the Woods" Mushrooms, Pomegranate, and Walnut, 104

Wouter's Birthday Brownies, 104

Cloudberry Jam with Coulommiers Cheese, Herb Salad, and Cloudberry Bread, 108

Cloudberry Bread, 109

Cloudberry Pavlova with Yogurt, 110

HERBS AND SPICES

Eccles Cakes with Remeker Cheese, 124

Poached Pear and Sabayon with Mulled Wine, 125

Broccoli Stalk with Toast and Parsley Salad, 129

Green Salad with Zucchini, Mint, Pistachio, and Parsley, 131

Tortellini with Ricotta, Pumpkin, and Sage Butter, 137

Sage "Opperdoezer" Potatoes with Mustard-Olive Sauce, 138

Tzatziki with Yogurt, Cucumber, and Snow Peas, 144

Juice of Fermented Honey with Pear, Sorrel, and Vervain, 144

Wouter's Oatmeal with Saffron, 148

Jeweled Rice with Candied Orange, Pistachio, and Saffron, 149

Flower Butter, 152

Hot Chocolate with Valerian, 154

LEAVES AND FLOWERS

Nettle Spring Roll with Sweet and Sour Mushroom, Carrot, and Avocado, 172

Stir-Fried Nettle Leaves with Avocado and Sesame Seeds, 173

Salad of Ginkgo with White Asparagus and Granny Smith Apples, 178

Rice Pudding with Ginkgo Nut, Red Date, and Cranberry Powder, 179

Turnip in Chamomile Salt Crust with Ravigote Sauce, 184

Cherries with Chamomile Granita and Oudwijker Lazuli Cheese, 185

Energy Balls with Seeds, Nuts, Dried Fruit, and Matcha, 189

Tempura of Shiso and Shiitake with Matcha Salt, 190

Feta with Peas and Meadowsweet, 196

Tempura of Meadowsweet with White Asparagus and Gribiche Sauce, 199

Bitter Salad Leaves, Dandelion, and Roasted Grapefruit, 204

Salsa Verde with Dandelion and Zucchini, 205

BULBS AND ROOTS

Candied Stem Ginger with Cream, 221

Ginger Beer with Strawberries, 222

Chawanmushi – Savoury Ginseng Custard, 228

Strawberries with Ginseng Mousse, 229

Caramelized Celeriac with Garlic, Mirin, Soy, and Soft-Boiled Egg, 233

Garlic Velouté with Roasted Carrots and Onion, 236

Turmeric Pancakes with Enoki Mushroom, Cilantro, and Spanish Pepper, 241

Tartlet with Vegetarian Rendang and White Asparagus Pickle, 243

Fennel Salad with Horseradish Buttermilk Dressing, 246

Glazed Eggplant with Horseradish Cream and Seaweed, 248

Pickled Black Radish, 253

Radish with Bread and Butter, 253

FOOD GLOSSARY

Aioli: cold Mediterranean sauce, which consists of an emulsion of garlic and sunflower or another neutral oil

Cilantro: leaves and stem of the coriander plant

Coulommiers cheese: a soft raw cheese with a bloomy rind similar to brie

Dashi: a family of stocks that serve as base for many Japanese dishes; a common one is a simple broth from kombu and bonito flakes

Furikake: Japanese seasoning, typically made with toasted sesame seeds, nori, salt, and sugar. It varies according to the region.

Kombu: a dried edible kelp that, in traditional Japanese cuisine, is used as seasoning in soup stock

Mirin: sweet rice wine; can be substituted by dry sherry or white wine

Opperdoezer potatoes: a round, firm boiling potato with delicate taste from the Dutch town Opperdoes; can be substituted with baby Dutch yellow waxy boiling potatoes

Ponzu: Japanese stock or dipping sauce made from soy sauce, citrus juice, mirin and other ingredients

Remeker cheese: a raw cheese from cowsmilk; in style similar to Gouda

Oudwijker Lazuli cheese: a soft Dutch blue cheese like Gorgonzola

INDEX

A

abdominal pain 161, 181
acne. See *skin*
adaptogens 209, 225, 226, 254, 262
addiction 151, 259
agaritine 41
aging 12, 14, 55, 82, 187, 262, 263, 264. See also *anti-aging*
ajo blanco with melon 86
alcohol macerate 26, 35, 36
alertness 96, 113, 187, 206
alkaloids 206, 212
allopathic medicine 22, 262, 42, 206
aluminum 42, 206
Alzheimer's disease 10, 61, 64, 102, 175, 239, 265
amino acids 14, 47, 55, 61, 262
analgesic 121, 122, 181, 193, 255, 258
anandamine 157
anemia 264, 266
anesthetic 82, 119, 121, 209, 255, 256
anthocyanin 10, 89, 107
anti-aging 22, 82, 89, 95, 107, 127, 175, 202
antibacterial 14, 51, 89, 121, 133, 141, 142, 181, 232, 239, 251, 262
antibacterial drug 157
antibiotic 11, 157, 231, 232, 245, 262
anticarcinogenic 10, 55, 82
antidepressant 21, 22, 69, 147, 262
antidiabetic 251, 262
antidote 51, 167, 209
anti-emetic 209
antimicrobial 82, 219, 245 , 262, 263
antimutagen 239
antinutrients 217
antioxidants 11, 12, 14, 35, 41, 55, 73, 81, 82, 96, 101, 102, 113, 127, 141, 142, 147, 157, 175, 187, 201, 202, 209, 219, 239, 251, 262, 263, 265
anti-rheumatic 167, 168, 193, 262
antiseptic 121, 133, 262
antispasmodic 121, 127, 142, 151, 181, 219, 245
antithrombotic 101
anti-tumor 51, 56, 61, 262
antiviral 14, 35, 47, 51, 55, 181, 239, 262
anxiety (inhibitory) 13, 68, 141, 142, 147, 151, 157, 255

aphrodisiac 121, 147, 160, 231, 261, 231
apiol 127
appetizing 89, 202, 219, 245, 251, 266
archeobotany 18
archeochemistry 18
arteriosclerosis 81, 82
arthritis 56, 102, 202, 264
ascorbic acid 266
astaxanthin 90, 262
asthma. See *respiration*
astromycologists 33
atoms 22
autoimmune diseases 11, 15
avocado with fermented-shiitake powder 56
ayahuasca 21, 119, 211, 258, 266
ayurveda 6, 12, 151, 219, 232, 239

B

Bacchus 81
bacteria 10, 11, 14, 82, 217, 232, 262. See also *antibacterial*
barium 206
beer 158, 159, 160, 161
bees 16, 82, 133, 141, 151, 201
beta-carotene 75
betulin 35, 262
biodiversity 22, 114, 165, 261
biopiracy 115, 119, 265
biotin 266
bilberry candy 91
bilberry pie 93
bitter salad leaves, dandelion, and roasted grapefruit 204
bitters 75, 96, 102, 113, 119, 142, 148, 160, 165, 245, 262
bitter-wood 203
blood 264
blood circulation 89, 187, 231
blood clots 96, 102, 133, 231
blood flow 55, 81, 82, 175, 202, 220, 225, 231, 245, 265
blood pressure 41, 56, 76, 96, 127, 134, 219, 231, 245, 264
blood purifying 127, 167, 203, 232
blood sugar 12, 47, 84, 202, 262, 264
blood supply 12, 82, 156, 266
blood vessels 81, 168, 175, 187, 219, 232
blood-cleansing 168, 201

blood-thinning 51, 89, 90, 175, 232
blue lotus 27, 82, 208, 266
bones 114, 133, 254, 264
Boniface 160
boron 51
bottles 26
brain 7, 10, 12, 14, 33, 41, 51, 61, 67, 82, 101, 102, 147, 157, 175, 210, 213, 257
breathing 51, 147, 175, 176, 231, 251
broccoli 10, 13, 15, 245, 257
broccoli stalk with toast and parsley salad 129, 130
bromine 263
Brugmansia 211
bruises 141, 142
burnout 147
businessman's trip 257

C

caffeine 22, 113, 187
calcium 55, 75, 127, 167, 187,
calendula 29, 110
calming 17, 133, 142, 151, 157, 181, 255, 263
candied stem ginger with cream 221
cannabinoid 28, 157
cannabis 27, 28, 95, 156, 157
capillaries 81, 84, 175, 225
caramelized celeriac with garlic, mirin, soy, and soft-boiled egg 235
carapa 114, 115
carcinogens 82, 107
cardiac tonic 22
cardiovascular diseases 55, 73, 81, 82, 95, 96, 102, 107, 127, 157, 187, 201, 232
cardiovascular system 61, 96, 231, 232
carnosic acid 133
cartilage 41
cell membranes 102, 262
cell-killing 245
ceremonies 7, 21, 68, 95, 113, 187, 210, 211,212, 239, 255, 256, 257, 258, 259
chaga 28, 33, 34-37, 39, 65
chagakombucha 37
chamomile 180-181, 183-185, 201
champignon á la grecque with artichoke and fennel seeds 44
chawanmushi, savory ginseng custard 228
cheese 49, 107, 108, 124, 137, 185, 196

INDEX

cherries with chamomile granita and Oudwijker Lazuli cheese 185
chlorine 264
cholesterol 55, 96, 202, 231, 262
choline 266
christianity 19, 65, 66, 81, 95, 101, 141, 151, 160, 210, 262, 266
chromium 51, 264
circulation system 187, 219
cloudberry 10-110
cloudberry bread 109
cloudberry jam with Coulommiers cheese, herb salad, and cloudberry bread 108, 109
cloves 102, 120, 121, 122, 124, 125, 220
cluster headache 69
cobalamin 266
cobalt 264
coca 51, 113, 119, 206, 207, 254, 255
cognitive functions 12, 61, 113, 187, 225
cold 55, 102, 133, 167, 181, 246
cold water extract 28, 152, 255, 256
comfrey 29
concentration 113, 187, 206, 225
connective tissue 41, 202, 265
constipation 76, 90, 96, 202, 209
copper 41, 42, 51, 55, 206, 245, 264
corns 201, 203
cortisol 13
cough 133, 201, 245, 246

D

dandelion 26, 200-205, 262
death cult 127, 208
defenses 6, 9, 12, 14, 22, 217, 231, 261, 264. See also *resistance*
dementia 61, 175, 225, 239
detoxifying 47, 51, 81, 96, 201, 202, 220, 231, 232, 239
diabetes 89
diarrhea 89, 90, 201
digestion 7, 75, 102, 113, 133, 141, 181, 202, 203, 219, 245, 251, 262
Dionysus 81, 101
diseases 14, 56, 95, 141, 263, 265
disinfecting 181, 232, 251
diuretic 127, 133, 201, 202, 245, 262
DMT 257, 258
DNA 41, 89, 119, 187, 226
dosage 22, 119, 211, 213, 251
drying plants 26
dye 82, 147, 201, 239

E

Eccles cakes with Remeker cheese 124
Eleusis 66, 101, 265
ellagic acid 107
endurance 7, 51, 206, 225, 254
energy balls with seeds, nuts, dried fruit, and matcha 189
entheogens 18, 21, 66, 258, 259, 263
enzymes 76, 245, 263, 266
epilepsy 151, 255
ethnobotany 7, 263
Eucharist 66, 101, 266
eugenol 121
eulorpein 96
extraction methods 26, 167
extracts 35, 61, 107, 113, 151, 176
eye 81, 82, 89, 90, 107, 156, 232, 264

F

fasting 14, 84, 213
fats 11, 73, 96, 206, 232, 251
fatty acids 10, 73, 82, 156
fennel salad with horseradish-buttermilk dressing 246
fertility 75, 101, 102, 167, 175, 254
Fesenjān with "chicken of the woods" mushrooms, pomegranate, and walnut 103, 104
feta with peas and meadowsweet 196
fever 142, 161, 181, 203, 212, 219
fiber 10, 102, 107, 255, 263
flavones 202
flavonoids 82, 121 127, 129, 133, 202
flavonol glycosides 175
flower butter 152
fluorine 264
fly agaric 32, 64, 65, 66, 266
focaccia with olives and sage 98
folic acid 127, 266
food 10, 11, 14, 15, 21, 23, 156, 262
food poisoning 113
forgetfulness 51
free radicals 10, 11, 12, 14, 55, 187, 209, 261, 263, 265
fruiting body 41, 263
fulvates 12
fulvic acid 12

G

gale 27, 158, 159, 160, 161
gallbladder 81, 95, 96, 201, 202, 239, 251
garden 115, 239
garlic 48, 51, 62, 86, 98, 104, 127, 129, 144, 173, 205, 220, 230, 231, 232, 235, 236, 243, 251
garlic velouté with roasted carrots and onion 236
gas 121, 202, 219, 262
gastrointestinal system 61, 76, 89, 102, 133, 147, 181, 201, 219, 232, 251
germanium 51
ginger 39, 53, 63, 78, 218-222, 225, 239, 243
ginger beer with strawberries 222
ginkgo 82, 174, 175, 178, 179, 225
ginseng 23, 51, 175, 224, 225, 228, 229,
giving birth 141, 181
glazed eggplant with horseradish cream and seaweed 248
glutathione 14, 262, 265
glycemic index 84
glycosides 175, 263
goji berry 22
gold 107, 141, 264
grapes 10, 80, 81, 82, 84, 85, 86
green papaya salad 78
green salad with zucchini, mint, pistachio, and parsley 131
gut flora 10, 11, 15, 73, 75, 81, 89, 96, 232

H

hallucinogens 21, 127, 134, 160, 161, 209, 210, 213, 259, 263
heart 22, 61, 81, 82, 96, 113, 201, 202, 231, 232, 245, 263, 266
heavy metals 14, 35, 264
herbal medicine 7, 17, 22, 26, 118, 265
homeopathy 22
hormesis 13
horseradish 244-248
horseradish cream, glazed eggplant with seaweed 248
hot chocolate with valerian 154
hot water extraction 28, 35, 36
huachuma cactus 210, 211
hypnotic 181, 255, 263
hysteria 151

279

I

iboga 259, 260, 266
inflammation 10, 11, 12, 13, 14, 41, 55, 61, 75, 82, 89, 96, 101, 102, 121, 133, 141, 147, 167, 175, 181, 193, 202, 219, 232, 239, 245, 261
immune cells 11, 14
immune response 11, 262
immune system 7, 10, 11, 12, 13, 14, 15, 35, 51, 61, 73, 76, 96, 107, 187, 262
immune weakness 13, 129
immune-boosting 35, 41, 55, 75, 107
immunomodulatory 47, 167, 262
immunostimulating 231, 254
incense 19, 121, 211, 257, 258
influenza 14, 56, 89, 167, 193, 246
ink cap 46, 47, 48, 49
inositol 266
inquisition 19, 47, 65, 159
insect repellent 115
insulin 47, 89, 264
iodine 264
iron 55, 75, 121, 127, 142, 187, 206, 219, 245, 264
isothiocyanate 245
itching 121, 167, 181, 183

J

jeweled rice with candied orange, pistachio, and saffron 149
joik 35
joints 115, 193, 212. See also *anti-rheumatic, arthritic, osteoarthritis, rheumatism*
juice of fermented honey with pear, sorrel, and vervain 144

K

kava kava 255, 256
kidneys 35, 102, 167, 201, 202
KOAG/KAG Inspection Board 22
kola nut 113
krappa 114, 115
Kukulcan 258
kykeon 66

L

laxative 75, 89, 95, 263
lectin 217
libido 102, 147, 209, 254
life-enhancing 55

lime 63, 78, 82, 84, 95, 206
liver 14, 51, 82, 127, 151, 161, 201, 202, 209, 226, 239, 256
lose weight 147
LSD 68, 213, 266
lungs 102, 161, 201, 207, 245, 252
lymph nodes 13

M

maca 254
macerates 26, 152, 203. See also *alcohol macerate, water macerate*
macralle 89, 160
macrophages 76, 263
magic mushrooms 41, 67, 68, 161
magnesium 55, 121, 127, 206, 219, 264
malaria 75, 119, 203
manganese 55, 121, 245, 264
master plant 206
matcha 10, 186–190
meadowsweet 192, 193, 194, 196, 199
medicine man 7, 114, 211, 212, 213, 256, 257, 258
meditation 13, 206
melatonin 13
memory 61, 147, 148, 157, 175, 225, 264, 266. See also *dementia*
menopause 133
menstruation 127, 133, 181, 219, 254
mescaline 210, 211, 212, 213
metabolism 246, 264
microbes 10, 14. See also *antimicrobial*
microbiome 232, 263
microdosing 18, 21, 61, 68, 210, 213, 260
microorganisms 10, 263
milk production 41, 76, 133
millefeuille of raw button mushroom, cocoa, apple, and avocado 42
minerals 11, 12, 47, 51, 55, 61, 75, 107, 127, 167, 187, 206, 219, 245, 251, 254, 263
mint, pistachio, and parsley with green salad and zucchini 131
Mithras cult 65
molecules 22
molybdenum 264
mood 10, 68, 101, 102, 113, 119, 148, 157, 256, 26. See also *antidepressant*
mouth freshener 121
movement 10, 12, 13, 14, 15, 127
mucus 141, 168, 181, 203, 245, 251

mung bean soup with chaga and souffléd naan 39
muscles 55, 127, 193, 202, 245, 255, 256, 262, 264, 265
mushroom 33, 40, 41, 42, 44, 55, 133
mycelium 33, 35, 51, 55, 66, 265
mycologist 56, 265
myristicin 127
myrtilus 10, 35, 73, 88, 89, 90,91, 93, 263
mystery schools 21, 142, 209, 231, 265
mysticism 118, 142, 167, 257, 263

N

nails 167, 262, 265
nausea 47, 157, 201, 202, 219, 220
nervousness 142
nervous system 41, 51, 55, 61, 67,68, 81, 82, 113, 133, 142, 151, 181, 187, 239, 263, 264, 265, 266
nettle spring roll with sweet and sour mushroom, carrot, and avocado 171, 172
neurodegenerative 96, 157, 265
neurogenesis 61, 68, 69, 265
neuroprotective 96, 175, 239
neuroregenerative 61, 68
neurotonic 141
niacin 41, 266
nutrients 11, 12, 14, 41, 72, 129, 202

O

oil pulling 96
ointment 29, 95, 96, 151
olive 94, 95, 96, 98, 139
omega-3, 6 & 9 fatty acids 10, 73, 82, 96, 101, 102, 107
Osiris 67, 142
osteoarthritis 167, 201, 219
oxalic acid 167, 217
oxidative stress 7, 113, 133, 262, 265
oxygen 127, 231, 254, 264

P

panacea 133, 225, 231
pantothenic acid 266
papaya 74, 75, 76, 78, 148
papayasambal 78
paralysis 212
parasites 47, 75, 114, 203, 262
parsley 48, 62, 86, 98, 126, 127, 129, 131, 178, 184, 196, 199, 202, 205, 232, 273

INDEX

parsley salad 129, 130
particulate matter 13
pasta aglio e olio 98
pathogen(s) 11, 231, 265
perseverance 231
peyote cactus 66, 212, 213, 266
pharmacognosy 7, 23, 193, 265
pharmaka 66, 81, 265
phosphate 206
phosphorus 55, 61, 75, 245, 263, 264
phytic acid 217
phytomedicine 22
phytonutrients 89, 217
phytotherapy 22, 142, 225, 263, 265
pistachio and jeweled rice with candied orange and saffron 149
plant ingredients 11, 18, 22, 55, 72, 82, 119, 122, 127, 142, 165, 225
poached pear and sabayon of mulled wine 125
poached pom pom blanc with ponzu and ginger 63
polyphenols 10, 96, 107, 127
polysaccharides 51, 265
potassium 55, 61, 127, 187, 201, 245, 264
prebiotics 11, 263
preventive medicine 15
probiotics 10, 11
procyanidin 82
proteins 11, 14, 33, 41, 55, 102, 187, 206, 245, 262
psilocybin 61, 67, 68, 69, 161, 265
psoriasis 64
psychedelic expression 66
psychedelic renaissance 21, 101
psychedelics 7, 18, 21, 101, 102, 156, 157, 208, 211, 213, 257, 263
psychoactive 18, 28, 66, 101, 127, 160, 161, 209, 255, 256, 263, 266
psychonaut 18
pyridoxine 266

Q

quassia amara 119, 203

R

radiation 13, 35, 51, 175, 226
radish, black 202, 250, 251, 252, 253
radish, black, pickled 253
radish, black, with bread and butter 253

rapé 211, 257
raphanusine 251
rastafari 156
red date and cranberry powder, rice pudding with gingko nut 179
reinforcing 101, 251, 263
reishi 33, 50, 51, 52, 53, 254
reishi chai latte 53
relaxant 151, 181, 225, 255, 256
resistance 35, 41, 75, 82, 133, 254, 264. See also *defense*
resveratrol 10, 82, 262
rheumatic disorders 56
rheumatism 201, 202, 245, 261. See also *anti-rheumatic*
riboflavin 41, 266
rice pudding with ginkgo nut, red dates, and cranberry powder 179
rituals 7, 18, 127, 133, 142, 156, 187, 206, 208, 211, 255
rubefacient 245, 265

S

sacrament 18, 66, 67, 68, 102, 157, 208, 211, 212, 213, 258, 259, 266
saffron 146, 147, 148, 149, 239, 266
sage 98, 132, 133, 134, 138, 139
sage "Opperdoezer" potatoes with mustard-olive sauce 138
salad of ginkgo with white asparagus and granny smith apples 177, 178
salad with kiwi, cucumber, verbena, and baked grapes 86
salsa verde with dandelion and zucchini 205
Sámi 20, 35, 66
sananga 90
seaweed 248
selenium 11, 51, 55, 61, 264
serotonin 10, 13, 102, 167
set 21
setting 21
shamans 21, 64, 66, 67, 119
shiitake 54, 55, 56, 58, 172, 190
shiitake dashi with furikake eggs 58
shilajit 12
silicon 127, 167, 264
skin 41, 81, 114, 115, 161, 187, 201, 203, 219, 231, 239, 240, 258, 261, 263, 264
sleep 13, 133, 141, 142, 147, 151, 181, 263

slug repellent 133
smudging 133
soap 14, 115
sodium 75, 264
sterile environment 11, 13
sterilizing jars or bottles 26
stimulant 219, 225, 251, 254, 266
stinging nettle 11, 166, 167, 168, 172, 173, 202
stir-fried nettle leaves with avocado and sesame seed 173
"stoned ape" theory 67
strawberries with ginseng mousse 229
stress 10, 13, 14, 51, 61, 115, 181, 209, 225, 254, 261, 263, 264
sugar 12, 254
sulforaphane 10
sulfur 167, 264, 265
sulfur compounds 232, 251

T

tartlet with vegetarian rendang and white asparagus pickle 243
teacher plant 157, 206, 210, 212
teeth 96, 121, 122, 142, 181, 264
temples 6, 67, 147, 175, 259
tempura of lion's mane mushroom with garlic powder and parsley aioli 62
tempura of meadowsweet with white asparagus and gribiche sauce 199
tempura of shiso and shiitake with matcha salt 190
tendons 55
tepezcohuite 257, 258, 266
The New Ark, LSP Paradise 115, 239
theine 187
theobromine 113, 187
throat 133, 134, 167, 245
thiamine 266
thujone 134
tiramisu with reishi coffee 52
toast with fried ink caps and parsley butter 48
tocopherol 266
tonic 84, 141, 202, 203, 210, 225, 231, 232, 251, 258, 266
tortellini with ricotta, pumpkin, and sage butter 138
trace elements 11, 51, 55, 167, 263
tree cult 66, 160, 259
tryptamine 257

tryptophan 13, 102
turmeric 29, 39, 238, 239, 240, 241, 243
turmeric pancakes with enoki mushroom, cilantro, and Spanish pepper 241
turnip in chamomile salt crust with ravigote sauce 184
tzatziki with yogurt, cucumber, and snow peas 143, 144

U

UV radiation 107, 265

V

vaccines 11
valerian 17, 26, 150, 151, 152, 154, 266
validation 15
vanadium 47
vegetarian pasta carbonara with ink cap and Remeker cheese 49
verbena 86, 140, 141, 142, 144, 193, 262
vervain. See *verbena*
vessel walls 81, 84, 89, 96, 175
vinegar 28, 82, 84, 245
virus 10, 13, 14, 55, 239, 265. See also *antiviral*
visions 21, 66, 68, 101, 134, 157, 210, 213
vitality 7, 12, 225, 263
vitamins 10, 11, 41, 47, 51, 55, 73, 75, 102, 107, 127, 133, 142, 167, 187, 201, 206, 219, 245, 251, 252, 254, 266

W

walnuts 10, 14, 73, 100, 101, 102, 104
warming 51, 102, 219, 225
war on drugs 66, 206
willpower 231
witch's salves 101, 142, 147, 266
witches 41, 64, 68, 89, 101, 141, 160, 167, 266. See also *macralle*
world wood web 33
worming agent 75
Wouter's birthday brownies 104
Wouter's oatmeal with saffron 148

Z

zinc 47, 55, 61, 121, 167, 206, 219, 245, 263, 265

Thank You

"This book is dedicated to the entire universe, the illusion that sustains reality."

With these words by Meher Baba I dedicate this work in particular to plants and mushrooms—it is an ode to these entities.

I want to thank everything and everyone I have ever met, or whose work I have read. You all have shaped me as much as this book.

We are as one.

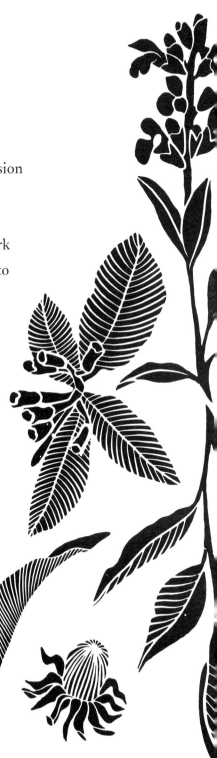

ABOUT THE AUTHORS

WOUTER BIJDENDIJK, M.Sc., is an anthropologist who specialized in ethnobotany and pharmacognosy. Following a degree in cultural anthropology from Amsterdam University, he studied pharmacognosy at the Utrecht Institute CAM and clinical herbalism at Herbal Constituents Inc. in Colorado, USA. Further studies took Wouter to gain insight into Siddha medicine, ayurvedic medicine, and Kalaripayattu at the Bhargava Kalari Sangam and C.V.N. Kalari in Kodhikode, India. He also holds a degree in museology from Amsterdam University of the Arts.

Growing up with his siblings in the city as well as in the countryside, Wouter's curiosity of and love for nature blossomed from childhood on. His special interest in performing arts lead to a career as renowned mentalist and magician Ramana, who captivates audiences worldwide with his brand-activating stunts, mentalism, and Indian magic.

For more than twenty years, Wouter traveled the world performing, while he continued to study herbal medicine from all corners of the globe. He also has been volunteering for more than ten years in Amsterdam Free University (VU) Botanical Gardens, Botanische tuin Zuidas, where he keeps almost extinct original European black bees (*Apis mellifera mellifera*). A creative author, lecturer, and TEDx speaker, Wouter has two daughters and lives in the Netherlands.

For more information visit his website
https://ramana.nl/en/ and *www.instagram.com/ramanamagic* or contact him on instagram via *@_plantkracht_* and *@greenmanpowerplants*, where he keeps a plant blog.

JORIS BIJDENDIJK is an award-winning Dutch chef renowned for redefining modern Dutch cuisine. As executive chef of RIJKS®, the restaurant of the Rijksmuseum, and Wils—both honored with a Michelin star—as well as Wils Bakery Café in Amsterdam, Joris is one of the leading culinary figures in the Netherlands. Beyond the kitchen, he is a columnist for Dutch newspaper *Het Parool*, founder of the Low Food Foundation, and author of several cookbooks. In February 2025, he was named "Chef of the Year" by Gault & Millau. He also holds the prestigious title of SVH Master Chef, the highest culinary recognition in the Netherlands.

Joris' love for beautiful products and good food developed early. Every weekend, the Bijdendijk family drove from Amsterdam to the Ardennes in Belgium, where they had a farm with a large vegetable garden. Together with his eldest brother, Wouter, they searched for mushrooms and other edible plants in the forest from an early age. Now in their forties, they combined their expertise and created this book together, their vision of the world of medicinal plants. The chef and the ethnobotanist. Joris lives with his family in the Netherlands.

For more information visit his website
www.jorisbijdendijk.nl or contact him on Instagram via *@Jorisbijdendijk*.

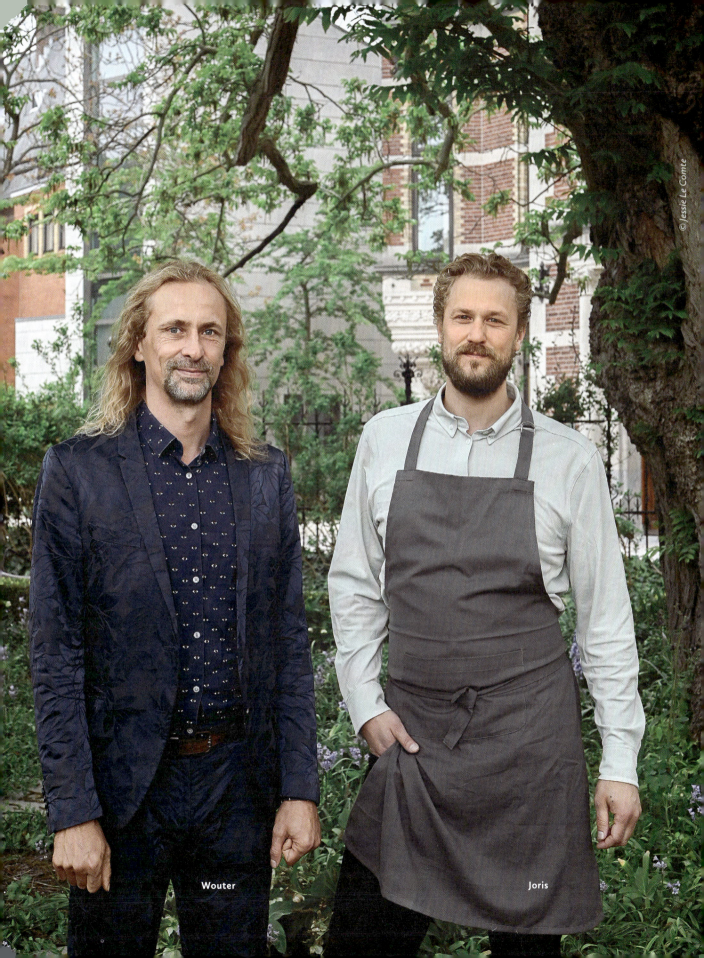

Findhorn Press
One Park Street
Rochester, Vermont 05767
www.findhornpress.com

Findhorn Press is a division of Inner Traditions International

Text copyright © 2022, 2025 by Wouter Bijdendijk
Recipes copyright © 2022, 2025 by Joris Bijdendijk

Originally published in Dutch in 2022 by Nijgh Atelier, Nijgh & Van Ditmar,
Amsterdam under the title *Plantkracht: Het Heilzame Plantenboek*

English edition published in 2025 by Findhorn Press

Nederlands letterenfonds
dutch foundation for literature

The publisher gratefully acknowledges the support
of the Dutch Foundation for Literature.

All rights reserved. No part of this book may be reproduced or utilized in any form or by any means, electronic or mechanical, including photocopying, recording, or by any information storage and retrieval system, without permission in writing from the publisher. No part of this book may be used or reproduced to train artificial intelligence technologies or systems.

Disclaimer

The information in this book is given in good faith and is neither intended to diagnose any physical or mental condition nor to serve as a substitute for informed medical advice or care. Please contact your health professional for medical advice and treatment. Neither author nor publisher can be held liable by any person for any loss or damage whatsoever which may arise from the use of this book or any of the information therein.

Cataloging-in-Publication data for this title is available from the Library of Congress

ISBN 979-8-88850-269-3 (print)
ISBN 979-8-88850-270-9 (ebook)

Printed and bound in India by Replika Press Pvt. Ltd.

10 9 8 7 6 5 4 3 2 1

Food and product photography, styling and illustrations: Jessie le Comte
Lifestyle photography: Saskia van Osnabrugge
Photos pages 83 and 90: Wouter Bijdendijk
Food styling: Joris Bijdendijk, Ivan Beusink, Yascha Oosterberg
Ceramics: The Bird Tsang Ceramics Studio, Corien Ridderikhof, and private collection
Botanical editor: Roxali Bijmoer
Culinary editor: Yulia Knol
Editor of English edition: Nicky Leach
Cover and interior design: Jelle F. Post and Damian Keenan (for the English edition)

This book was typeset in Newsreader Text and DF-Dejavu Pro

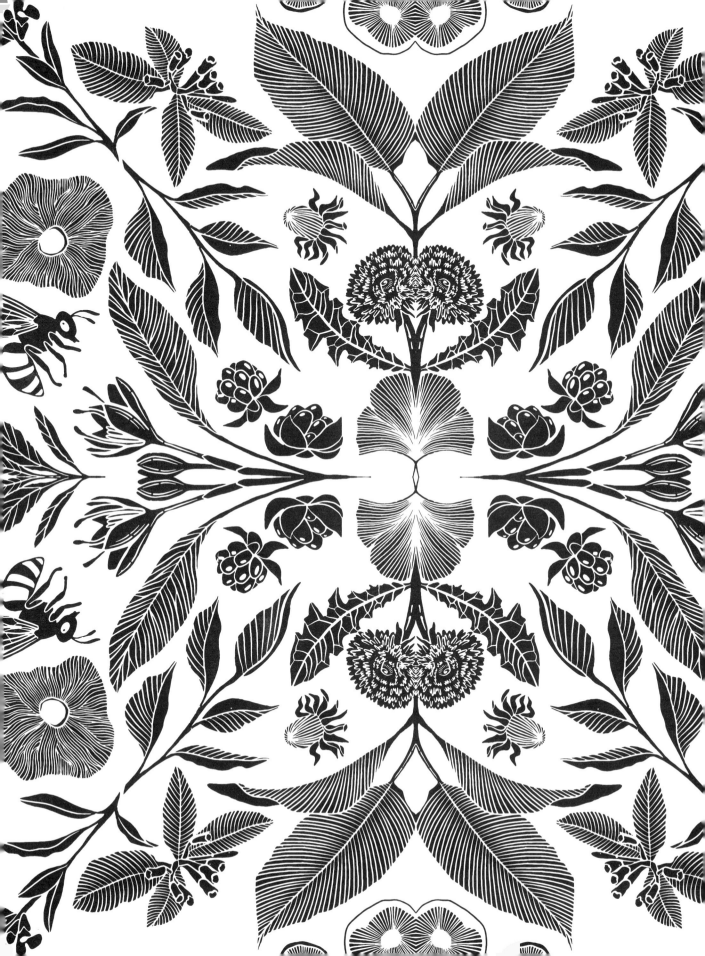

FINDHORN PRESS

Life-Changing Books

Learn more about us and our books at
www.findhornpress.com

For information on the Findhorn Foundation:
www.findhorn.org

Scan the QR code and save 25% at InnerTraditions.com.
Browse over 2,000 titles on spirituality, the occult, ancient
mysteries, new science, holistic health, and natural medicine.

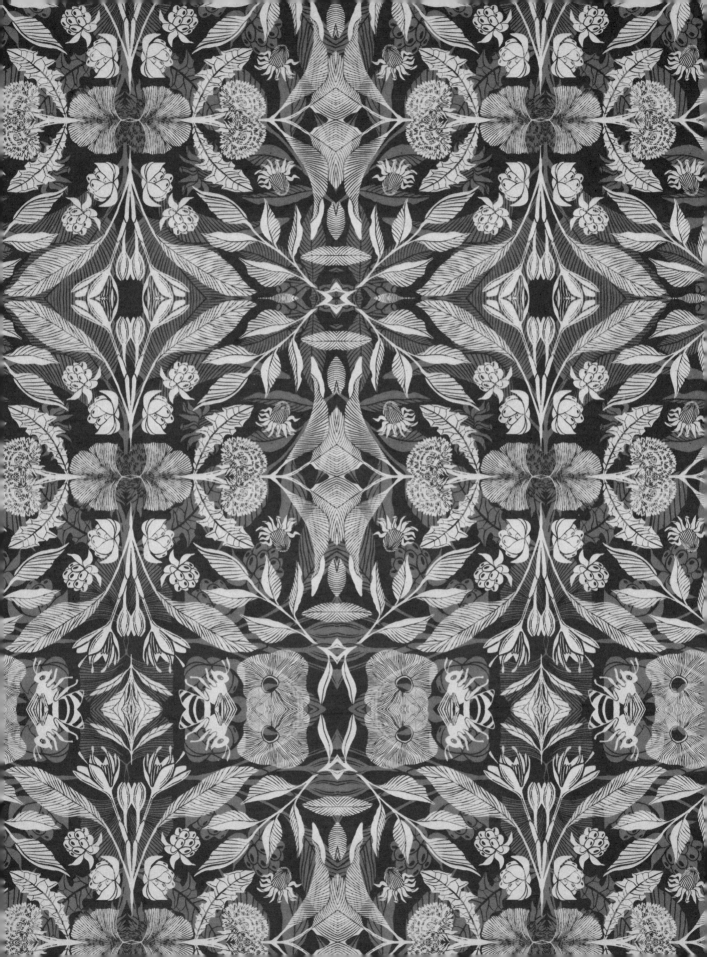

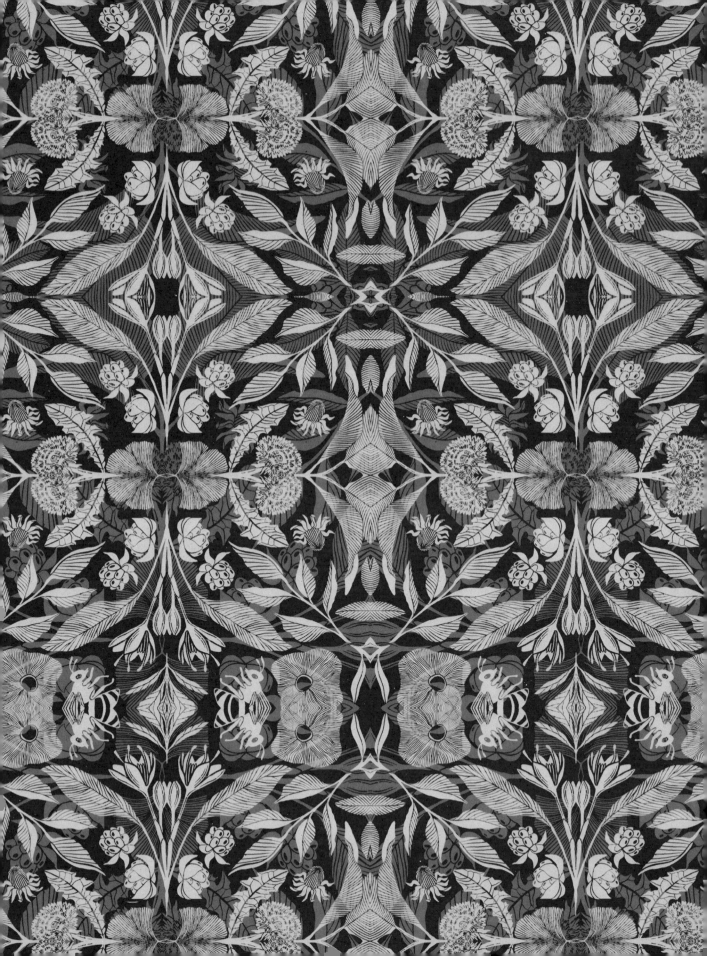